Veterinary Acupuncture

Veterinary Acupuncture

Alan M. Klide, V.M.D.

Shiu H. Kung, Ph.D.

PENN

UNIVERSITY OF PENNSYLVANIA PRESS

First paperback printing 2002
Printed in the United States of America on acid-free paper

Published by
University of Pennsylvania Press
Philadelphia, Pennsylvania 19104-4011

Library of Congress Cataloging-in-Publication Data

Klide, Alan M.
  Veterinary acupuncture.
  Includes index.
  ISBN 0-8122-7721-X (cloth) —
  ISBN 0-8122-1839-6 (pbk. : alk. paper)
  1. Acupuncture, Veterinary. I. Kung, Shiu H., 1939– joint author. II. Title.
SF914.5.K58   636.089'5'892   77-22703

DEDICATED TO

Folly*
Charlie (Abracadabra)**
Donna***

whose responses to acupuncture therapy provided continual amazement and stimulation during the writing of this book.

* Labrador Retriever
** Thoroughbred
*** Morgan

Contents

Tables

Acknowledgments

I would like to thank the people and animals who helped during my acupuncture studies and the writing of this book:

Carolyn Arnold, who worked laboriously to transfer my handwritten cryptic notes to typed manuscript. Art Siegel, who transformed sketches and illustrations to finished photographs;

All of the people who graciously allowed the use of their various materials: S. H. Chen, O. Kothbauer, T. Matsumoto, M. Okada, T. Okada, A. Shores, J. M. Sobin, E. C. Wong, and H. G. Young;

The National Association for Veterinary Acupuncture: R. E. Glassberg, J. Ottaviano, S. H. Shin, and H. E. Warner.

The McCabe Research Fund, which provided funds for my acupuncture research;

All of the companies who permitted the use of their material: Ack Laboratories, Inc.; American Journal of Chinese Medicine; Brethren Corporation; B.X.&L. Industries, Inc.; East Wind Medical Instruments Company, Ltd.; Intertronic Systems, Ltd.; Nikka Overseas Agency, Ltd.; Professional Medical Distributors, Inc.; Sobin Chemicals, Inc.; Wright-Okada, Inc.;

The University of Pennsylvania Press for their willingness to undertake this project;

Janice Heald for her remarkable assistance in locating obscure references from all over the world and printed during two centuries;

The International Veterinary Acupuncture Society and its members whose case reports were used: R. Buchli, M. J. Cain, M. Chaney, D. Darlington, W. J. Davis, J. Finkelstein, G. Fox, J. A. Garon, L. Gideon, W. Grogen, W. J. Hankins, R. M. Heath, G. R. Holt, R. A. Jaeger, D. H. Jaggar, D. K. Johnson, H. R. Johnson, J. Landholm, S. L. Maas, S. C. Miller, M. S. Newman, G. A. Petkus, J. A. Purvis, R. F. Reichard, S. Stern, W. R. West, B. J. Woodruff, H. G. Young, J. P. Young, Jr.;

J. Beech, L. Cushing, D. Freeman, D. Koch, M. Mackay-Smith, D. Marks, W. Moyer, and C. W. Raker for their help with clinical cases;

C. Baetjer, J. Kritchevsky, and J. Sherman for their help with my acupuncture projects;

R. Cimprich, K. Homer, and E. Ledyard for their confidence and interest;

"Mo-Daddy", "Junior" and "Snow" for their patience and understanding during my early probings.

ALAN M. KLIDE

I would like to acknowledge the assistance of the following people: 1) Martin Cummings, MD, Director of the National Library of Medicine for permission to make the collection of the library available; 2) Ms. Mary E. Corning, Assistant Director for the International Program of the Library of Medicine for arrangements with other libraries where there are collections; 3) Mr. Lawrence Black, Chief Librarian of the Institute of Basic Research in Mental Retardation for help in literature search; 4) Ms. Anna Krauthammer for editorial assistance; 5) Vivian Cheng, MD, Wai Y. Kwok, DCM (Doctor of Chinese Medicine, China), and Kun, C. Lem, DMV (China), for discussion during the preparation of the manuscript.

SHIU H. KUNG

Foreword

Acupuncture, in the mind of the American public has always been accompanied by a certain mystique. What is acupuncture all about? What does it do? If it is effective as stated why do not more physicians and veterinarians in the United States routinely employ acupuncture? These and many similar questions have arisen in the minds of the American public, especially since the visits to China beginning this decade by western scientists, physicians, and high officials in the government. Acupuncture in the United States is now receiving serious attention as evidenced by the development of National and International organizations of acupuncture, both of which are headquartered in the United States, the presentation of many seminars and short courses on the subject, and the appearance of numerous scientific publications.

This text by Drs. Klide and Kung reviews in depth the ancient Chinese art of acupuncture and explores and describes the theories upon which the therapy is based. The Yin-Yang and the Meridian Theories, wherein all organ systems and tissues are defined and classified, are two of the most significant theories upon which acupuncture is based.

Dr. Shiu H. Kung is a scientist and a scholar of the classics of traditional Chinese medicine, including acupuncture. His collaborator, Dr. Alan M. Klide, Associate Professor and Chief, Section of Anesthesia, University of Pennsylvania, School of Veterinary Medicine, has an intense interest in acupuncture both as a form of anesthesia for surgical procedures and for the relief of signs of disease. The training and experience of the two coauthors compliment each other, resulting in an interesting and useful text on veterinary acupuncture.

Reading through the text gave me the opportunity to begin an understanding of the history of the Chinese art and science of acupuncture. This review was interesting and useful as an introduction to this method of therapy. The in-depth information on the physiologic action and effects of acupuncture helps prepare the reader for a first attempt at clinical application.

The application of the principles of acupuncture depend upon an accurate and in-depth knowledge of the designated acupuncture points as determined for each species of animal and man. In veterinary medicine these have been worked out well for some species, but are incomplete in others. The text summarizes and supplies all available information, especially graphic in the many figures. Activation of these points is said to restore a more normal balance of action and interaction between tissues and organs leading to a relief of signs of disease. Several techniques by which acupuncture is applied are described, such as the insertion and manipulation of needles, supplementation by stimulation with electric current, and the use by some acupuncturists of heat or fire. To effectively accomplish the various forms of acupuncture, sources of equipment and their use is covered in detail.

The authors have compiled an impressive number of case reports that illustrate the use and effects of acupuncture in veterinary medicine. As a colleague of Dr. Klide, I have had the opportunity to observe the application of acupuncture to some of my equine patients. My experience has stimulated an interest in acupuncture as some of my patients have shown marked clinical improvement. I am also aware of other horses with clinical signs of chronic pain that were relieved and restored to a state of usefulness following acupuncture therapy. On the basis of this knowledge and experience, I anticipate that in time acupuncture will prove useful in the management of some diseases of our animal population. Acupuncture alone or in combination with western medicine should improve our ability to manage disease, reduce suffering, and restore the animal to a state of health. From my observations, chronic pain seems to be one of the areas in which acupuncture holds great promise as effective therapy.

This book will serve as a very useful source of information for veterinarians and other qualified persons who now employ acupuncture as a method of therapy as well as for those who contemplate doing so in the future. To better understand the merits and applicability of acupuncture, and to remove it from the area of mystique to one based upon sound medical principles, extensive research must be done. In general, the basic Chinese work lacks scientific control as we know it in the western world. Controlled studies are now in progress, and additional ones will be required for scientific documentation. Clinical results and experiences strongly support some of the basic Chinese claims. Acupuncture should not be thought of as a "cure-all," but rather as a method of treatment of disease that may supplement and on occasion replace western medicine to improve our ability to render effective therapy. As additional information becomes available through research and experience, it should be possible to develop a definite set of guidelines with indications and contraindications for the application of acupuncture.

Drs. Klide and Kung are to be complimented for the preparation of this useful and interesting textbook.

CHARLES W. RAKER, V.M.D.
Lawrence Baker Sheppard
Professor of Surgery

Introduction

ACUPUNCTURE was brought to the attention of the western world in the early 1970s through newspaper accounts, magazine articles, and movies made by people visiting China. Discussions about acupuncture were occurring daily. The techniques, equipment and theories concerning this ancient practice were difficult to understand or believe. Many people began promoting acupuncture as a panacea for the ills of the world.

At present, the wave of intense interest has passed studies from the very basic to completely clinical have been started; some are just beginning to be reported. Many of the studies are providing much needed information in pain control and pain mechanisms. People have been helped by acupuncture therapy who were not being successfully treated by standard medical means; others have been hurt physically, emotionally, and economically by people who offered claims for acupuncture that were unfounded, or by people who were not qualified to administer acupuncture therapy. Much more work must be done before the value of acupuncture as a treatment or method of analgesia can be known with any degree of certainty.

A similar sequence has been followed in the use of acupuncture in animals, although information on acupuncture in animals has been much more difficult to obtain. Through the efforts of people like H. Grady Young and Marvin J. Cain, and the two veterinary acupuncture societies (the International Veterinary Acupuncture Society [IVAS] and the National Asso-

ciation for Veterinary Acupuncture [NAVA]), much information on this subject has been brought to the United States. However, intensive, careful investigation at both the very basic and the very clinical level must be carried out before any attempts can be made to suggest what conditions (and in which species) might respond to acupuncture therapy, what treatment schedules should be used and, which type of stimulation is best for a specific point or a specific disease. There is no question that unscrupulous individuals may tout acupuncture and their ability in this field as a panacea and that some individuals with little or no training will treat some animals. It is hoped that these few individuals do not give acupuncture such a bad reputation that interest will decrease and legislation be directed against it before the factual information has been collected and proof presented that will demonstrate the benefits acupuncture can offer to animals and their owners.

It is the authors' intent to provide a book that presents the available world's information on acupuncture in animals: to make available a starting point from which basic or clinical investigators can begin to devise studies for sorting out the riddle of acupuncture; to make available to animal owners the information on this subject that will help them to better understand acupuncture and the possible benefits it may offer their animals; to make available a source from which veterinarians can find out what has been done in the theory and practice of veterinary acupuncture. We hope the book will be informative and useful to anyone interested in the subject of acupuncture.

The writing of this book began with the contributions of Dr. Kung in New York, using materials of Chinese in origin (chapters 1, 2, 3, 4, 5, 6, and 8); this was subsequently merged with the contributions of Dr. Klide (chapters 2, 3, 4, 6, 7, and 8). Dr. Kung's contribution was edited by Miss Anna Krauhammer in New York; while Dr. Klide did the overall editing. We hope that this co-authorship has produced a book that will be informative and useful to anyone interested in the subject of acupuncture.

Many sources of information were used for this book: the English literature; the newsletters and pamphlets of the International Veterinary Acupuncture Society and the National Association for Veterinary Acupuncture; case reports from members of the International Veterinary Acupuncture Society; charts and information from various authors and publishers; the clinical and research experience of Dr. Klide; equipment manufacturers' brochures and letters; translations of Chinese, French, German, and Japanese books, chapters, and journal articles; and a Chinese veterinary handbook.

Most of the translated material is presented "as is" so that the reader can get the feeling and flavor of the material as it was originally written. Transliterating, or "Romanizing," of Chinese characters presents a particular problem in that there are several transliterating systems, each producing words that are spelled differently. The system used in this book is Wade Giles, a British system that is the most widely accepted and is used for catalogues in most libraries in the English-speaking world.

1

Basic Principles of Traditional Chinese Veterinary Medicine

The Yin-Yang Theory*

The Yin-Yang Theory describes the principle underlying the laws governing the universe in its physical and metaphysical aspects. The theory is based on observations of natural phenomena. It was formulated during the Chou Dynasty, when it was published in *Shang Shu* (*The Ancient Book*). During the Spring and Autumn Period, it was applied as a guideline for the practice of Chinese medicine in humans and animals. It was incorporated into a book called the *Nei Ching*, which is the most important book of traditional Chinese medicine. Its compilation began some time after 722 BC. The purpose of the book was to set standards of acupuncture for the benefit of later generations. It is a timeless work to which each successive generation has left its mark (see page 281).

After observing the pattern and the regularity of movement of the stars, the Chinese assumed that the heavens moved and the earth was stationary. They classified the heavens as *yang*, or having an active, positive quality and the earth as *yin*, or having a

negative, passive quality. Other natural phenomena were classified in the same way. The sun was classified as yang, because its heat and light made things grow and it was considered active. The moon was classified as yin, because it represented diminished light and it was considered passive. The seasons and directions were also classified: The north and west were yin, the east and south were yang; autumn and winter were yin, summer and spring were yang. According to this theory, every organic and inorganic thing in the universe was classified either predominantly yin or yang.

The basic principle of the Yin-Yang Theory is that yin and yang constantly interact with, and react to, each other in order to achieve a balance; thus, one cannot exist without the other, and each constantly affects the other. According to the theory, the universe is always in a dynamic state, trying to achieve an equilibrium between yin and yang. The interactions and reactions of all the organs and functions of humans and animals are thought of in the same way.

The Yin-Yang Theory separates organs in the body into the categories of *ts'ang* and *fu*. The ts'ang organs are yin, and the fu organs are yang. Each organ of the body and its functions interact with and react to other organs to maintain a balance. According to

---

* From "Shu wen", *Nei Ching*, in the chapter "Yin yang ying hsing ta' lun" ("The relationship of yin and yang and diseases"). Also in "Shu wen", *Nei Ching*, in the chapter "Yin yang p'ieh lun" ("Further discussion of yin and yang").

traditional Chinese medicine, diseases occur when the yin-yang balance in the body is upset. Chinese medicine therefore attempts to cure disease by re-establishing the body's natural balance of yin and yang.

According to the Yin-Yang Theory, yang is active and yin is passive, but these categories are not absolute. The assignment of the basic characteristic is relative. For example, the ts'ang organs are considered essentially yin because they are less active and are more reactive than the fu organs. However, this does not mean they can't be active under certain circumstances. These categories only describe the dominant characteristics of the organ or function when the body is in balance.

The term *balance* in reference to the body is also a relative one, because according to the theory, the body is never completely balanced. That would imply stasis. Rather, the body is constantly in a state of attempting to achieve balance, as indicated by the interdependence of yin and yang in their reactions and interactions.

The physiological process of digestion illustrates the concept of the interdependence of yin and yang. The animal must ingest food to absorb the nutrients that enable the organs to function. Conversely, the absorption of food depends on the functional activity of the visceral organs that process the food so that the body may be nourished. The function itself is yin; and the nutrient is yang. Without nutrients, functional activity cannot exist, nor can it continue. Without functional activity, the nutrients cannot be absorbed and utilized. Thus, yin and yang are intrinsically interdependent in humans and other animals.

If either yin or yang goes to extremes in interacting or reacting, the opposite state results; that is, an excess of yin will produce yang, and vice versa. This can be illustrated by the relationship between the inhibitory and stimulatory mechanisms of the body, which are also known as the "feedback" mechanism. If there is an undersupply of a specific hormone (yin), production of the hormone will increase (yang). Conversely, if the body produces too much hormone (yang), the feedback mechanism will inhibit and reduce the production (yin).

Acupuncture attempts to correct the imbalance caused by an extreme of yin or yang when the body itself can no longer correct it. However, acupuncture does not correct the imbalance by directly manipulating yin or yang. It manipulates *ch'i*, the basic dynamic energy of the universe, which flows in a specific pattern throughout the body. Ch'i is an ex-pression of the interaction between yin and yang. It flows in the meridians, which link all the body organs to each other and to the surface of the body. Yin and yang flow in the form of ch'i within the meridians, and acupuncture tries to keep the balance of yin and yang in the body through the manipulation of ch'i by the needle.

The Theory of Five Elements, the classification of the tsang and fu organs, the "Ching Lo", or Meridian Theory, the concepts of *ch'i, wei, ying, hsueh, spirit* and *fluid*, the classification of *Chi Heng Chih Fu* and the four methods of diagnosis all extend the basic principles of the Yin-Yang Theory.

The Ts'ang and Fu Organs

An organ in traditional Chinese veterinary medicine differs from its Western counterpart in that its definition includes more than the function of the isolated organ itself. An organ is defined as the physical organ itself, including all its functions, the relationship of its functions to the other organs, and the functions of the other organs that specifically interact with it. It has a specific yin or yang characteristic, and it possesses a specific and individual ch'i that interacts with the ch'i of the other organs and the total ch'i of the body.

The six ts'ang and six fu organs are visceral organs. The ts'ang organs are yin; the fu organs, yang. Each is assigned an element as well as a specific function. In general, the ts'ang organs are responsible for the absorption, transformation, and transportation of nutritive elements; the fu organs are responsible for storage and excretion. The visceral organs mediate between the ch'i of the universe and the ch'i of the body. They absorb the ch'i of the universe as the nutrients and excrete the ch'i of the organisms back into the universe as waste.

The ts'ang organs, which are relatively solid, are the heart, pericardium, lung, liver, spleen, and kidney. The fu organs, which are hollow, are the gall-bladder, small intestine, stomach, large intestine, triple-burner, and the urinary bladder.

The ts'ang and fu organs interact with each other to form a closed and balanced system in which all life-sustaining functions take place. Each ts'ang organ has a corresponding fu organ, with which it has a permanent relationship and with which it must be in balance in accordance with the theories of Yin-Yang and of Five Elements. Because of the close relationship of these organs, pathologic changes in one organ influence and are reflected in other organs. The signs

TABLE 1-1. *The Five Categories in Nature and Living Beings*

Five elements	Wood	Fire	Earth	Metal	Water
Five stages of life	Embryo	Adolescence	Adulthood	Old age	Death
Five seasons	Spring	Summer	Late summer	Autumn	Winter
Five directions	East	South	Center	West	North
Five ch'i	Wind	Fire, heat	Moisture	Dryness	Cold
Five tsang organs	Liver	Heart	Spleen	Lung	Kidney
Five fu organs	Gallbladder	Small intestine	Stomach	Large intestine	Urinary bladder
Five t'i	Muscle	Blood vessels	Fat	Skin and hair	Bone
Five ch'ao orifices	Eye	Tongue	Mouth	Nose	Ear
Five fluids	Tear	Sweat	Saliva	Mucus	Urine
Five pulses	Taut (hsien)	Full (huang)	Slow (ch'ih)	Light (fu)	Deep (ch'en)
Five colors	Green	Red	Yellow	White	Black
Five tastes	Sour	Bitter	Sweat	Spicy	Salty
Five functional processes	Germination	Growth	Maturation	Fruit production	Dormancy

of disease are both on the surface and readily apparent, and subsurface and not readily apparent. In diagnosis, if disease of a ts'ang organ is suspected, its corresponding fu organ is checked and vice versa. Generally, diseases of the fu organs are less severe and are more responsive to treatment; diseases of the ts'ang organs are more severe and less responsive. Each organ manifests its pathologic condition through a specific orifice, color, pulse, taste, and fluid secretion, all of which are checked when disease is suspected. Basically, Chinese medicine assumes that an animal is a harmonious unit and that imbalances inside the body are manifested as diagnostic characteristics on the surface of the organism and vice versa. (See Table 1-1).

THE T'SANG ORGANS

The Heart

Blood converges in the heart, and is sent out to various parts of the body. The pulse reflects the characteristics of blood flow and the state of circulation.

Because the heart is the main organ of circulation, any changes in heart function affect the physiological activity of the blood and pulse. The physiological conditions of the heart, blood, and pulse are reflected by the condition of the inside of the mouth and the color and brightness of the hair, because the ch'i that carries the nutritive elements of the blood makes the hair smooth and shiny, and the mouth red. When the heart is overworked or weak, the blood does not transport nutrients properly, and the hair looks dry and dull, and there are changes in the color of the mouth.

Clinical practice has proven that if the tongue is scarlet red, it is a symptom of an excess of fire (see

The Theory of Five Elements, p. 9). If the tongue is light red, it is a symptom of an insufficient amount of blood and ch'i*; furuncle on the tongue is a symptom of heat accumulation in the heart meridian.†

The heart is related to the small intestine, a fu organ.

The Pericardium

The pericardium surrounds the heart and has two functions: to protect the heart and to enable the blood to flow to and from the heart.

When disease invades the body, the primary function of the pericardium is to fight the invasion and protect the ch'i of the heart from being destroyed, because the heart by controlling the blood flow, controls the life-sustaining activities of the organism.‡ The pericardium may be considered a separate ts'ang organ (bringing the total number to six), or part of the heart. When counted as a separate organ, it is related to the triple-burner, a fu organ. The pericardium is also known as "circulation-sex", "heart constrictor", and "envelope of the heart."

The Liver

The liver supports and nourishes growth and promotes the ch'i related to all growth functions. It is most important for the liver ch'i to avoid congestion

* In *Yuan Heng Liao Ma Chi*, in the chapter "Wang Liang hsien shih t'ien t'i wu ts'ang lun" ("The theory of five ts'ang organs according to my late teacher Wang Liang"), the relationship of heart and tongue is explained.

† In *Yuan Heng Liao Ma Chi*, in the chapter "Shui ching wu ts'ang lun" ("Collections of important facts of the theory of five ts'ang organs").

‡ In "Ling shu" section of *Nei Ching*, in the chapter "Hsieh k'e p'ien" ("The evil and uninvited visitors").

3 *Traditional Chinese Veterinary Medicine*

and retardation.* Liver diseases produce yin symptoms. The signs include an upward gaze and dazed expression, unstable gait, foaming at the mouth, tight jaw, stiff neck, distended abdomen, dsypnea, and conjunctivitis.*

The liver and kidney are related (see The Theory of Five Elements, p. 9). If the kidney cannot nourish the liver, a disease resulting in an excess of liver yang will occur. Herbal medicine or acupuncture points are used to promote the strengthening of the kidney yin and the moderation of liver yang.†

The liver retains the most nutritive elements of the blood and regulates the quantity of blood in the body. When the animal is quiet and at rest, part of the blood flows into the liver and is stored there. During activity, when the energy of the body is being spent at a faster rate, the rate of blood flow increases, and the blood stored in the liver is released into the meridians to be circulated through the tsang and fu organs to provide nourishment for the body.‡

Nourishment of the eyes originates in the liver.§ Under normal conditions and with proper nourishment, the eyes are sharp, bright, and clear. With improper nourishment, the eyes appear dull and are dried and irritated. Also vision seems to be impaired and dizziness occurs. When animals are infected by disease, the symptoms of the eyes differ according to the type of resulting imbalance. For example, if there is excessive wind and heat of the liver and its meridian, the eyeballs protrude, there are congestion, opacity, and sticky eyelids. For excessive cold, the eyes are hypersensitive to external irritation.‖

The liver supplies blood to the muscles for their activities, and is related to the flexion and extension of the joints. Under normal conditions, the liver nourishes the muscles by providing them with nutrient-laden blood, resulting in normal muscular activities. If the liver is not functioning properly, nourishment of the muscles and joints is not normal. The following symptoms may appear: convulsion, opisthotonus, stiff neck, and muscle spasm.¶ An insufficient amount of the blood from the liver results in softness and thickness of hoof and paw keratin, and retardation and disturbance of their development.*

The liver is related to the gallbladder, a fu organ.

The Spleen

After food is absorbed and digested in the stomach, some ch'i must be absorbed for use and some ch'i may be excreted. The function of the spleen is to extract the useful (nourishing) ch'i from the useless ch'i and dispatch it to the lungs, where it combines with the ch'i of the universe to form *ching ch'i*. The ching ch'i enters the meridians and is transported to the rest of the body. Also, the spleen sends the gaseous ch'i to the lung to be excreted.†

If the spleen is weak and digestion of water, grain, and grass is insufficient, the symptoms are abdominal

---

* The pathologic manifestations of the liver, described in this paragraph of the text are found in *Yuan Heng Liao Ma Chi*, in "The 25th section of the 81 question-answer sections by Chao Fu", and in the 19th section discussing the liver "wind".

† The "mother" of the liver "wood" is the kidney "water", and insufficiency of kidney "water" cannot nourish the liver "wood" and in a disease due to an imbalance of yin and yang, an excess of yang will occur (See The Theory of Five Elements, p. 9).

‡ In *Nei Ching*, "Ling shu" section, in the chapter, "Pen shen p'ien" ("The origin and preservation of the spirit"); also in *Nei Ching*, "Shu wen" section, in the chapter, "Wu ts'ang shen tsang lun" ("Discussion on the development of five ts'ang organs").

§ Ancient Chinese classics of veterinary medicine emphasize the close relationship of the liver and eyes. In *Nei Ching*, "Shu wen" section, in the chapter "Mo tu p'ien", ("On pulse measurement"), it says, "Liver communicates with the eyes." In *Nei Ching*, "Shu wen" section, in the chapter "Ching kuei chen yen lun" ("The truth of medicine"), it says, "The orifice of the liver is the eyes." In *Yuan Heng Liao Ma Chi*, in the chapter "Ku yen lung" ("The theory of bones and eyes"), it says, "The liver is the origin of the eyes." In *Nei Ching*, "Shu wen" section, in the chapter "Wu ts'ang shen tsang lun", it says, "Liver receives blood and makes vision possible." In *Szu Mu An Ch'i Chi*, in the chapter "Ma Shih Huang wu ts'ang lun" ("Ma Shih Huang's theory of five ts'ang organs"), it says, 'The exterior correspondence of the liver is the eyes; in good coordination, the eyes produce proper lacrimation."

‖ From *Yuan Heng Liao Ma Chi*, in the chapter "Shui ching wu ts'ang lun" ("Collection of important facts on the theory of five ts'ang organs").

¶ From *Szu Mu An Ch'i Chi*, in the chapter "T'ien huang chih 36 ping yuan ke", ("The 36 origins of yellow diseases").

* The relationship of the liver and paws is found in many classics of Chinese veterinary medicine. In Chao's *Chu Ping Yuan Hou Lun* (*The Etiology of Various Diseases*), it says, "The paws are the extension of muscles." In *Nei Ching*, "Shu wen" section, in the chapter "Liu chieh ts'ang hsiang lun" ("Six segments of the phenomena of the ts'ang organs"), it says, "The cream of the liver, . . . is found in the paws." In *Ch'uan Ch'i T'ung Hsien Lun*, it says, "The substance of the liver . . . appears in the paws and scales." Discussion of these liver disorders is found in two chapters of *Yuan Heng Liao Ma Chi*; in the chapter "Ku yen lun" and in the chapter "Chao fu 81 nan ching", in the 30th question and answer.

† In *Nei Ching*, "Shu wen" section, in the chapter "Ching mo pieh lun" ("Discussion of ching and mo"), it says, "The stomach stores the ingested food that is full of nutritive essence and Ch'i; the spleen collects these and transports them to the lung."

distension and diarrhea. The sick animals are skinny, suffer general malaise; and their limbs are fatigued and weak.

The spleen functions to transform water and moisture into the ch'i of the body. A weakness in splenic ch'i decreases the efficiency of this water and moisture transformation. In mild disorders, there is a loose stool. In severe disorders, water and moisture overflow below the umbilicus, becoming edema and ascites.*

If wind and cold invade the body and affect the spleen, coldness of the ears and nose, excessive motions of the head and tail, lying on the ground with body bent, twisting limbs, rumbling intestines, and diarrhea may result. These symptoms are caused by extended periods of exposure to cold winds and rain during feeding, exposure to frost and snow, excessive thirst, and excessive drinking of cold water on an empty stomach.†

The growth of the muscles of the mouth and lips depends on the nutrients (which are the essential parts of the water, grains, and grass) transformed by the spleen. With insufficient nutrients, the animal becomes skinny and weak, and the hair coarse and loose. In clinical practice, it is possible to appreciate the relationship of the mouth and tongue muscles to the spleen—for example, when splenic function is normal, the muscles are rich and full, and the interior of the tongue and lips (oral mucosa) is moist and shiny. When splenic function is abnormal, muscle bulk is lean and the oral mucosa is pale. If the spleen is cold, the lip is twisted; if the spleen is poisoned, the lips become swollen.‡

The Lung

Ch'i may be understood in two ways: one is the functional ch'i of respiration; the other is the ch'i of the animal. The ch'i for respiration is the process in which the lung continuously inhales uncontaminated ch'i of the universe and exhales the unwholesome ch'i. Thus, under normal conditions, the lung is able to distinguish the clear from the contaminated ch'i of the body, and the lung provides swift and com-fortable respiration. If the lung is sick, the clear ch'i cannot be inhaled and the contaminated ch'i cannot be readily exhaled; and cough, shortness of breath, and purulent nasal discharge result. This demonstrates that the lung controls the ch'i of respiration.§

The ch'i of the animal is composed of the vital elements of the body, without which the body dies. The ch'i of the body is constantly renewed from the intake of ch'i from the water, grains, and grass. However, without the ch'i of respiration to inhale the clear and exhale the contaminated portions, the ch'i from water, grass, and grains cannot sustain the life of the animal. In the process of respiration, the contaminated ch'i is exhaled and the clear ch'i is inhaled, combining with the ch'i of the water, grass, and grains to become the ch'i of vitality. Thus, the life processes are maintained. Clinically, the high and low levels of lung ch'i determine the strong or weak physical condition of animals.

The lungs control the ch'i of breathing, but inhalation and exhalation take place through the airways of the nose, clearly indicating an intrinsic relationship between the nose and the lungs.‖ Clinically, the signs from the nose are related to the functional state of the lungs. For example, in pig diseases where there is a shortness of breath, and in horses and donkeys with asthmatic lung disorders, noisy breathing, flaring of the nostrils, purulent discharges, and offensive odors from the nose are evident. These can be treated by needling the lung meridians.¶

Some of the usable ch'i derived from undigested food collects in the lungs. After combination with the clear ch'i of respiration, it is transported from the surface of the lungs to the surface of the body, where the skin and muscles are located. It then becomes *wei ch'i*, which protects and fortifies the body surface against the invasion of diseases. If the ch'i from the lung is weak, the wei ch'i is insufficient. The defense mechanism is then weakened, and disease may invade the body. The sick animals may develop fever, chills, fu pulse, and nasal discharges. If these disorders are not treated soon enough, symptoms such as coughing, shortness of breath, and redness of the mouth appear.*

Treatment consists of cleaning the lung and fortify-

---

* In *Szu Mu An Ch'i Chi*, in the chapter "Ching chu wu ts'ang lun" ("The discussion on usable and unusable"), it says, "The spleen digests all kinds of rice."

† In *Nei Ching*, "Shu wen" section, in the chapter "Chen yao ta lun" ("Discussion of the truth and essentials"); also in the chapter "Hsuan ming wu ch'i p'ien" ("Clarification of five ch'i").

‡ In *Szu Mu An Ch'i Chi*, in the chapter "Ma Shih Huang wu ts'ang lun".

§ In *Nei Ching*, in the chapter "Tung ping shu lun" (Discussion on deficiency and fullness").

‖ In *Szu Mu An Ch'i Chi*, in the discussion of the lung.

¶ In *Yuan Heng Liao Ma Chi*, in a discussion of the offensive odor and its relation to the lung.

* In *Yuan Heng Liao Ma Chi*.

ing the body surface to prevent further influence by the wind. The skin must also be cleaned. If domestic animals are not bathed in the summer, dirt may obstruct the hair orifices, causing an imbalance between the temperatures of the interior and exterior of the body (yin and yang). Thus, heat accumulates in the heart and thorax, affecting the lung; and the heat of the lung produces the wind that causes itchy skin. Sick horses may be itchy over the entire body surface, or they may have small extremely itchy papillary rashes. The sick animal loses normal appetite, becomes skinny, loses hair, and has crusted skin.*

The larynx, located the upper end of the trachea, is the passage of inhalation of lung ch'i. It is also the organ of vocal function. When the lung malfunctions, vocal changes occur. For example, after shortness of breath has affected the pig for a considerable time, vocalization is weak and hoarse. Other symptoms such as laryngeal edema and frequent hemorrhage of the larynx and lung are related.

Diseases of the larynx also spread to the lungs; for example, if laryngeal edema is not diagnosed and treated early enough, coughing and purulent nasal discharges will develop.* Treatment for this type of disease expels the heat of the lung, cleans the larynx, and relaxes the respiratory muscles, thus opening the thorax and creating a favorable condition for the diaphragm by managing the fire.*

The Lung is related to the fu organ, large intestine.

The Kidney

The kidney stores the surplus ching ch'i. The water, grain, and grass possess their own ching ch'i when they enter the body. This, plus the surplus ching ch'i not used by the body, is stored in the kidney. The ching ch'i is stored in fluid form and is called *kidney fluid*. There is a constant conversion of the body ching ch'i into stored ch'i and a simultaneous conversion of the stored ch'i for the use of the whole body.† The kidney also controls the flow of excessive water for excretion and therefore regulates the quantity of water retained by the body.

A coordination of the right and left kidneys catering to the need of the individual depends on the balance of yin and yang. An insufficiency of yang causes diarrhea, and an insufficiency of yin causes constipation and oliguria. Treatment for the former

is "warm strengthening" of the kidney; treatment of the latter includes the nourishment of kidney yin. Furthermore, when kidney function is disordered, a disturbance of the transformation of ch'i makes it impossible for the ch'i to condense into kidney fluid and may cause an accumulation of the fluid, resulting in edema, ascites, and bladder retention.

For treating these diseases, it is necessary to strengthen the kidney yin and kidney yang so that the two may properly regulate the fluid of the body. The kidney has its own ch'i, which is also referred to as *kidney yin*. This ch'i controls reproduction.

The ch'i stored in the kidney includes the ch'i for copulation. When domestic animals become mature, they have a sufficient amount of ch'i for reproduction. When they grow old, the production of ch'i diminishes or even stops and reproductive ability is reduced or lost. Clinically, reproductive disorders include an insufficient sex drive in the male animal, sterility, and an inconspicuous and inaccurate mating period in the female. The treatment for this type of disorder is to strengthen the kidneys.

The kidney produces and regulates water. The kidney fluid is yin; and where there is yin, there is yang. If physiological condition is to be normal, yin and yang must be in balance. Therefore, a balance of water and fire is mandatory to maintain good health (see The Theory of Five Elements, p. 9). The fire of the kidney is the fire of the "gate of life", the manifestation of which is the sex drive. If the fire of the gate of life is insufficient, impotency and other symptoms of reproductive disorders will appear. If the fire of the gate of life is in excess, the sex drive will be hyperactive. Therefore, the treatment of the former disorder is tonification (see pp. 21–22) of the kidney and strengthening of the yang; treatment of the latter is tonification of yin and lowering of the fire.

THE FU ORGANS

Because each fu organ has a relationship to one of the ts'ang organs, illness in a fu organ is first manifested in a ts'ang organ. These manifestations are easily recognized.

The Gallbladder

The gallbladder stores bile.‡ It is considered the "pure" organ§ because, while the other fu organs

---

* In *Yuan Heng Liao Ma Chi.*

† In *Nei Ching*, "Shu wen" section, in the chapter "Shang ku t'ien lun" ("Ancient theory of the constituents of the universe").

‡ In *Szu Mu An Ch'i Chi*, "Liver is the ts'ang organ of wind and gallbladder is the fu organ of clearness."

§ In *Lui Ching (Treatise of Classification)* and in *Yuan*

store the nutrients and residues of the digested water, grass, and grains, bile from the gallbladder is a pure product that is secreted into the small intestine to help digestion.

The liver is yin and the gallbladder is yang. In clinical practice, it is not uncommon to see gallbladder disorders. In most cases they are a pathological sign that the yang of the liver has overflowed.*

The Stomach

The structure of the stomach is different in different animals; for example, cattle, goats, and camels have four stomachs. Chinese veterinary medicine considers these stomachs a single organ.

The stomach absorbs water, grain, and grass, and separates them into usable and unusable nutrients. The ch'i of the stomach is essential to life because it aids in transforming the nutrients into ching ch'i, which supports the ch'i of the body, in turn maintaining and perpetuating the life-sustaining functions. If the gastric ch'i is weak, the capacity of the stomach for storage and separation is reduced, and splenic function is impaired. The supply of nutrients to the other ts'ang and fu organs and other parts of the body is reduced, and illness results.†

The Relationship Between Spleen and Stomach

The spleen and the stomach cooperate to supply the body with nutrients as far as the functional characteristics are concerned. The spleen is yin and the stomach is yang. Under normal conditions, the characteristics interact with each other, establishing an equilibrium. However, under pathologic conditions, disorders of one organ adversely affect the other.

If the yang of the stomach is insufficient, and there is an excess of cold, there will be cold symptoms. For example, if the animal has a stomach cold, salivation becomes excessive. If a pig has a stomach cold, vomiting occurs. In disorders of this nature, the pulse is slow and weak, and the colors of the mouth are green and yellow.‡

To treat this disease, the spleen should be strengthened, the stomach and the intestine should be warmed, and the ts'ang organs should be tonified. For acupuncture treatment, hot needle insertion is made into pi shu (T10).

If horses are excessively labored and heat accumulates and spreads in the stomach, the fire of the stomach is distributed throughout the six ts'ang organs, resulting in heat syndrome. The symptoms are general malaise, loss of appetite, lung weakness, and dislike of water. Treatment of this disease includes prescriptions for clearing stomach heat, cooling the spleen, and sweeping away the accumulation.

Indigestion in horses, camels, and goats are diseases of stomach heat.

The Small Intestine

The small intestine extracts the ching ch'i originally in food and sends it to the kidney for storage. It also separates the ch'i to be excreted into fluid and solid parts and sends the fluid to the urinary bladder and the solid to the large intestine.§

If the basic function of the small intestine is impaired, diseases result. If more fluid than normal stays in the large intestine, less urine will be secreted and diarrhea will result. If an excessive amount of fluid is retained by the urinary bladder, there will be excessive urine secretion and constipation; therefore, in treating diarrhea, diuretic medicine is used so that more water will enter the bladder.‖

The Relationship of the Heart to the Intestine

The heart is related to the small intestine, a fu organ. The clinical signs that illustrate this relationship are a red, swollen, ulcerated tongue and the production of sparse, colored urine. The tongue is related to the heart, and symptoms related to the tongue may indicate excessive heat in the heart. Symptoms of abnormal urine provide evidence that the fire of the heart is so excessive that it runs downward into the small intestine. As a result, the nutrients, ch'i, and blood are not in harmony, causing production of urine with a bloody color. The principle for treating the disease is to clear the heat of the heart using the diuretic method.¶

Heng Liao Ma Chi, in the chapter "Wang Liang hsien shih t'ien t'i wu ts'ang lun".

* In *Szu Mu An Ch'i Chi*, in the chapters "Ma Shih Huang wu ts'ang lun" and "Ching chu wu ts'ang lun".

† In *Szu Mu An Ch'i Chi*, in the chapter "Ma Shih Huang wu ts'ang lun", it says, "The stomach is the fu organ for water and rice". Also, see the chapter "Ma Shih Huang pa hsieh lun" ("Eight evils by Ma Shih Huang").

‡ In *Szu Mu An Ch'i Chi*, in the chapter "Shui ching wu ts'ang lun"; the identical chapter is found in *Yuan Heng Liao Ma Chi*.

§ In *Szu Mu An Ch'i Chi*, in the chapter "Ma shih huang wu ts'ang lun".

‖ In *Yuan Heng Liao Ma Chi*, in the chapter "Che wor yieh sou lun" (The management of common diseases").

¶ In *Szu Mu An Ch'i Chi*, in the chapter "Ma shih huang wu ts'ang lun".

The Large Intestine

The large intestine is the fu organ for transporting material to be excreted. Different animal species have structural differences in the large intestine; for example, the cecum of the horse is better developed. The principles of Chinese veterinary medicine, however, apply to these variations in structure.

The large intestine is related to the lung, a ts'ang organ. The large intestine consolidates, clears, and dries the residue passing from the small intestine and reduces it for passage from the body.

The large intestine is the main thoroughfare by which contaminated ch'i is excreted, expelling the portion of the contaminated ch'i not excreted by respiration. The contaminated ch'i is then excreted through the anus in the form of solid waste.

Diseases of the large intestine are shown by the state of the solid waste. For example, if the large intestine is excessively dry, constipation is evident. If the organ is excessively moist, diarrhea results. The large intestine is responsible for the excretion of the contaminated ch'i. When there is no obstruction, descendence of the contaminated ch'i is rapid, corresponding to the rapid ascendence of the contaminated gaseous ch'i from the lungs. The excretion of the gaseous ch'i is in balance with the excretion of the solid ch'i. If the lung is not functioning properly, the gaseous ch'i will descend to seek excretion, causing intestinal difficulties. If the excretion of solid waste is inefficient, the contaminated ch'i will try to ascend and invade lung ch'i, causing respiratory ailments. These conditions further cause the heat of the lung and asthmatic disorders. Treatment should focus on sweeping away the obstructions for the swift flow of ch'i and to disperse the accumulation of heat. For constipated animals without asthmatic disorders, it should aid the lung to resist ascendence of ch'i and help contaminated ch'i to descend.

Treatment of large intestine ch'i deficiency is by tonification of the lung ch'i.* In horses and donkeys, the deficiency type of anal prolapse syndrome is mostly caused by the overlaboring of the lung. The effect of the lung injury is transmitted into the large intestine, causing weakness and loss of large intestine function.

The Urinary Bladder

The urinary bladder stores polluted fluid for excretion. Because the quantity of water in the body of an animal is constant, and excessive water is excreted through the surface of the body as sweat and through the urinary bladder as urine, there is a close relationship between fluid, sweat, and urine.

Body fluid is depleted rapidly when perspiration and diarrhea are excessive. Thus, the amount of urine output is diminished. Conversely, urine output is increased as the body fluid increases; for example, when the animal does not perspire after drinking a large quantity of water.†

The yang ch'i of the kidney is necessary for the formation of urine. Therefore, if kidney yang is weak, ch'i formation is insufficient. The fluid does not become urine, causing diarrhea and edema. Reduced urine secretion caused by kidney ch'i insufficiency can be treated by tonification of the kidney ch'i and strengthening of the original yang.

Urinary bladder disorders are manifested by abnormal urine. The accumulation of moisture and heat disrupts urinary bladder function, causing an accumulation of sand and stones, and thus blocking the ureter.

The Triple-Burner

The triple-burner is one of the six fu organs and the only fu organ without a fixed anatomic location and morphology. Two theories about this fu organ are widely accepted today. The first theory proposes that the triple-burner has a definite morphology and performs specific functions. The second theory proposes that the triple-burner represents a group of specific functions. The triple-burner as an organ in itself is physically nonexistent.

The sphere of functional influence of the triple-burner includes the whole trunk and the six ts'ang and six fu organs. It facilitates and synchronizes the physiologic activities and pathologic changes of the whole organism. It facilitates the flow of fluid, blood, and ch'i; promotes the circulation; and aids digestion, excretion, and other vital functions. It is a medium of transportation and exchange.

The organ is divided into three parts: the upper, middle, and lower portions.‡ The upper burner includes the area cephalad to the diaphragm or pylorus. Included are the head, neck, thorax, heart, and lungs. The middle burner includes the region between the umbilicus and the diaphragm, including the cranial abdomen, the spleen, and stomach. The lower burner

---

* In *Nei Ching,* it says, "Lung is the master of ch'i; when there is a deficiency of ch'i, there is deficiency of the lung."

† In Ch'ao's *Chu Ping Yuan Hou Lun.*

‡ In *Szu Mu An Ch'i Chi,* in the chapter "Ching chu wu ts'ang lun".

includes the region caudad to the level of the umbilicus, including the caudal abdomen, the liver, large and small intestines, and urinary bladder.

Although the triple-burner consists of three separate portions, these are closely interrelated. In a general sense, the function of the triple-burner is to facilitate the circulation of ch'i, blood, and fluid in the skin and muscle and in and between the ts'ang and fu organs.

The upper burner includes the lung. Although the movement of ch'i is regulated by the lung, the origin of ch'i is the middle burner, where grain and water are digested before being transformed into minute elements that condense in the lung to form ching ch'i. In this way, the muscle and skin get the nutrients needed to form the *wei ch'i,* or defense mechanism. The upper burner also serves as the passageway for grain, water, and grass to pass through to the stomach. Disorders of the upper burner are caused by the accumulation of heat in the lung. An example of the disorder in the horse is a cough and serous nasal discharge.

The middle burner includes the spleen and the stomach. These organs receive food, which is then digested. The ch'i, blood, and fluid thus produced then nourish the whole body. The function of the middle burner, therefore, is to facilitate the distribution of ch'i, blood, and fluid throughout the body. To assure that the stomach and spleen function properly, the middle burner has a regulatory and moderating effect. Thus, disorders of the middle burner cause indigestion. In the horse this is manifested by loss of appetite, and in cattle, by gaseous distension.

The main functions of the lower burner are to ensure the proper drainage of fluid, to separate the clear from the contaminated ch'i, and to ensure the excretion of the contaminated ch'i as fluid and solid wastes. Disorders of the lower burner disrupt the formation of fluid in the urinary bladder, and edema, ascites, and reduction in urine production are found.*

The Theory of Five Elements†

The Yin-Yang Theory and the Theory of Five Elements were established as independent branches of Chinese physiology during the time of the Spring and Autumn and the Warring States periods. After the Ch'in and Han dynasties, these two theories were combined as basic concepts underlying Chinese medicine.

The Theory of Five Elements postulates that five elements—Wood, Fire, Earth, Metal, and Water—make up the fundamental materials of the universe. The individual properties and interrelationships of these five elements form the basis of the theory to explain the workings of the universe.

Everything of the earth is considered to belong to one or several of the five elements. The Theory of Five Elements categorizes all materials of the universe, living or nonliving, into the five categories and then postulates their interdependence in terms of stimulation or inhibition, creation or destruction.

The basic implication of the Yin-Yang Theory—that people and animals are microcosms of the universe—was integrated into the Theory of Five Elements so that it could be used to explain the physiological and pathologic characteristics of both. Every organ of the living organism is assigned an element that interacts with elements of other organs in the same way as the elements in the universe interact with each other. The Theory of Five Elements postulates that the environment affects the physiologic and pathologic characteristics of animals, and it explains motion and change, not only in the universe but also in animals, by considering the animal as a whole unit, and by describing the interdependence and self-regulatory mechanism of each organ.

The five elements refer to categories that are euphemistic and symbolic for a set of characteristics and functions. They are not to be taken literally.

CHARACTERISTICS OF THE FIVE ELEMENTS

The five elements are not static; they are always dynamically in motion through the processes of growth and transformation.

There are two aspects of change in the universe—the changes resulting from the growth and development of living organisms and the transformation of nonliving materials, and changes in the environment. Environmental changes directly affect the growth and transformation of living and nonliving materials. Chinese philosophy postulates five fundamental changes that take place in nature. These are related to the five elements of the universe and to environmental changes. Human beings and animals also go through five fundamental changes corresponding to the changes in nature. The relationships are shown in Table 1-1. The interaction of the five elements serves as a description of the rule that regulates the

---

* In *Nan Ching,* the 31st question and answer.

† In *Shang Shu,* in the chapter "Hung fan" ("Grand dimension"). Also in "Shu wen", *Nei Ching,* in the chapter "Yin-yang ying hsing ta lun".

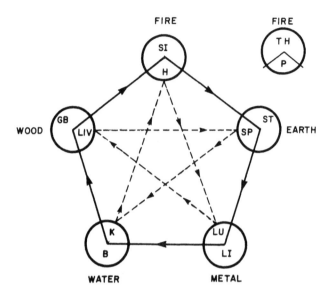

FIGURE 1–1. Diagramatic representation of the Theory of Five Elements. The solid line is the creation cycle and the broken line is the destruction cycle. SI—small intestine; H—heart; ST—stomach; SP—spleen; LU—lung; LI—large intestine; K—kidney; B—bladder; GB—gall bladder; LIV—liver; TH—triple burner; P—percardium.

universal pattern of changes. This interaction is duplicated in the organisms.

The basic rule governing the interaction of the five elements is that of mutual creation and mutual destruction—both of which occur simultaneously in the universe and in the organism to maintain equilibrium. Pathologic conditions occur when the regulated relationship of creation and destruction is disrupted.

The order of mutual creation is shown in Figure 1–1: wood creates fire; fire creates earth; earth creates metal; metal creates water; and water creates wood.

Wood may be burned; therefore, it creates fire. The materials, being burned in the fire, become ash; therefore, fire creates earth. Earth is where the minerals are located from which the metal is extracted; therefore, earth creates metal. The moisture of the air condenses on metal to become water drop—therefore, metal creates water. Water provides the moisture necessary for the growth of vegetation; therefore, water creates wood.

At the same time, mutual destruction takes place. Mutual destruction, or inhibition, is designed to limit overdevelopment and excessive creation. The order of mutual destruction is also shown in Figure 1–1: wood destroys earth; earth destroys water; water destroys fire; fire destroys metal; and metal destroys wood.

The roots of the tree stretch into the earth and absorb the nutrients; therefore, wood destroys earth. An earthen dam can limit the flow of water; therefore, earth destroys water. Fire melts metal; therefore, fire destroys metal. Metal can be an axe to cut down the tree; therefore, metal destroys wood. It can be seen that each element creates and destroys another simultaneously, while it is being created and destroyed by another element. For example, wood creates fire and destroys earth while it is created by water and destroyed by metal.

The same principles are applicable to the ts'ang and fu organs. Each ts'ang organ stimulates and inhibits another ts'ang organ and stimulates and inhibits a fu organ, and at the same time it is being created and destroyed by another ts'ang organ and another fu organ. The same is true for the fu organs. (Fig. 1–1).

There is what is called the *mother-and-son relationship* in mutual creation and destruction. Because water creates wood, it is said that water is the *mother* and wood is the *son*.

The mother-and-son relationship is also important to the concept of mutual destruction. Both creation and destruction are normally unidirectional; however, under pathologic conditions, there is a phenomenon of reverse inhibition. For example, when the relative strength of the water diminishes, fire will destroy water. This concept is also applicable to the ts'ang and fu organs.

MUTUAL REGULATION OF THE FIVE ELEMENTS

Mutual regulation is the state of equilibrium having a balance of creation and destruction. Equilibrium is the fundamental rule of the universe. If creation or destruction dominates, the animal cannot maintain a normal, well-balanced development. For example, water destroys fire; however, water creates wood, and wood creates fire. Therefore, equilibrium is gained through the well-coordinated processes of mutual creation and destruction. None of the categories defined by each of the five elements is absolute or static. Under certain conditions, all of these categories are in the state of transformation.

THE RELATIONSHIP OF THE YIN-YANG THEORY AND THE THEORY OF FIVE ELEMENTS IN CHINESE MEDICINE

The Theory of Five Elements utilizes all the basic concepts either stated or implied by the Yin-Yang

Theory: (1) the need for balance, (2) the interdependence between living organism and environment, and (3) the relationship of the destruction of imbalance (due to excess or deficiency) to pathologic conditions. Diagnosis and therapy in Chinese medicine utilize the Yin-Yang Theory as a framework, and the Theory of Five Elements for specific guidelines to recognize pathologic conditions.

Etiology

In Chinese veterinary medicine, disease results from an imbalance in yin and yang to such an extent that the body, by itself, cannot reestablish the balance. Thus, the veterinarian attempts to reestablish the balance by strengthening the healthy, or the normal, signs of the organism and destroying the unhealthy or abnormal, signs. These signs are called *chen*, or *hsieh.**

Diagnosis

In order to treat successfully, the Chinese veterinarian attempts to diagnose by going through a series of steps. He first checks the color of the mouth and tongue, the type of pulses, and the condition of the orifices (eyes, mouth, nose, ears, and tongue) (see Table 1-1). Each of these may manifest abnormal signs of the ts'ang or fu organs.

Each abnormal sign may be classified as hot or cold (yin or yang in nature),† deficient or full (due to deficiency or overabundance of ch'i and blood),‡ and superficial or deep (in accordance to its severity, its relationship to ts'ang or fu organ, or its actual location).§ After he has determined all that is abnormal, he ascribes the signs as belonging to one or several syndromes: moisture, dryness, heat, cold, wind, fire. These names are euphemistic and serve only to categorize certain signs, for acupuncture prescriptions also include these categories. These names, rather than describing the nature of the disease, refer to an internal or external factor causing the disease because it is believed that diseases are caused by environmental factors that influence internal weakness or abuses.

---

* In *Yuan Heng Liao Ma Chi,* in the chapters "Chen chen lun" (Chen syndrome), and "Hsieh chen lun" (Hsieh syndrome).

† In *Yuan Heng Liao Ma Chi,* in the chapters "Han chen lun" (Han syndrome) and "Je chen lun" (Je syndrome).

‡ In *Yuan Heng Liao Ma Chi,* in the chapters "Shu chen lun" (Shu syndrome) and "Ssee chen lun" (Ssee syndrome).

§ In *Yuan Heng Liao Ma Chi,* in the chapters "Piao chen lun" (Piao syndrome) and "Lei chen lun" (Lei syndrome).

Four Procedures to Determine the Abnormal Signs

There are four steps in the diagnostic procedure: observation, listening, questioning, and palpation.

OBSERVATION

Observation, vital signs, color, posture, actions, and other external signs are observed by the veterinarian and combined with other information in order to find a proper diagnosis and determine a prescription.

According to the concepts of the ts'ang and fu organs, observation of the external features of the domestic animal provides information on the physiological conditions of the internal organs; for example, the tongue corresponds to the heart and the eyes correspond to the liver. From the urine, it is possible to determine diseases of the urinary bladder; from stool examination, pathologic changes in the stomach and intestine. From observation of the limbs, diseases of the legs and hooves can be found. Skin diseases such as furuncles, pustules, and carbuncles, indicate conditions of the blood and ch'i.

Because different species of animals have different morphologies, to properly notice the abnormal signs it is essential that the normal signs of the individual animal are known.

Observation emphasizes different factors. For example, in the pig, behavior during feeding, urine, and stool excretion should be noted; in cattle, normal or abnormal sweating on the nose; in horses, the standing and lying postures because they indicate painful spots; in sheep, whether it stays with the flock; in chickens, the condition of the crown and the wings. Observation of the color of the mouth is a very special feature of Chinese veterinary medicine, because the state of ch'i and blood is shown by the color of the mouth.

The relationship of color to the various parts of the mouth and the intestines is described in the following paragraphs.

1. The lips. The spleen corresponds to the lips, and the spleen is related to the stomach. Therefore, changes in the lips reflect diseases of the spleen and stomach.

If the sick animal has red lips, excessive "heat" is present in the spleen. Yellow lips indicate excessive "cold-moisture" of the spleen meridian. White lips indicate "cold" in the spleen and stomach. Green lips indicate a poor prognosis.

2. The teeth. The gums of the teeth are related to the stomach and intestines; therefore, changes in the gums occur if the stomach and intestines are sick.

If the gums are scarlet and dry, there is "heat" in the stomach and intestines; if white, moist and slippery, there is "cold" in the stomach and intestine. If the gums and the tip of the tongue are scarlet, there is "heat" in the heart meridian, as in cases of hematuria. If the gums are white and the tongue is a faint yellow with additional difficulty in the movement of the low back region, back pain caused by "cold" is present; if the gums are ulcerous and bleeding, with bad breath and thirst, there is a "fullness" type of "heat".

3. "Silkworms." There are elevated areas on both sides of the base of the tongue, said to resemble silkworms, the left one corresponds to the liver (golden gate); the right corresponds to the lung (jade house). These two areas reflect diseases of these two organs.

If the golden gate is green, there is "wind" in the liver meridian; if yellow or in combination with a yellow color of the inside membranes of the eyes, mouth, and nose, jaundice is present; if red, there is liver "heat". The jade house corresponds to the lung. If it is white, there is "cold" and deficiency in both ch'i and blood.

4. The tongue. The cornified coating of the tongue reflects the functional state of the heart. Clinically, observations of changes in color, temperature, and moisture of the tongue provide evidence of the conditions of ch'i and blood, the type of syndrome ("cold" or "hot", "fullness" or "deficiency", "external" or "internal") and the prognosis.

There are two categories of changes in the tongue: cold or hot. In cold syndromes, circulation of ch'i and blood is slow. If this condition is mild, the tongue is dark red; if severe, it is green-purple. If the tongue is dark green, an emergency is indicated. In hot syndromes, the circulation of ch'i and blood are accelerated. If the condition is mild, the color is red; if severe, scarlet; if dark purple, an emergency is indicated.

Different techniques are used for observing mouth color in different animals. The emphasis is also different. In the pig, the color of the tongue, gum, lips, silkworm and mouth corner is most important (the characteristics.are the same as for the tongue). In cattle, the tongue and silkworm are emphasized; in goats and camels, the color of the tongue.

LISTENING (INCLUDING HEARING AND SMELLING)

The sounds the veterinarian should listen for are crying, coughing, heavy breathing, shortness of breath, belching, grinding of teeth, and a rumbling stomach. Heavy breathing and shortness of breath are related to lung disorders; belching, to disorders of the spleen and stomach; the grinding of teeth and moaning, to kidney disorders; rumbling, to intestinal disorders. The ability to distinguish the nature of sound is helpful in determining the nature of the organ in disorder.

Under healthy conditions, the ch'i and blood of the animal are well-regulated, and the animal does not have any particular odors except its own. When the animal is sick, the circulation of ch'i and blood is not properly regulated and metabolism is abnormal, thus producing changes in secretions, such as those from the mouth, nose, anus, and skin, and changes in odor.

QUESTIONING

In this diagnostic procedure, the case history of the animal is taken from its owner. Understanding the management and feeding of the sick animal and the course of the disease is necessary to form a correct diagnosis. The age, sex, and history of the sick animal must be recorded.

The owner should always be questioned about signs, appetite, respiration, abdominal pain, feces, and urine. For example, if the sick animal has lost its appetite and also drinks very little water, there is a deficiency or weakness of stomach ch'i. If the sick animal has a good appetite, the disease is mild. If there is a complete loss of appetite, the disorder is severe.

PALPATION

In addition to ordinary palpation, pulse readings on the medial side of the femur, characteristic changes in sensory response, and changes in body surface temperature and condition must be checked. Pulse diagnosis is the most important part of palpation, because changes in pulses explain the rise and fall of the levels of ch'i and blood in the body.*

Sites for taking the pulse vary in different species, and even within a species several sites can be used.

Horse—Most veterinarians agree that the preferred site for pulse diagnosis is on the chest, lateral to the trachea. The points are located cephalad and dorsad to the sternum, at the depression lateral to the trachea. This is the passageway of the ch'i and blood. Each area (one on each side of the trachea) is divided into three sections. On the right side, there

* In *Yuan Heng Liao Ma Chi,* in the chapter "Mo sse lun" (On pulse and color).

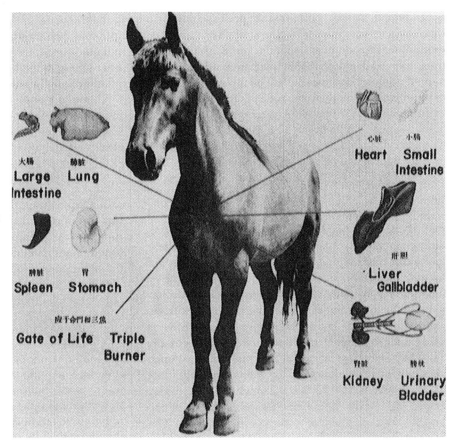

FIGURE 1–2. Location of the pulses in the horse.

Large Lung
Intestine

Spleen Stomach

Gate of Life Triple
Burner

Heart Small
Intestine

Liver
Gallbladder

Kidney Urinary
Bladder

are three "gates". On the left, there are three "portions".

The three portions are the upper, middle, and the lower. The three gates are the *feng gate*, the *ch'i gate* and the *ming gate*. The three portions and the three gates correspond to the various ts'ang and fu organs. The left upper portion corresponds to the heart and the small intestine; the left middle portion corresponds to liver and gallbladder; the left lower portion corresponds to kidney and urinary bladder; the right feng gate corresponds to the lungs and large intestine; the right ch'i gate corresponds to the spleen and stomach; the right ming gate corresponds to the triple-burner and the ching ch'i of the kidney (Fig. 1–2).

In pulse diagnosis, the animal should be kept calm, and diagnosis should start on the left side of the animal. The veterinarian stands on the right side of the animal and uses his right hand in the diagnosis. The index finger presses the upper portion; the middle finger presses the middle portion; the ring finger presses the lower portion. Then, the veterinarian turns to the left side of the animal and uses his left hand to palpate the right side of the animal.

The index finger presses the feng gate; the middle finger presses the ch'i gate; the ring finger presses the ming gate.

The method just described is used by those practicing Chinese veterinary medicine. However, a few practitioners use the submandibular area of the horse in diagnosing the right side. The veterinarian stands on the anterior right side of the animal; the right hand on the head. The index, middle, and ring fingers of the left hand are pressed on the facial artery of the sub-mandibular area. Then, the veterinarian turns to the other side; the left hand fixes the head of the animal; the index, middle, and ring fingers of the right hand press the artery of the left submandibular area.

In each of the portions or gates, there are three levels of pulse diagnosis—that is, three levels of pressure are applied to the pulse. The light level of pressure is the fu, or "superficial," level; the medium level of pressure is the chung level; and the ch'en level is the deep pulse taken by heavy finger pressure.

Pulse diagnosis should be done when the animal is calm. The thumb is first pressed hard on the side contralateral to the pulse-taking position, and the three fingers for pulse-taking are slightly curved to determine the accurate position for measuring the pulse rate and pulse phenomena, such as "large" or "small", "hung" or "hsien", "fu" or "ch'en" and "hua" or "sse" (see Types of Pulse, below).

The practitioner carefully examines the individual pulse phenomena. First, the index finger takes the fu level of the heart pulse. He then presses harder to take the chung or the medium level. Finally the veterinarian uses the middle finger to concentrate on the fu, chung, and ch'en sections and gates.

Swine—The site for taking the pulse is at the medial side of the posterior thigh. When the pulse is being taken, the owner of the pig must keep the sick animal calm and at rest, and the veterinarian should stay on the lateral side of the pig, with his hand inserted along the abdominal wall toward the posterior, to press on the artery at the medial side of the thigh.

Cattle—The site for taking the pulse in cattle is usually the tail artery at the root of the tail near the anus. When taking the pulse, the veterinarian stands at the immediate posterior of the animal; the left hand slightly raises the animal's tail with the index finger, the middle finger, and the ring finger on the middle of the proximal three segments of the tail. The various pressures of the fingers will help locate the correct position for taking the pulse. Other locations—such as the root of the ear and the leg—are seldom used.

Goat—The site for taking the pulse is at the artery of the medial side of the thigh. The method is the same as that used in swine.

A skillful technique is very important in pulse diagnosis. To achieve an accurate diagnosis, it is necessary for beginners to practice frequently. During pulse-taking, it is necessary for the practitioner to stay calm and concentrate.

Changes in pulse phenomena in domestic animals occur not only in diseases, but also in healthy animals when there are weather changes. In hot weather, the circulation of ch'i and blood is comparatively faster. "Hsien" and "huang" types of pulse appear. However, in colder weather, the circulation of ch'i and blood is slower. "Mao" and "shik" types of pulse appear.

Changes in pulse phenomena may be related to poor management in feeding and labor. For example, in a fully fed horse, hung pulse may be found. If the horse is improperly fed, deficiency types of pulse appear. After galloping, the shu pulse is usually found.

Pulse phenomena are also related to the age and physical condition of the animal. For example, in healthy adults the pulse is strong and conspicuous. Fat, strong animals have strong pulses; skinny, weak animals usually have weak, thready pulses.

Types of Pulse—There are only four types of pulse for pigs, cattle, and goats; they are fu, ch'en, shu, and ch'ih. Horses have all the different types of pulse discussed below (Fig. 1–3). In general, the nature of the pulse can be divided into p'ing (normal), fan (reversed), and yie (changed):

1. P'ing mo (normal pulse). This pulse is peaceful and moderate. In healthy domestic animals, the number of pulse beats are: pigs, 50–80/minute; cattle, 60–80/minute; horses, 36–44/minute; goats, 70–80/minute; and camel, 32–52/minute.

Pulse phenomena in the healthy animal change with the weather: spring, hsien mo; summer, mao mo; and winter, shih mo. However, whatever the variation, the pulse must flow evenly without interruption.

2. Fan mo (reverse pulse). This pulse is the opposite of the normal pulse, a sign that the animal is sick. For example, in spring and summer, the temperature is relatively high. Physiological activities in the animal are at their peak and the pulse should be hsien and hung. If the pulse is fast and strong, it is an indication of an excess ch'i, and the animal is sick. Different types of reverse pulse are described in the following paragraphs.

Fu mo is a light, flowing pulse, the nature of which is yang, indicating wind, and a deficiency syndrome. The symptoms are for cold (see pp. 11 and 12): hair on the end, fever and cough, gaseous distension and nasal discharge. This pulse may be divided into *floating firm,* or *floating infirm.* The floating firm pulse indicates superficial heat syndromes; the floating infirm pulse, superficial and deficiency syndromes.

Ch'en mo is a deep pulse that can be felt only if the veterinarian presses deeply. The ch'en mo indicates deep syndromes. It appears in indigestion and overlabor. It is divided into "deep firm" or "deep infirm" types. If it is deep and firm, there is a deep and fullness syndrome. If it is deep and infirm, there is a deep and deficiency syndrome.

Ch'ih mo is a slow pulse, mainly indicating cold syndromes. Ch'ih mo appears in sick animals with excessive labor producing weakness of ch'i and in deficient and cold syndromes of the spleen and stomach. Ch'ih mo also has firm and infirm types. If the ch'ih mo is firm, excessive cold syndromes are

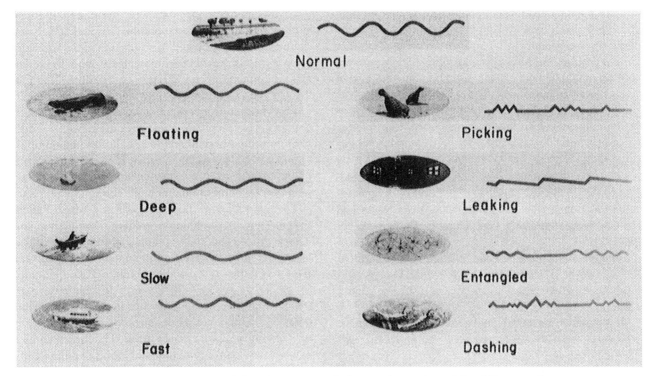

FIGURE 1–3. Diagramatic representation of the characteristic feeling of the quality of the different pulses.

most likely indicated—for example, gastroenteritis and gastrointestinal spasmodic pain. If the ch'ih mo is infirm, deficient cold syndromes are indicated—for example, drooling and anal prolapse.

Shu mo is a quick pulse, which can be felt with a light, superficial pressure. Shu mo indicates mainly excessive heat syndromes. The sick animal has a dry mouth and tongue, oligurea, and constipation, and heat accumulation of the ts'ang and fu organs. Shu mo may be firm or infirm. If the shu mo is firm, an excess and heat syndrome is indicated. If the shu mo is infirm, a deficient and heat syndrome is indicated.

Hsien mo is a taut pulse, the feeling of which is like a tremulous musical string. Superficial syndromes are indicated by the hsien mo, and it is found in animals with wind and obstruction of the circulation of ch'i and blood, as, for example, in tetanus. Furthermore, it also indicates a liver disease, such as in liver heat (influenza).

Huang mo is a full, overflowing pulse, bounding and forceful. Huang mo is yang in nature and indicates heat, as in an accumulation of heat in the triple-burner, oral sores, abscesses, and other syndromes of excessive heat.

Hua mo is a slippery pulse. The pulse is strong and forceful, yet rolling (like rolling pearls in the tray). The slippery pulse indicates that the animal is full of ch'i, and it is an indication of the competition of the ch'i of the body and the invading ch'i. Hua mo is often found concomitantly with the shu mo pulse. Hua mo is equivalent to shu and firm pulse phenomena, and it indicates a fullness syndrome or fullness and heat syndromes.

Sse mo is a feeble and intermittent pulse. It is caused by a deficiency of blood and fluid, or an obstruction of the flow of ch'i and blood. The animal shows a general malaise, chronic diarrhea, and a coldness of ears and nose. It indicates a deficiency and cold syndrome.

K'ou mo is a large, hollow, superficial, soft pulse. It feels like one is squeezing an onion stalk. It indicates deficiency and feebleness, and is caused by a sudden loss of blood and floating and dispersion of the yang type of ch'i. This pulse is usually found in animals with excessive bleeding due to traumatic injury, hematuria, a deficiency of ch'i, and a weakness of blood.

Hsi mo is a small, slender, feeble pulse. It feels perceptible and thin, like a silk thread. It is found in chronically debilitated animals.

3. Yie mo (changed pulse). There are five kinds of yie mo. The pulse phenomena indicate signs of critical stages of the life of the animal.

The *picking pulse* is irregular with a missing beat in every three of four beats. It is found in the late stages of gangrene.

The *leaking pulse* has an irregular time interval between feeble beats. It is found in late stages of acute heart failure. A descriptive feature of the pulse is that it is like leaking water drops from the ceiling.

The *entangled pulse* is fast and feeble; the beat is irregular and intermittent. It is found in horse gangrene.

The *dashing pulse* is very superficial; it may suddenly disappear and reappear. It is found in gastrointestinal rupture in horse, and has been described as a shrimp swimming very close to the surface of water.

The *puffing pulse* is like puffing bubbles from boiled water. It indicates the terminal stages of a disease resulting from a failure of the five ts'ang organs.

If properly mastered, pulse diagnosis in Chinese veterinary medicine is supposed to be of great prognostic value.

Acupuncture Points and the Meridian Theory

An acupuncture point is a specifically designated location on the body surface. It is sometimes called the *stimulating point*. According to Chinese medical concepts, the points are not isolated sites on the surface of the body of humans and animals, but are linked with visceral organs.*

The relationships between the acupuncture points on the surface of the body and the viscera inside are as follows: From the inside of the body to the outside—disease of an area causes local points on the surface of the body to become tender. From the acupuncture points on the surface of the body toward the viscera—stimulating the acupuncture point on the surface of the body causes healing of the problem. When a person or animal is sick, certain sites on the surface of the body demonstrate sensitivity or a local tenderness with applied pressure. For example, in human stomach disease, there are local "tender points" in the regions of the skin corresponding to the heart; in human appendicitis, the tender points appear on the surface of the lower right abdomen and on the lateral surface of the tibia. The tender points are the basis of the location of acupuncture points.

An accumulation of clinical experience indicates that many acupuncture points are found to have healing effects not only on localized or adjacent areas, but also on distant areas.† In order to explain this relationship, the Ching Lo, or the Meridian Theory, was established.

For thousands of years, diagnosis and treatment using herbal medicine or acupuncture depended heavily on the Meridian Theory. The practical application of the Meridian Theory is late in coming to Chinese veterinary medicine compared with its application in Chinese human medicine.

The *ching lo* in Chinese are the channels where the ch'i and the blood circulate. The Ching Lo Theory states that, in the human body is a series of large and small pathways interconnected on the surface and in the interior of the body. These channels are called *ching mo* and *lo mo*. The ching mo are the main trunks, and the lo mo are the small tributaries branching out in the form of a weblike structure among the large main trunks. The large channels have a large quantity of ch'i and blood flowing inside, and the smaller channels have smaller quantities. The large channels are sometimes called *meridians*; thus, the Ching Lo Theory, or Meridian Theory.

Whenever there is a disturbance in the flow of ch'i and blood in the ching and lo, there is disease. The site at which the regulation or readjustment of the flow of ch'i and blood can be achieved is mainly, but not exclusively, on the 14 classic meridians.‡ The regulation of ch'i and blood is necessary in the treatment of disease.

The ching lo provides a communicating network, linking individual acupuncture points on the body to the visceral organs. Specific groups of acupuncture points belong to a specific meridian and provide a link to a particular visceral organ through the distribution of the large channels.

Essentially, the Ching Lo Theory explains the relationship between different areas of the body surface, the relationship between the body surface and the internal viscera, and the relationship between one

* In *Nan Ching*, the "23rd question and answer", it says that the twelve meridians belong to the organs in the interior of the body, and the meridians communicate with joints and limbs.

† In *Yuan Heng Liao Ma Chi*, in the chapter "Hsing chen lun" (The syndromes). Also in the "Shu wen" section of *Nei Ching*, in the chapter "P'i pu lun", (On the skin). Literally, it says, "The skin and the hair are sites from which diseases may originate. The etiologic factors of disease first invade the hair, skin, and subcutaneous tissues, entering the ching and lo, then into the ts'ang and fu organs and at last they accumulate in the stomach and intestine. The twelve meridians are distributed on the surface of the skin."

‡ The "Ling shu" section of *Nei Ching*, in the chapter "Ching mo p'ien" (The meridian channels) says the "meridians determine the diagnosis and treatment of diseases".

visceral organ and another. These relationships provide the most important rule in the use of the Meridian Theory for therapeutic purposes: the acupuncture points are prescribed on the meridian in the area where disease symptoms are manifested.

THE STRUCTURE OF CHING LO

The ching lo has a physiologic and a pathologic function. The six ts'ang organs and six fu organs and other tissues and organs have different physiologic functions. The ching and lo form a network interconnecting all organs to maintain an equilibrium.* The ching and lo not only passively serve as an interconnecting pathway, but also have the function of promoting the circulation of ch'i and blood, so that the ts'ang, fu, and other tissues and organs can be properly nourished, maintain normal physiologic activities, and sustain an equilibrium of yin and yang.

There is always a close relationship between the organic body of the domestic animal and changes in the surrounding environment. Because the ching and lo provide a network between the interior of the body with the exterior surface, an equilibrium must also be maintained between the physiologic activities of the body and the external environment.

Under normal physiologic conditions, the meridian facilitates the flow of ch'i and blood, so that when the disease invades the body, the ching and lo regulate the level of activities of the defense mechanism (wei) and physiologic activities of the organs so that the body is defended against disease. If the natural defense mechanism of the organic body is weakened, yin and yang lose equilibrium, and disease enters through the surface to the channels of ching and lo. For example, "wind" and "cold" cause abdominal pain and diarrhea. They enter the body through the skin, and using the channels of the ching and lo, they reach and accumulate in the intestine.† On the other hand, diseases of the intestine are manifested on the surface through ching and lo.

THE APPLICATION OF
CHING LO THEORY TO DIAGNOSIS‡

Because the ching and lo provide the network between the internal viscera and the skin surface, a disease can affect the visceral organs through these channels. When a visceral organ is diseased, symptoms occur in the form of tender points along the related meridian. According to the case history, symptoms, and the diagnostic examination of the tender points, it is possible to determine whether the disease is related to one meridian or to several meridians. From the relation of the meridian to the organs, it is then possible to determine the affected organ(s).

Pathologic changes in the acupuncture points (or the site of tenderness) have an important diagnostic significance. For example, a cough may be caused by disorders of the lung meridian and the kidney meridian. To distinguish to which meridian the disorder belongs, observation of changes in the local tenderness of acupuncture points is essential. Furthermore, systematic knowledge of the symptoms of the two meridians is useful. For example, the asthmatic cough of the lung meridian indicates emphysema. The animal walks slowly with the front limb fully extended. On the other hand, the cough of the kidney meridian is a cold cough—that is, the type of cough that is more severe at night and is associated with other symptoms. During this cough, the hindlimb may be flexed to reduce the pain of the low back region.

THE APPLICATION OF
THE CHING LO THEORY IN THERAPY

In therapy, medicinal herbs and acupuncture adjust the ching and lo that are not functioning properly. There are many ways to treat the disease of one organ because more than one meridian may affect the organ. In other words, the same disease may be treated by using herbs on different meridians.

The pharmacologic characteristics of herbs differ, so that the meridian routes that the pharmacologic effect will take to reach the diseased organ and to regulate the obstructed ch'i of the organ differ. For example, an orally administered herb or drug can treat the diseases of a ts'ang organ; the pharmacologic property of a drug may reach the area of pathologic change of the property of ching lo—that is, transportation. Therefore, the nature of the drug in Chinese

* The "Ling shu" section of Nei Ching, in the chapter "Ching mo p'ien" (The meridian channels) says "Meridians determine the diagnosis and treatment of diseases."

† In Yuan Heng Liao Ma Chi, in the chapter "Hsing chen lun" (The syndromes). Also in "Shu wen" section of Nei Ching, in the chapter "P'i pu lun" (On the skin). Literally, it says "The skin and the hair are the sites on which diseases may originate. The etiologic factors of disease first invade the hair, skin, and subcutaneous tissues, entering the ching and lo, then into the ts'ang and fu organs, and at last they accumulate in the stomach and intestine. The twelve meridians are distributed on the surface of the skin."

‡ The "Ling shu" section of Nei Ching, in the chapter "Ching mo p'ien" (The meridian channels) says "Meridians determine the diagnosis and treatment of diseases."

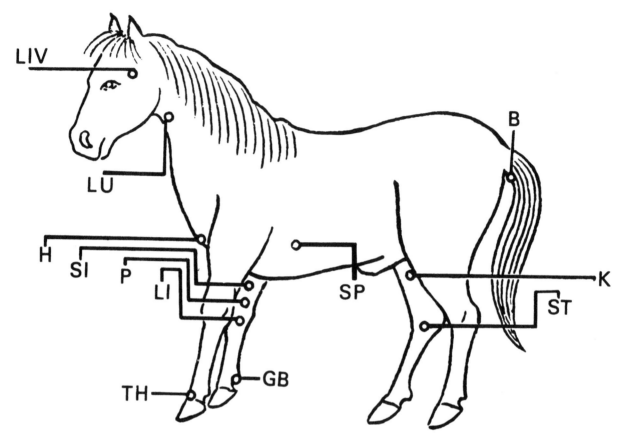

FIGURE 1-4. Drawing of a horse showing the location of the twelve meridian points. LIV–Liver, HN6; LU–Lung, HN18; H–Heart, FL16; P–Pericardium, FL24; SP–Spleen, T13; K–Kidney, HL15; TH–Triple Burner, FL20; ST–Stomach, FL18; GB–Gall Bladder, FL19; LI–Large Intestine, HL16; B–Bladder, HL19; SI–Small Intestine, front leg, Tung Chin (cephalic vein, just ventral to the sternum).

medicine is classified according to its interaction with the meridians, in addition to the kind of disease against which it is effective. In other words, to properly prescribe the herbal medicine for a particular disease, knowledge of the Meridian Theory is fundamental.

In acupuncture treatment, some diseases are treated using acupuncture points close to the site of disorder. In other diseases, the prescription of acupuncture points follows the location and flow of the meridian. In the horse, for example, acupuncture point HN6 is used in heat syndrome of the liver meridian, being transmitted from the liver to the eyes; for the heat syndromes of the heart meridian, FL16 is used; for the cold syndrome of the spleen meridian, T10 is used; for the pain syndrome of the lung meridian, T12 is used; and for the heat syndromes of the kidney meridian, HL15 is used.

In *Yuan Heng Liao Ma Chi*, the definitive work on veterinary medicine, the names of twelve acupuncture points representing each of the twelve

meridians are mentioned (Fig. 1-4 and Fig. 3-12). The Institute for Research in Chinese Veterinary Medicine of the Chinese Academy of Agricultural Science took the position, in June 1972, that further effort is necessary to determine to which meridians the unassigned acupuncture points belong.[1]

The Meridian Theory is fundamental to the application of the Yin-Yang Theory and the Theory of Five Elements for the prescription of acupuncture points following the flow of meridians in diagnosis and treatment.

THE CLASSIFICATION AND NOMENCLATURE OF CHING LO OR MERIDIANS

In horses, there are three yin and three yang ching in each of the forelimbs and a similar arrangement in the hindlimbs. The three yin are: lesser yin, absolute yin, and greater yin. The three yang are: sunlight yang, greater yang and lesser yang. The six yin and six yang vessels are sometimes called the *twelve mo*. Meridians are sometimes called *ching mo*.

The classification and nomenclature of meridians are based on the relationship of particular meridians to specific organs. Because there are six ts'ang and six fu organs, and there is a meridian, or ching, responsible for the linking of these organs to each other and to the surface of the body, the twelve meridians link the four limbs and the ts'ang and fu organs together as a unit.

The meridians are distributed in the limbs, and they are located either in the forelimb or in the hindlimb; there are forelimb meridians and hindlimb meridians. Furthermore, the ts'ang meridians flow on the medial surface of the limbs; the fu meridians flow on the lateral surface. Therefore, the ts'ang meridians are interior or subsurface; the fu meridians are exterior or superficial. The relationships between exterior and interior meridians, respectively, are as follows: forelimb greater yin lung meridian and forelimb sunlight yang large intestine meridian; hindlimb greater yin spleen meridian and hindlimb sunlight yang stomach meridian; forelimb lesser yin heart meridian and forelimb greater yang small intestine meridian; hindlimb lesser yin kidney meridian and hindlimb greater yang urinary bladder meridian; forelimb absolute yin pericardium meridian and forelimb lesser yang triple-burner meridian; and hindlimb absolute yin liver meridian and hindlimb lesser yang gallbladder meridian.

The meridian theory is not as well developed for animals as it is for humans. *Yuan Heng Liao Ma Chi* was the only source that describes any relationship of individual points to a specific meridian, and it only indicates one point for each meridian (in the horse) (Fig. 1–4 and Fig. 3–12).

"The point HN6 (yan mai) is in the absolute yin meridian, good for the moderation of liver fire. The point HN18 (ching mai) is in the lung greater yin meridian, good for distinguishing the heat of the five ts'ang organs. The point FL16 (hsiung t'ang) produces lesser yin; needle insertion into the point extinguishes the fire of the heart. The point FL24 (yeh yan) is not for needle insertion; it is related to absolute yin and the pericardium. The point T13 (tai mai) drains the greater yin; it drains the fire of spleen. The heat of the kidney produces swelling of the kidney meridian; the point HL15 (shen t'ang) of the lesser yin meridian is the one to use. For the obstruction of lesser yang and the triple-burner, the point FL20 (t'i t'ou) is good to clear the passage of drainage. The point FL18 (hsi hai) is in the greater yang meridian, good to absorb the heat of sunlight yang. The point FL19 (ch'an wan) is to attain balance of the gallbladder meridian. To extinguish the fire of the sunlight yang, the point HL16 (chu chih) is the one. For the drainage of the urinary bladder of the greater yang, the points HL18 (wei ken) and HL19 (wei pen) are the choice. The point S53 (tung chin) drains the small intestine, extinguishing the heart fire of the greater yang."[*] The location of these points is described in Chapter Three.

There is considerable controversy over modern charts that group many points on specific meridians for the horse. Chapter Three contains an extensive discussion of this problem. Classics of Chinese Veterinary Medicine have no information on meridians in any other domestic animals.

REFERENCE

1. Anon. 1972. "The meridians." In *Chung Sau I Chiang Dun Tsueh (Diagnosis in Chinese Veterinary Medicine)*, ed. Chinese Academy of Agriculture, Research Institute of Chinese Veterinary Medicine. Peking: Agriculture Press.

[*] In *Yuen Heng Liao Ma Chi*, in the chapter "Pai Lo ming tong lun" (Acupuncture points of General Pai Lo).

2

Acupuncture Techniques
and Equipment

Methods of Stimulation of Acupuncture Points

Acupuncture therapy requires the stimulation of one or more acupuncture points. There are many methods of producing this stimulation. A few are commonly used, some are rarely used, and some new ones are being investigated.

Needle. Needles are placed through the skin to the level of the acupuncture point. The needle is usually then manipulated to stimulate the point. This is the most commonly used technique and will be described in great detail.

Bleeding. This method uses various types of needles to cut or pierce the skin, with the intention of causing a variable but controlled amount of bleeding. Many of the points in farm animals, described in the Chinese literature, are points that are supposed to be stimulated by bleeding. This technique is also used in humans, but it has not received much popular attention in North America.

Injection. A variant of the traditional needle technique is the injection of various materials near the acupuncture point; some of the substances injected have been 5% dextrose, vitamin B_{12}, local anesthetic, sterile water, methylphenidate, volatile bases from *Sarracenia purpurea*, epinephrine in oil, and camphor in oil.

Implantation. There are several variants of this technique: (1) An acupuncture needle (usually very small with a round handle) is positioned and left in place for a period of days or weeks. (2) An acupuncture needle is positioned, and the shaft cut so that part of the shaft remains in the animal. (3) A small stainless steel or gold ball is placed subcutaneously either through a surgical incision or a large bore needle. (4) A piece of stainless steel or gold wire is placed through a needle and left in the site. (5) One of the several surgical staples or clips is implanted at the site through a surgical incision.

Temperature. Heat or cold can be used to stimulate the points.

Electromagnetic radiation. Various forms of light and sound have been used, such as ultraviolet light, visible light focused by a lens, laser beams, and ultrasound. Electric fields and magnetic fields have also been used.

External pressure. Pressure is applied to the skin by several methods: (1) finger; (2) tei-shin, which is a spring-loaded, blunt metal probe; and (3) granules, which are very small stainless steel balls applied to the skin with a small piece of tape.

Sedation and Tonification

Regardless of the method chosen for stimulating the points, two different levels of stimulation are

TABLE 2–1. *Techniques for Tonifying and Sedating Acupuncture Points*

METHOD	TONIFICATION	SEDATION
Needle	Slow movement	Fast movement
	Gentle movement	Rough movement
	Rotate clockwise	Rotate counterclockwise
	Insert or manipulate during exhalation	Insert or manipulate during inhalation
	Insert in the direction of the flow of ch'i	Insert in the direction opposite to the flow of ch'i
	Gold needle	Silver needle
	Bleeding—small quantity	Bleeding—large quantity
	Injection—small volume	Injection—large volume
	Injection—vitamin B_{12}	Injection—local anesthetic
Electric	Low frequency: 0.5–1 Hz	High frequency: 1–3 Hz
	Positive electrode	Negative electrode
All Methods	Gentle	Strong
	Short duration: 5–10 min	Long duration: 15–30 min

classically described—one is to tonify the point, and the other is to sedate it. Tonification is produced by the gentle stimulation of the acupuncture point; sedation is achieved by a more vigorous stimulation (Table 2–1). In general, tonification techniques are used in chronic conditions, and sedating techniques are used in acute conditions.

VETERINARY NEEDLE ACUPUNCTURE

The first part of this section will be almost a direct translation of a recently published veterinary book from China.[1] The tables giving dimensions were made by measuring commercially available Chinese needles.

Different types of acupuncture needles have traditionally been used to treat animals in China (Fig.

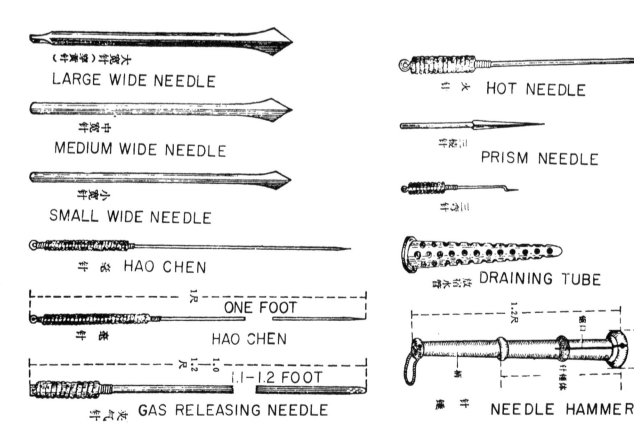

FIGURE 2–1. Drawings of commonly used Chinese veterinary needles.

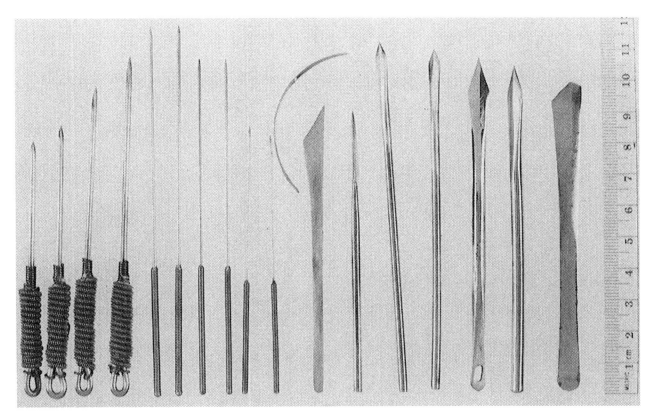

FIGURE 2–2. Set of Chinese veterinary needles (variety).

2–1). The acupuncture needle, or hao chen, is widely used in both the East and West. Other needle types are of limited use; for example, the piercing jaundice needle may be replaced by surgical instruments.

Several different sets of veterinary needles are commercially available in China at present. One set consists of only hao chen of various sizes. Other sets contain several different types of needle, including hao chen, wide needles, prism needles, hot needles, and piercing jaundice needles (Figs. 2–2, 2–3) (Tables 2–2 to 2–4).

Owing to the large diameter of many of the Chinese veterinary acupuncture needles and the thickness of the skin of some species, a device known as a needle hammer is sometimes used to place the needle (Figs. 2–1, 2–9 to 2–11). The hammer is basically a wooden handle (like an axe handle) in which the needle is inserted. The handle is then used like an axe, impaling the needle at the chosen site. The hammer is then removed from the needle.

Needle Types and Uses

Hao chen—This is the most commonly used needle and consists of two parts—the handle and the shaft (Figs. 2–1 to 2–4). The diameter ranges from 22- to 19-gauge, and the lengths vary from about 2 to 12 inches. The longer needles are used for insertion into several points at once.

Four major techniques are used for insertion of this needle (Fig. 2–5):

1. Pressing with the fingernail—the fingernail of the index finger or the thumb of one hand is used to apply digital pressure at the site immediately adjacent to the site of the acupuncture point. The needle is held between the index finger and the thumb of the other hand for forceful whirling. The middle and ring fingers support the needle. The needle is then directed toward the locus of the acupuncture point and is inserted through the skin to the desired depth. Coordination is essential.

2. Holding the handle of the needle with the thumb and the index finger of one hand, the needle is pressed down. At the same time, the thumb and index finger of the other hand hold the needle at the acupuncture point. This method is also useful when a long needle is used where the skin or musculature of the site is thick—for example, HL3 and HL4 in the horse.

3. Spreading the skin over the point—the skin is spread by using the thumb and index finger of one

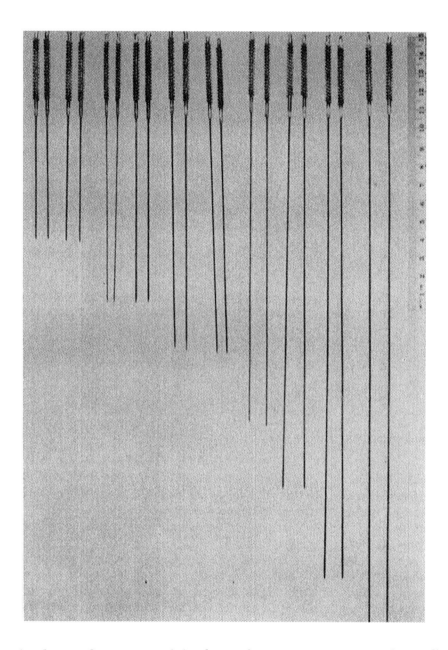

FIGURE 2–3. Set of Chinese veterinary needles (hao chen only).

hand to produce tension of the skin at the acupuncture point, to facilitate needle insertion. The other hand holds the needle between the thumb and the index finger and inserts the needle. The technique is used in area where the skin is loose—for example, points on the abdomen.

4. Lifting the skin up with the thumb and index finger of one hand, the needle is introduced with the other hand from a lateral direction. This technique is used in areas where the skin is thin—for example, points over the face.

Different angles of needle insertion are used, depending on the requirements of individual acupuncture points and needles used (Fig. 2–6). In *straight in-*sertion, the needle is perpendicular to the skin. This method is suitable for most acupuncture points in domestic animals. In *slanting insertion,* a 45-degree insertion is used for acupuncture points located in the depth of bony joints, or where vital organs are located underneath. In *lateral insertion,* a 15- to 25-degree angle for slanting insertion is used where the skin is very thin and the point is superficial.

Insertion may be slanting or perpendicular for methods 1, 2, and 3. Method 4 always requires slanting insertion. Needle insertion for any of the techniques just described may be done in two ways: In *quick insertion,* with the initial act of insertion, the needle reaches the subcutaneous tissue. The needle

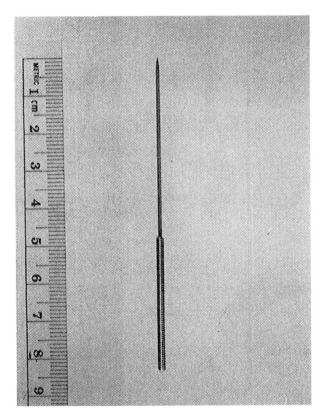

FIGURE 2–4. Hao chen.

is then twirled to a desired depth. In *twirling insertion*, after a quick initial insertion through the epidermis, gentle pressure is applied, and the handle is continuously twirled. The needle then finally reaches the desired depth.

A successful needle insertion will elicit a certain response from the animal known as *te ch'i*. The needle operator will feel a sinking and tightening of the needle. The animal will, in time, raise the limb, bend the back, swing the tail, and/or have muscular contractions. It is most likely that the point has not been hit if the acupuncturist feels a loose needle without any resistance. If this is the case, the needle is raised to the subcutaneous location and inserted again in the correct direction.

The purpose of the following procedures is to provide stimulation of the acupuncture point after the act of insertion is successful, as indicated by the state of te ch'i:

1. In sedation (suspension) and twirling, periodic and alternating clockwise and counterclockwise twirling and vibration of the inserted needle are used until the needle is very tightly grasped by the surrounding tissue. The needle then remains undisturbed for 2–3 min before this procedure is repeated.

2. Outward-inward movements of the inserted

TABLE 2–2. *15-Needle Chinese Veterinary Acupuncture Set*

DIAMETER (INCHES)	APPROX. GAUGE	LENGTH (INCHES)	NUMBER IN SET	NEEDLE TYPE
.035	20	1	1	Hao chen
.040	19	1½	1	Hao chen
.038	19	2	1	Hao chen
.0425	19	2½	1	Hao chen
.042	19	3	1	Hao chen
.042	19	3½	1	Hao chen
.0775	14	2	1	Hot
.077	14	3	1	Hot
.203	NA	2¾	1	Wide
.270	NA	2⅞	1	Wide
.125	11	2¾	1	Prism
.18	NA	3½	1	Cutting
.2	NA	3-3/16	1	Cutting
NA	NA	NA	2	Spay hooks

NA—Not applicable.

TABLE 2–3. *18-Needle Chinese Veterinary Acupuncture Set*

DIAMETER (INCHES)	APPROX. GAUGE	LENGTH (INCHES)	NUMBER IN SET	NEEDLE TYPE
.268	NA	4	1	Wide
.268	NA	4⅛	1	Wide
.180	NA	4¼	1	Wide
.2015	NA	4½	1	Wide
.032	21	2	2	Hao chen
.0375	19	2¾	2	Hao chen
.0455	18	3	2	Hao chen
.075	15	1⅞	1	Hot
.0765	14	2	1	Hot
.071	15	2⅛	1	Hot
.0745	15	2½	1	Hot
NA	NA	NA	1	Piercing jaundice
.025	NA	3-5/16	1	Cutting
			1	Unknown

NA—Not applicable.

TABLE 2–4. *20-Needle Chinese Veterinary Acupuncture Set*

DIAMETER (INCHES)	APPROX. GAUGE	LENGTH (INCHES)	NUMBER IN SET	NEEDLE TYPE
.037	19	2⅞	4	
.022	24	3-15/16	2	
.0365	19	4	2	
.0365	19	5	4	All hao
.0285	22	6½	2	chen
.037	19	8⅛	2	
.036	19	10	2	
.037	19	11	2	

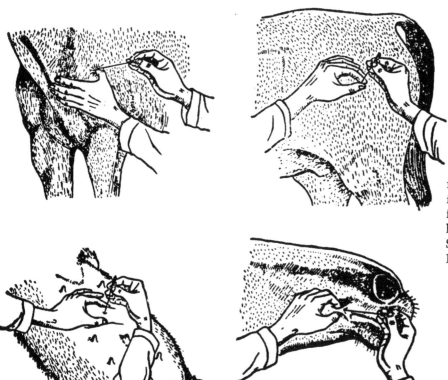

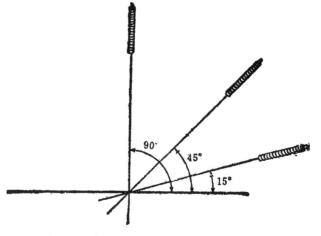

FIGURE 2–5. Techniques for needle insertion. *Upper left,* Pressing with fingernail. *Upper right,* Holding handle and point. *Lower left,* Spreading the skin. *Lower right,* Lifting the skin.

needle. When the needle is at the desired depth in the acupuncture point, it is withdrawn lightly and slowly, then inserted inward back to the desired depth of the acupuncture point forcefully and rapidly. This method provides a much stronger stimulation than sedation and twirling, and it is generally used at points with well-developed musculature. The operation lasts 2–5 min, and it is used every 2 or 3 days.

After the treatment with any needle and method, the needle is gently withdrawn by whirling. After withdrawal, the locus of the acupuncture point is sterilized.

If the needle is long, special precautions should be taken to prevent bending or breaking. The veterinarian should minimize any movement of the animal and also avoid exciting it. If the needle bends during treatment, it is slowly withdrawn by gentle twirling. If the needle is broken during treatment, the skin surrounding the point of insertion is pressed hard, and if possible, the broken segment is withdrawn with the help of a pair of forceps. If that is unsuccessful, a surgical operation is necessary.

Hot Needle—The use of the hot needle is similar to that of the hao chen; however, it provides a

stronger stimulation than the hao chen (Figs. 2–1, 2–2, 2–7). Hot needles cause more tissue destruction and therefore require a longer recovery period. In hot needle treatment, the prescription of points should be planned so that not more than three to five acupuncture points are used at one time. The same acupuncture points should not be used more than once a week. Improper sterilization, insufficient burning, or dampening of the needle hole may cause

FIGURE 2–6. Angles of needle insertion.

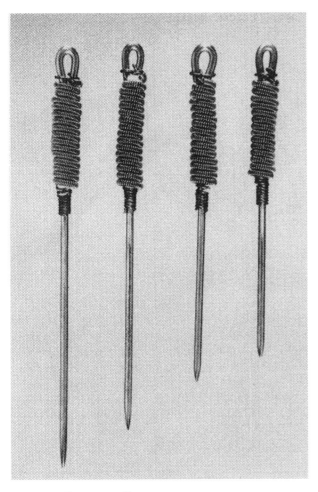

FIGURE 2–7. Hot needles.

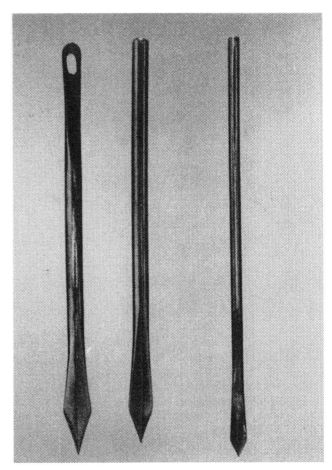

FIGURE 2–8. Wide needles.

abscesses when the hot needle is used. It is, therefore, essential that precautions are taken.

The procedure of hot needle insertion is as follows: The needle is cleaned, wrapped in a cotton ball, and then immersed in vegetable oil or alcohol, and burned until the cotton ball contracts and becomes black. When the fire becomes dim, the burnt cotton is removed with forceps, and the needle is then ready for use.

Before the needle is heated, the site of the acupuncture point is shaved and sterilized. As soon as the needle is ready, it is inserted to the required depth; the needle should stay in place for 2–5 min. The therapeutic effect can be achieved without having the needle stay in after insertion.

The needle is withdrawn, and the site is sterilized with iodine.

Wide Needle—This needle has a wide, spear-shaped tip, and it is 2.5–3 inches long (Figs. 2–1, 2–2, 2–8) (Table 2–2, 2–3). There are three sizes: small, medium, and large, with widths of 0.15, 0.20, and 0.25 in. They are used primarily for drawing blood and frequently called *blood needles*.

The needle is tightly grasped during insertion. If a needle hammer is used, the needle is secured tightly in accordance with the depth of insertion. Insertion should be fast and accurate, and the needle blade should be parallel with the blood vessels (Fig. 2–9). The build and size of the animal, characteristics of the disease, and seasonal factors determine the amount of blood to be drawn. For example, more blood can be drawn from a strongly and bulkily built animal than from a thin and weak animal.

The color and viscosity of the blood should also be taken into consideration—a change from dark brown to brilliant red is an indication that enough blood has been drawn to achieve a therapeutic effect. In general, less blood should be drawn in the winter than in the summer. After blood is drawn from acupuncture points, bleeding will stop. If bleeding continues, it is appropriate to stop it. If the blood involves the carotid artery or vessels of the temporal region, a rod should be attached to the neck of the sick animal. As

27 *Acupuncture Techniques and Equipment*

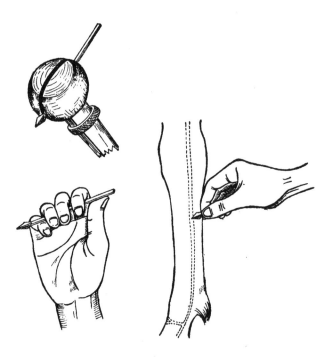

FIGURE 2–9. Use of wide needle. *Upper left,* Wide needle inserted in the needle hammer. *Lower left,* Wide needle held by hand. *Right,* Wide needle being inserted into and parallel with a large vein.

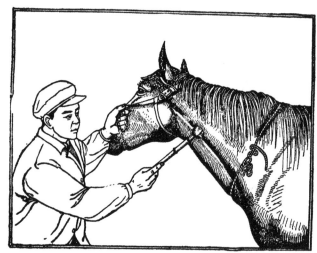

FIGURE 2–10. Wide needle, held by needle hammer, being inserted into HN18.

soon as a sufficient amount of blood has been drawn, the rod is used as a tourniquet to stop the bleeding. If the bleeding involves other parts of the body, a sterilized piece of cotton soaked with iodine is pressed for 5–10 min on the site, or a bandage is used.

If the needle is applied to the acupuncture points of the limbs, animals should be kept dry in order to lessen the chance of infection. The blood needle should not be used for animals who have lost large quantities of blood because of illness or late stages of pregnancy.

In the horse, the large, wide needle is used to bleed HN18 and FL20, where large blood vessels are located (Fig. 2–10). The medium, wide needle is used to bleed HN5, FL16, FL19, HL15, HL19, and FL20 of the baby donkey (Fig. 2–11). The small, wide needle is used to bleed HN4 and HN15 at the location of venules or venous plexuses (Fig. 2–12).

In using the large or medium, wide needle to bleed HN18 or FL16, a hammer, fitted with the appropriate needle is sometimes used. However, a hand-held needle is still a practical alternative. The insertion technique for different points is found in Figures 2–9 to 2–12.

Prism Needle—This needle with a triangular or prism-like head is also used for drawing blood (Figs. 2–1, 2–2, 2–13). The thumb, index, and middle fin-

gers are used to insert this needle (Fig. 2–14). The needle is used in the horse for HN16, HN15, HN4, and HN14, where there is dense connective tissue (Fig. 2–14). If there is bony tissue underneath, caution should be used to prevent needle breakage.

Piercing Jaundice Needle—This needle is used only at ch'uan huang (piercing jaundice, T14) (Figs. 2–2 and 2–15). The skin of the thoracic region of the animal is squeezed from the underlying connective

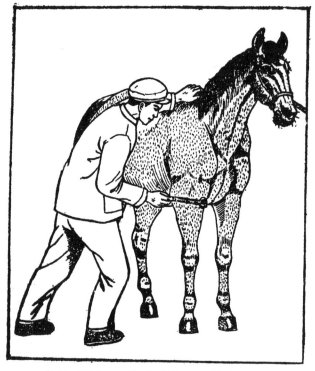

FIGURE 2–11. Wide needle, held by needle hammer, being inserted into FL16.

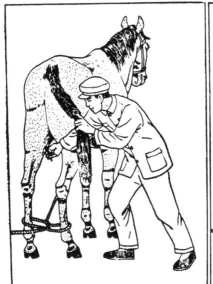

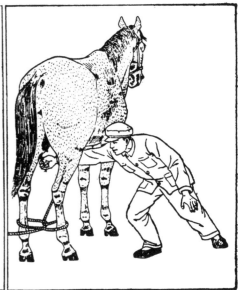

FIGURE 2–12. Two methods of inserting wide needle into HL15.

tissue by using the index and middle fingers and the thumb, and a large wide needle is used to pierce two holes in the skin, approximately one inch apart. The piercing jaundice needle, which is threaded, directs the thread through the holes. The two ends of the thread are then tied to some heavy object to avoid occlusion of the wound and to allow satisfactory drainage, until local swelling due to edema improves. The thread is made of horse tail, hair, or hemp. The diameter of the thread is about the combined thickness of 20 hairs of the horse's tail. The thread is soaked with a drug like secretio bufonis or arsenicum sublimatu.

Gas Releasing—This needle is used only for chia ch'i (gas releasing, FL15) (Fig. 2–1). It is a long needle with a round, dull end, 0.15 inches in diameter and 1–1.5 ft long. It is made of bamboo or a metal alloy. After the needle and the site of insertion are sterilized, the skin is cut, using a large wide needle;

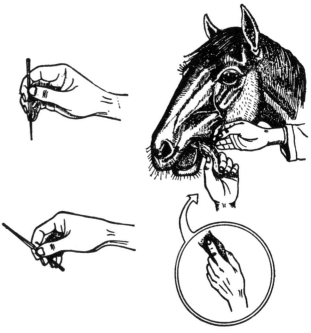

FIGURE 2–14. Use of prism needle. *Left*, Holding prism needle. *Right*, Inserting prism needle into HN16.

FIGURE 2–13. Prism needle.

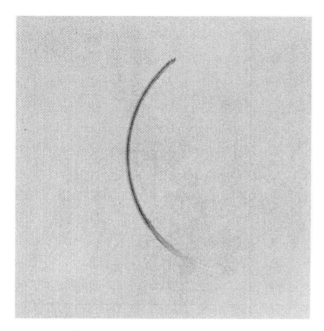

FIGURE 2–15. Piercing jaundice needle.

then the gas-releasing needle is inserted into the loose connective tissue between the arm and the shoulder (Fig. 2–16). The direction of needle insertion must be dorsal and lateral, a medial direction perpendicular to the skin surface would produce pneumothorax.

Commonly Used Methods of Stabilization

A suitable stabilization method is essential for ensuring the safety of the animal and the accuracy of needle insertion:

1. *Head-lowering stabilization method.* The forelimb is encircled with the rein, which is then tied around the bridle, underneath the mandible. It is then pulled up from between the two limbs. The head of the horse is lowered when the rein is pulled. The blood vessels of the head will swell and be clearly seen. This method is suitable to draw blood from, for example, the san chiang point (three rivers, HN4) and the t'ai yang point (greater yang, HN5) (Fig. 2–17).

2. *Double hindlimb stabilization method.* A 15-ft rein is used to tie around the neck of the horse. It is also knotted. The long end of the rein is then used to circle the lumbar area and then is pulled out between the two hindlimbs. The rein is then moved around the abdomen, and backward, around the thigh to the stifle. The rein is pulled tight, and the animal then remains calm and cannot kick. After the needle insertion operation, the rein around the neck and other areas is unfastened. This method is suitable

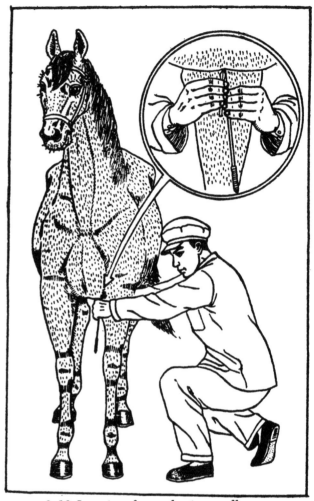

FIGURE 2–16. Insertion of gas-releasing needle.

for points on forelimbs and the lumbar and thigh regions (Fig. 2–18).

3. *The two pole stabilization method.* The neck rope is first tied up and then the circumference rope and the two hang ropes (Fig. 2–19). (End of Chinese translation)

Composition of Needles

In the past, needles were made from stone flints, sharpened bamboo, fish bones, iron, gold, and silver. The most widely used material today is stainless steel. There are many types of stainless steel, each of which has different characteristics. Some of the necessary properties of stainless steel used for acupuncture needles are: machinability, workability, corrosion resistance (tissue fluid and some sterilizing techniques are very corrosive), and strength without brittleness.

Stainless steels are alloys of iron to which a minimum of about 12% chromium has been added to

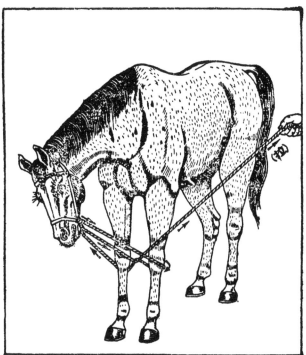

FIGURE 2–17. Head-lowering stabilization method.

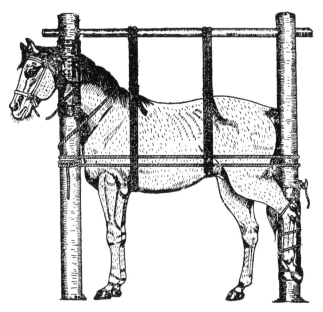

FIGURE 2–19. Two-pole stabilization method.

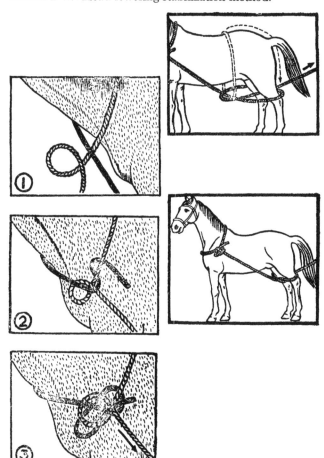

FIGURE 2–18. Double-hindlimb stabilization method.

impart corrosion resistance. A 12% chromium stainless steel will not corrode or "rust" when exposed to the weather. To obtain greater corrosion resistance, more chromium is added to the alloy. Corrosion resistance is the result of an invisible, self-forming and self-healing passive film (nonreactive chromium oxide), which forms in the presence of oxygen.

Along with iron and chromium, all stainless steels contain some carbon. It is difficult to get much less than about 0.03% carbon, and sometimes it is deliberately added up to 1.00% or more. The more carbon there is, the more chromium must be used, because carbon can take from the alloy about 17 times its own weight of chromium to form carbides. The chromium in the form of carbides is of little use for resisting corrosion. The carbon is added for the same purpose as in ordinary steel, to make the alloy stronger.

Other alloying elements are added for improved corrosion resistance, variations in strength, and special modifications for optimum fabricability. Some of these added elements are nickel, molybdenum, copper, titanium, silicon, aluminum, and selenium. The most important of these is nickel; if enough nickel is added, the entire nature of the alloy changes and corrosion resistance is considerably enhanced.

Type 304 stainless steel is most commonly used in the production of medical hypodermic needles and contains the following: carbon, 0.08% max.; manganese, 2.00% max.; phosphorous, 0.045% max.; sulfur, 0.030% max.; silicon, 1.00% max.; chromium, 18.00–20.00%; and nickel, 8.00–10.50%.

TABLE 2–5. *Manufacturers of Acupuncture Needles*

| MANUFACTURERS | TYPE OF STAINLESS STEEL | | TAPER RATIO | GAUGE |
	NEEDLE	HANDLE		
Trueline, Inc. P.O. Box 1357 Englewood, Colorado 80110 303-781-6621	302	321	4:1	25, 28, 30, 32
J. M. Dean, Inc. Peter & Mechanic Sts. Putnum, Connecticut 06260 Attn: P. J. Lamont 203-928-7701	316L	316L	any	28 and special order
Acu-Tube Corp. 3211 W. Bear Creek Dr. Englewood, Colorado 80110 303-761-2258	304	321	6:1–7:1	25, 28, 30, 32

Corrosion and oxidation resistance is provided by the 18% minimum chromium content. The alloy's metallurgical characteristics are established primarily by the nickel content (8% min.), which also extends resistance to corrosion caused by reducing chemicals. Carbon, a necessity of mixed benefit, is held at a level (0.08% max.) that is satisfactory for most service applications.

This stainless alloy resists most oxidizing acids and can withstand all ordinary rusting. It is immune to foodstuffs, sterilizing solutions, most of the organic chemicals and dyestuffs, and a wide variety of inorganic chemicals. Type 304, or one of its modifications, is the material specified more than half the time whenever a stainless steel is used.

Type 316 is more resistant than 304, especially to sodium chloride. It contains the following: carbon, 0.08% max.; manganese, 2.00% max.; phosphorous, 0.045% max.; sulfur, 0.030% max.; silicon, 1.00% max.; chromium, 16.00 to 18.00%; nickel, 10.00 to 14.00%; and molybdenum, 2.00 to 3.00%. By virtue of the molybdenum addition, Type 316 can withstand corrosive attack by sodium and calcium brines and is used extensively for surgical implants within the hostile environment of the body. 316L is similar except that it has lower carbon content.

Gold and silver needles have been used in the Orient. In contemporary France and Germany, stainless steel needles with a layer of gold or silver electrically applied to them are commonly used.

Sources of Veterinary Acupuncture Needles

There are now several manufacturers and many distributors of acupuncture needles in the United States of America. There are also many importers of Chinese, Korean, and Japanese needles. There are, of course, many needles for use in humans, but there are also sources for needles made specifically for animals (Table 2–5).

The basic acupuncture needle is composed of a handle and shaft with a point. The handle enables more ease of handling and manipulating. Handle lengths vary but one long enough to allow two, preferably three, fingers is best. The length of the shaft varies because acupuncture points are at different depths. The diameter varies and is increased to add strength for greater ease of insertion into thick or tough skin. The point of the needle is important and can be described by its taper ratio; this is the length of the point divided by the diameter of the shaft (Fig. 2–20). It seems that penetration is easier using points with a high taper ratio.

Hypodermic needles could be used for acupuncture but have several drawbacks: (1) They are hollow; thus, they can fill with a core of tissue or cause bleeding. (2) The cutting edges of the needle could do much damage. (3) Many sizes are not available as disposable needles, and the cost of regular and especially special-order hypodermic needles might be more expensive than acupuncture needles. (4)

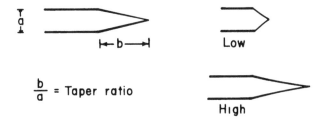

$$\frac{b}{a} = \text{Taper ratio}$$

FIGURE 2–20. Taper ratios of needle points. The taper ratio is the length of the point divided by the diameter of the needle.

The hollow needles might be less resistant to bending than the same diameter solid needle. (5) Once bent, the hollow needles are more distorted at the bend and would be more difficult to straighten without breaking.

Acupuncture needles for use in humans can be used in small animals, especially the dog, and in parts of large animals. It is very difficult to get a 30-gauge needle through the skin over the rump of the horse; however, it could be used on the legs. Chinese needles usually have wound-wire handles. Japanese needles usually have a very narrow smooth cylinder-shaped handle; it is made narrower than others to permit the use of a needle tube (see p. 34). Korean needles are usually one-piece and have been noteworthy in that relatively fine needles can penetrate tough skin. (Fig. 2–21). American-made needles usually have a cylindrical handle that is wider than the Japanese needle. Some handles are soldered on; some are compressed on.

Needles for humans are available in many lengths, from ¼ in. to 8 in. and in several gauges, from 32 to 28 gauge (Fig. 2–22). The taper ratio varies between the different manufacturers, from about 7:1 to 4:1. Most have smooth or cylindrical handles, and one has wire wound handles. Several manufacturers now have a line of veterinary needles that are from 1 in. to 4 in. and 25 gauge (Fig. 2–23). Some manufacturers will supply specially made needles of longer lengths and heavier gauge (Table 2–5).

In describing the diameter of needles, several methods may be used—gauge or diameter in inches or millimeters. The use of gauge has been somewhat confusing. There are at least two different gauge systems—one for hollow tubing and the other for solid wire (Table 2–6). Some manufacturers and authors used the hollow-needle gauge to describe the acupuncture needles; others used the solid-wire gauge to describe the needles. As a result of this, it is pos-

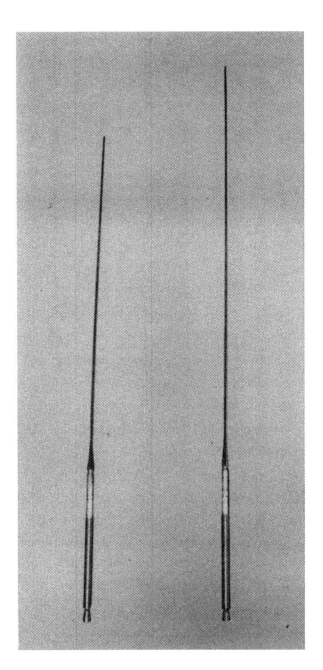

FIGURE 2–21. Korean needles.

sible to buy two 28-gauge needles that are different diameters.

Sterilization of Needles

Needles used for acupuncture should be sterilized. This can be done any of the several common ways—cold sterilizing solutions, autoclaving, or gas sterilizing with ethylene oxide. Gas sterilization is probably the best method, because it will have the least effect

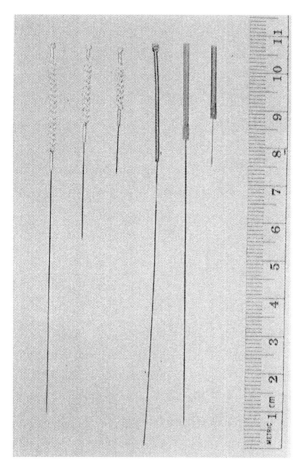

FIGURE 2–22. Human needles.

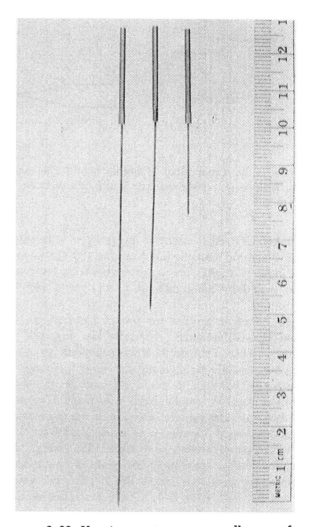

FIGURE 2–23. Veterinary acupuncture needles manufactured in the United States.

on the sharpness of the point and the needles will be dry when used.

Insertion of Needles

In general, the insertion of acupuncture needles is more time-consuming and difficult than insertion of hypodermic needles used for injection. There are several reasons for this: acupuncture needles are usually finer gauge than hypodermic needles; acupuncture needles may be longer than the common hypodermic needles; the site of insertion in acupuncture is more critical; some of the sites for acupuncture are difficult in terms of restraining the animal; and the longer time for insertion may make restraint more difficult, which may, in turn, increase the time for insertion.

The basic technique for insertion is to apply gentle pressure from the handle, and at the same time, rotate the needle along its long axis, clockwise and counterclockwise. When the needle is very thin, the needle long, or the skin very tough, the pressure applied must be small or the needle will bend. This can be overcome in several ways: (1) Don't press too hard. (2) Use a needle tube—a small diameter hollow tube that is a little shorter than the needle. Place the tube on the site; insert the needle to the skin (about ⅛ to ¼ in. of the handle is above the tube). Now tap the needle handle, causing the point to penetrate the skin. Then remove the tube and advance the needle to the desired level. (3) Use a heavier gauge needle. (4) Support the needle with the fingers of the other hand at the level of the skin. (5) Insert the needle by applying the pressure on the shaft close to the skin.

Techniques 4 and 5 are very useful but present sterility problems that can be overcome in several ways, the easiest of which is to use alcohol swabs to hold the needle for those two techniques.

Needle Manipulation

The stimulation of acupuncture points by a needle can be done in many ways. The classical literature contains elaborate descriptions of needle manipulation to produce certain effects and treat different conditions such as inserting needles during specific phases of the respiratory cycle.

To tonify a point, the needle is inserted at the end of exhalation to the required depth without rotation. The needle is then rotated slowly until the tissue clings to it; the needle is then quickly withdrawn during inspiration while it is being rotated. The hole is rubbed firmly with the finger (called "closing the hole"). The entire procedure takes less than 30 seconds.

To sedate a point, the needle is inserted rapidly while being rotated during inspiration. The needle is usually left in position for about 10 min, but it should be left in place until the tissue lets go and no longer clings to the needle. The needle is withdrawn slowly during exhalation; do not "close the hole".

Other directions for manipulation include: twirling of the needle with emphasis on clockwise direction for tonification and on counterclockwise direction for sedation; slow twirling for tonification, rapid twirling for sedation; and manipulating the needle in and out with emphasis on the push in for tonification and emphasis on the pull out for sedation. In general, gentle techniques are used for tonification and vigorous ones for sedation (Table 2–1).

The need or efficacy for these various manipulations has been questioned by some practitioners of acupuncture. However, there certainly are measurable differences in the type of neurophysiological effect produced by strong and weak stimulation, and the Chinese literature stresses that it is the "quantity" of stimulation that is of importance in the treatment of various conditions. Other methods for stimulating points with the use of needles involve the application of electric current or heat to the needles. Electric devices and their use are described in the section on electroacupuncture (p. 36). Generally, points are tonified by the application of low-frequency alternating current, with the needle being connected to the positive side of the circuit (Table 2–1), and sedated by the application of high-frequency alternating current, with the needle being connected to the negative side of the circuit.

In the Japanese system of ryodoraku (see p. 22), direct current is applied to the needle for a very short

TABLE 2–6. *Gauge versus Diameter of Hollow and Solid Wire Needles*

GAUGE	HOLLOW TUBING (INCHES)	SOLID WIRE (INCHES)
14	0.083	0.080
15	0.072	0.072
16	0.065	0.0625
17	0.059	0.054
18	0.05	0.0475
19	0.0425	0.0410
20	0.0355	0.0348
21	0.032	0.0317
22	0.028	0.0286
23	0.025	0.0258
24	0.022	0.0230
25	0.020	0.0204
26	0.018	0.0181
27	0.016	0.0173
28	0.014	0.0162
29	0.013	0.0150
30	0.012	0.014
31	0.010	0.013
32	0.009	0.012

time, 7 sec generally being recommended; the negative side of the circuit is usually connected to the needle.

The points can also be stimulated by the application of heat to the needles. The source of heat usually is burning moxa (dried plant, *Artemesia vulgaris*). Moxa and moxibustion are described on page 40. Electrical moxa devices are now available that essentially are batteries connected to a high-resistance wire. This wire heats up and is held near or touched to the needle. Prolonged stimulation with direct current may be painful.

BLEEDING

The piercing of a blood vessel strongly stimulates the nerve endings (receptors) in the connective tissue coat of blood vessels. Other factors such as tissue repair and hematoma may increase the quantity of stimulation. The needles most often used for this purpose are the wide needle and the prism needle (see p. 28). Many bleeding points are very close to large nerve trunks, such as FL19 (medial and lateral) in the horse being adjacent to the medial and lateral volar nerves. Because of this proximity of nerves and bleeding points, the possibility of inadvertent neurectomy must be considered in the mechanism of action and/or complication of this technique. There are many bleeding points in animals. Because animals cannot communicate any te ch'i, or needle sensation, bleeding indicates that receptors in the blood vessel wall have been stimulated. There are bleeding points and techniques for the human, but these techniques are generally not necessary because the achievement of needle sensation can be communicated to the acupuncturist by the patient, and adequate stimulation can usually be achieved by needling close to the vessel without actually puncturing it.

One common method of enhancing the bleeding is the use of cups. Essentially, these are small metal or glass cups in which ignited paper or alcohol-soaked cotton has been placed. The mouth of the cup is placed on the skin, and the oxygen consumption due to the fire produces a vacuum that holds the cup to the skin and increases the bleeding of the previously needled point. The cup is applied with its mouth upward so that the burning material does not fall on the skin.

INJECTION

Another technique used to stimulate acupuncture points is the injection of various materials into the acupuncture point. Many materials have been injected; the most common are sterile solutions of water, saline solution, dextrose, local anesthetics, vitamins (especially B_{12}), internal blisters, and camphor in oil. The volume of liquid can cause pressure that stimulates the point, and the material in solution can have an effect on the point.

IMPLANTATION

Various materials have been implanted under the skin to continuously stimulate acupuncture points, the most common being gold wire, stainless-steel wire, surgical staples or clips, and BB's. There also is an appliance called a granule. The BB from it has been used for implantation, either through a surgical incision or a large-gauge hypodermic needle.

PRESSURE

Several systems utilize external pressure (massage) applied to the skin over acupuncture points as the method of stimulation. The most common of these is the Japanese system (*shiatsu*) and the Chinese system of finger acupuncture (*tui nar*). Another common method of stimulating points by external pressure is the use of granules. These are small metal BB's held onto the skin (over a point) by a small piece of adhesive tape.

ACOUSTIC ENERGY

The most common type used is ultrasound.

ELECTROMAGNETIC ENERGY

Various types of electromagnetic-energy sources have been used to stimulate acupuncture points, the most common being ultraviolet light.

ELECTROACUPUNCTURE

This technique involves the use of electricity to stimulate acupuncture points. Most commonly, the source of electricity is connected to needles in the acupuncture point. An alternative, used by some, is the application of electricity to the skin surface. Electroacupuncture is especially useful where one might want to stimulate several needles continuously for a long time, such as during the technique of acupuncture analgesia. Many types of electric energy can be applied, and many types of equipment are available in the United States, Canada, China, Japan, and other countries.

Basic Electronics

Electricity is the flow of electrons through a material. This system can be quantified in several ways. The rate of flow of electrons per unit time is called the *current* and is measured in amperes (A); the force controlling this flow is called the *voltage* and is measured in volts (E or V); and the resistance of the material to the flow of electrons is called the *resistance* and is measured in ohms (R or Ω). The primary law relating these factors is called *Ohm's Law* and has three forms: $E = IR$, $I = E/R$, and $R = E/I$. Given any of the two factors, it is a simple matter to calculate the third. These basic parameters can be modified by the appropriate scientific notations to make them more convenient to write—for example, microamperes instead of 0.000001 A (Table 2–7). For the range of these parameters found in

TABLE 2–7. *Electrical Conversions*

1 Ampere = 1000 milliamperes (ma)
1 Ampere = 1,000,000 microamperes (μa)
0.001 ampere = 1 milliampere
0.000001 ampere = 1 microampere
1 ohm = 0.001 kilohm (kΩ)
1 ohm = 0.000001 megohm (mΩ)
1000 ohms = 1 kilohm
1,000,000 ohms = 1 megohm

acupuncture equipment, it is most convenient to use milli- or microamperes, volts, and kilo- or megohms—that is, in the Ohm's law calculations, use volts, milliamperes, and kilohms or volts, microamperes and megohms.

There are two types of current flow: direct current (dc) and alternating current (ac). Direct current is one in which the electrons flow through a circuit continuously in one direction, the type of current produced by a battery. The amplitude of the current may be positive or negative, and the flow is usually continuous.

Alternating current is one in which the electron flow through a circuit periodically changes direction. Two reversals of direction constitute a cycle, and the number of cycles, in hertz (Hz), occurring in one second is called the frequency. The shape of a plot of current versus time is called the waveform—for example, sine wave, square wave.

Electronic Equipment

The two basic pieces of acupuncture electrical equipment are point finders and stimulators.

Point Finders

It is reported that the skin above acupuncture points has a much lower resistance to the flow of current than the rest of the skin. If a large indifferent electrode is attached to the body and a source of current at constant voltage is applied to a searching electrode, the resistance can be measured by the change in current flow. This change can be read from an ammeter or may be indicated by the lighting of a lamp or an increase in frequency of an audible sound (Figs. 2–24, 2–25). These finders may seem to be a very simple way to find acupuncture points, but they are not. There are many problems associated with their use, especially in animals.

The pressure at which the searching electrode is applied to the skin can markedly affect the resistance, and a point can be indicated at any site merely by pressing the electrode firmly on the skin. The rate at which the electrode is moved over the surface of the skin will markedly affect the resistance and, if the searching electrode is left at one place on the surface of the skin for a few seconds, the resistance will fall dramatically, resulting in the creation of a pseudoacupuncture point that may remain for several hours.

If the applied voltage is too high, there may be many false points. If the voltage is too low, many points will not be indicated. If the voltage is too high,

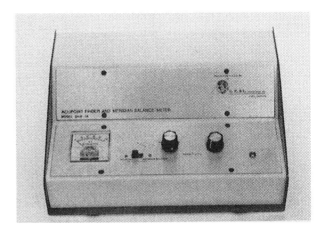

FIGURE 2–24. Acupuncture point finder and meridian balance meter. Model DHW–1A. (Courtesy of BX&L Industries, Inc., Irvine, California.)

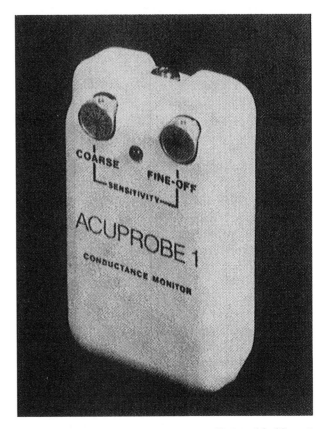

FIGURE 2–25. The Acuprobe I—a small, hand-held, unit for point location by skin conductance measurement, capable of sensing with very low currents in the region of 0.5–1.0 microamperes. Indication is by means of an audible sound plus a visual red light output. Probe-sensing is adjustable by means of two sensitivity controls, coarse and fine, for a full range of skin resistances. The power source is a standard 9-volt transistory battery. (Courtesy of Intertronic Systems, Ltd., Ontario, Canada.)

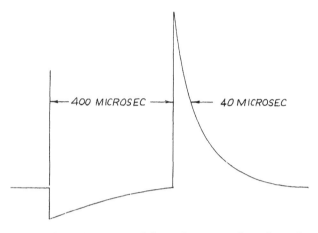

FIGURE 2–26. Drawing of the voltage waveform from the Chinese 626–1 stimulator. The negative portion of the wave has a duration of 400 msec and the positive portion has a duration of 40 msec at 50% of the peak amplitude. (From Babich. 1974. The American Journal of Chinese Medicine, 1:341–50. By permission of The American Journal of Chinese Medicine.)

the skin will be burned, and a blister may appear. If the animal is sweating, there will be many more points than when the skin is cold and dry. If the hair coat of an animal is very dense, there will be no response—these instruments do not work on unshaved cats but do on dogs. If the skin is irritated due to diseases or hair clipping, there will be points all over the area.

It appears that the low-resistance points are in the skin. If a point is found and the skin is then moved several inches, the point moves with the skin. If the skin is removed from the animal, the point remains in the skin—that is, the area of low electrical resistance can often be located in a piece of skin lying on a table.

The mobility of the skin of animals in relation to the underlying tissue, and the fact that the point to be stimulated is often in the deeper tissues, provide further complication in the use of point finders in animals. A system of diagnosis and treatment based on the actual values of current flow for certain points is called *ryodoraku* (see p. 22). This method, which originated in Japan for the treatment of humans, is being examined there and in other countries for possible application to animals.

Stimulators

These devices have many basic features in common; some models are very simple while others are very elaborate. Their basic function is to produce a current to stimulate acupuncture points.

Most of the stimulators used are battery-powered, usually with several 1.5-volt D batteries, several 9-volt transistor radio batteries, or with rechargeable batteries.

CURRENT TYPE

There are two basic groups of stimulators—those whose output is dc and those whose output is ac.

WAVEFORM

The ac stimulators may have one waveform or a choice of several waveforms. The most common waveform used is some variation of a spike (Figs. 2–26 to 2–28). Other possible waveforms are square wave, sine wave, and so on.

FREQUENCY CONTROL

Most machines have some method of controlling the frequency of stimulation. One common system is a continuously variable frequency control, from about 0.5–2 Hz to 100 Hz. Some devices have only preset frequencies that can be dialed.

MODE AND MODULATION

Many devices have controls that can vary the time between burts of stimuli—for example, the frequency of stimulation may be 10 Hz, but these stimuli may occur for only 3 sec and then no stimuli occur for a 3-sec period. During the periods of stimulation, the frequency of stimulation is 10 Hz. On many machines, another control varies the amplitude of the signal in a continuing consistent manner—for example, a signal may occur with a frequency of 10 Hz. The amplitude of this signal may be 20 volts. Normally, all the signals have the same amplitude; however, with this control, this may be varied. For example, a train of impulses can be generated with increasing amplitude, decreasing amplitude, or both.

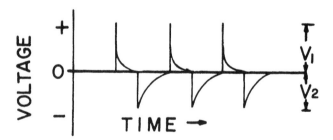

FIGURE 2–27. Drawing of a photograph of an oscilloscope screen display of the voltage waveform from an Acuflex CZ–110 Dual Neur-Metron. (Courtesy of Professional Medical Distributors, Wixom, Michigan.)

The manner in which these amplitude changes can occur can be varied in some machines.

There is always a control that varies the voltage applied and therefore the current flow, because the resistance remains constant. In many devices, the voltage controls are connected to each other so that as the voltage to one pair of needles is increased, the voltage at another pair of needles decreases. The opposite also occurs, so that when the voltage between one pair of needles is decreased, the voltage at another previously connected pair of needles increases. Therefore, great care must be taken to decrease the voltage control in small steps and to decrease the voltage to all the pairs of needles sequentially instead of just turning each control completely off before changing the next control.

Use of Electric Stimulators

Great care must be exercised when using electric stimulators. Before the connectors from the device are attached to implanted needles, the voltage controls must be checked to determine that they are in the *off* position or lowest possible setting. The voltage is then slowly increased to a maximum that the patient will comfortably tolerate. When needles are placed in or near muscle or appropriate nerves, the muscle will contract. When the stimulus is such that the muscles are gently contracting, the animal will usually tolerate the procedure; however, some animals are very sensitive and become agitated even with a stimulus that only causes barely perceptible muscle contractions.

When the stimuli are applied at sites that do not cause muscle contraction, it is more difficult to determine if the stimuli are reaching the site, if the animal feels the stimulus, and if the stimuli are as strong as the animal will comfortably tolerate. If the applied votage is slowly increased while the animal is carefully observed, it is usually possible to determine if, when, and to what extent the animal is feeling the stimuli. The person restraining the animal should be aware of what is going on and the possibility that the animal may react vigorously if the applied stimulus is too great.

In the horse, needles placed in some muscular sites, especially when electrically stimulated, may be expelled by the voluntary local twitching of the area by the animal, which often occurs—that is, the horse responds as if an insect were bothering it. Taping the needles in place usually overcomes this problem.

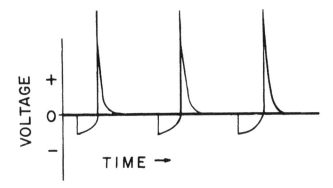

FIGURE 2–28. Drawing of a photograph of an oscilloscope screen display of the voltage from an Akupunctuer 71–6. (Courtesy of Ack Laboratories, New York, N.Y.)

Care should be taken to make sure the stimulator is in a relatively safe place, protected from the animal jumping on it or pulling it off a table because the leads are too short to accommodate movement of the animal.

It is generally thought that a pair of needles should not be connected across the chest because of the possibility of causing cardiac arrhythmias. The negative electrode is usually connected to a more important point. When decreasing the voltage or disconnecting leads, care must be exercised as described under "Amplitude" (above).

The discussion of the use of the stimulator so far has applied only to alternating-current stimulators. Direct-current stimulators are commonly used in the Japanese system of ryodoraku and must be used differently. The application of direct current may be painful and will be tolerated only for a short period so generally the stimulus is applied to one needle at a time and for 7 sec. (see p. 38).

When using high-frequency ac stimulation, the feeling is more uncomfortable at a particular voltage setting than that same voltage would be applied at a lower frequency. Therefore, if an animal is being stimulated at a low frequency and the frequency is going to be increased, the applied voltage should be reduced first. After the frequency has been increased to its new higher rate, then the voltage can be increased to a comfortable level.

Commercial Acupuncture Stimulators

There are many electric stimulators sold. Some are precision instruments and well constructed; others are very poorly designed and constructed. The original and the most well-known equipment worldwide comes from China and Japan (Figs. 2–29 to 2–32). Many devices are now manufactured in the United

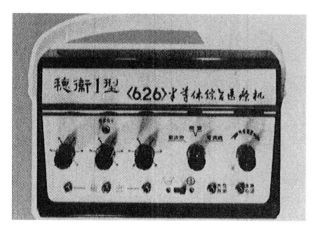

FIGURE 2–29. Chinese model 626–1 multipurpose electrotherapeutic apparatus. This equipment is manufactured by the People's Republic of China; sole distributor, East Wind Medical Instruments Company, Ltd., 589 Nathan Road, Kowloon, Hong Kong. (Courtesy of East Wind Medical Instruments Co., Ltd.)

States (Figs. 2–33 to 2–38). Importation of acupuncture equipment is strictly controlled by the Food and Drug Administration (see also "Importation of Equipment", p. 55).

To exemplify the operation and uses of electric acupuncture equipment, the instructions for use of several devices are reproduced in the appendix to this chapter. The inclusion of these specific models should not be construed as an indication of superiority or inferiority but merely examples of available equipment. The multiple Chinese examples are to provide an insight into the methods of operation and the equipment used by the Chinese.

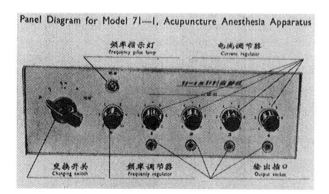

FIGURE 2–30. Panel diagram for Chinese model 71–1. This equipment is manufactured by the People's Republic of China; sole distributor, East Wind Medical Instruments Company, Ltd., 589 Nathan Road, Kowloon, Hong Kong. (Courtesy of East Wind Medical Instruments Co., Ltd.)

MOXIBUSTION

There are several variations of the technique called moxibustion. All use heat to stimulate acupuncture points or the local site of a disease problem. Several of the techniques are very similar to the common practice of firing and blistering known to veterinarians throughout the world. Moxa moxibustion is also used in treating humans.

The following description of the various techniques of moxibustion is from a modern Chinese veterinary textbook and is presented below without change or editorial comment.[1]

Moxibustion is the use of heat to stimulate acupuncture points. Several methods are used: cauterization, oat vinegar method, vinegar liquor method, cupping, and moxa moxibustion.

Cauterization. This technique is commonly used in chronic diseases of the limbs, and in diseases not responding to drug or needle treatment.

The assistant to the veterinarian should be responsible for the fire and the branding iron. The animal should be stabilized. In the two-pole stabilization method, the neck is first tied up and the circumference rope and the two hang ropes are then tied. According to the site of cauterization, the limbs should be further stabilized (Fig. 2–17). Twelve hours before the operation, feeding of the animal should be stopped so that it will not feel discomfort during therapy.

The first step of cauterization employs a sharp, pointed, knife-like branding iron to imprint a diagram of the cauterization. Then, the squared head branding iron is used to augment the branding effect (Fig. 2–39). The branding iron should move toward the wave of hair, and should be pressed lighter initially, and heavier gradually. The branding iron should be flat against the skin, to avoid cutaneous injury that would affect the operation. The sequence of the operation is from medial to lateral, and from cranial-dorsal to ventral-caudal. As soon as the branding area becomes a golden yellow, the branding iron should not be pressed too hard.

Precautions should be taken to get the right cauterization temperature. The branding iron should be of sandy yellow color. If the flame is too hot, the branding iron becomes a yellowish white color. It burns the skin, and the purpose of cauterization is not fulfilled. Possible injury to large nerve trunks and blood vessels should be avoided. The area of the joint, for example, or the medial side of the four limbs or an area of traumatic injury should not be cauterized. After cauterization, the sweat of the body surface is cleaned. The animal should not drink water after cauterization and should be fed before any liquid is allowed.

The cauterized surface should be kept clean and dry, and no soft paste should be used. The animal may itch during the recovery period. Precautions should be taken to protect the animal from biting the wound to avoid possible infection or ulceration.

The cauterized animal should work as usual. If it is being kept in the stable, without physical labor, the therapeutic effect will be reduced.

In general, cauterization is performed only once to effect a cure. If it is necessary to cauterize twice at the same site, it is essential to avoid the area altogether or wait until the wound fully heals.

In cold weather, hot weather, or during rainy or windy days, cauterization should not be performed. This method should not be practiced on old, very young, weak, or pregnant animals. The animal should be strong and fully mature.

Oat Vinegar Method. This is used mainly for arthritis pain in the lumbar region. Twenty pounds of oats fried in four pounds of vinegar is used. The preparation is then divided into two packs used alternately as hot packs, and it is applied to the affected area once every day for one or two hours.

Vinegar Liquor Method. This is used mainly for lumbar or hindlimb arthritis. The animal is first stabilized. The hair is moistened with warm vinegar, from the withers, along the spine, toward the lumbosacral region. This area is then covered with vinigrated paper. The liquor is then poured to create flame. If the flame is not sufficient, liquor is added; if there is excessive flame, vinegar is added. Cauterization is continued until the thorax and the upper limb area of the affected animal begin to sweat. The quantity of liquor and vinegar used varies in accordance with the disease; however, approximately 2–3 lb of liquor and 5 lb of vinegar are necessary. After the operation, the animal is covered with blankets for warmth and placed in a warm room to rest. If the weather is nice, the animal may be taken out in the sun. This method is, again, not suitable for weak, very old, very young, or pregnant animals.

Cupping. This can be used in rheumatoid and paralytic diseases of the limbs in combination with acupuncture. There are many kinds of cups: ceramic, bamboo, and glass. A ceramic cup 2–3 in. deep with a diameter of 2 in. is the type commonly used. First, the area around the point is moistened. A cotton ball soaked with alcohol is then lit and put inside the cup. When heat is felt, the acupuncture point is covered quickly. The cup is left in position 5–10 min before release. At the time of this operation, the sucked area is seen to swell. If cupping is performed after use of the needle, a small amount of blood may be sucked out.

Moxa Moxibustion. This is used mainly in chronic pain diseases. The leaves of the moxa tree are used as a raw material. There are two methods. In the direct moxibustion method, moxa is rolled in the form of a cigarette with a length of 5 in and a diameter of 0.6 in. The end of the moxa is burned at a distance of 0.5–1 in. from the skin where the loci of the acupuncture points are located.

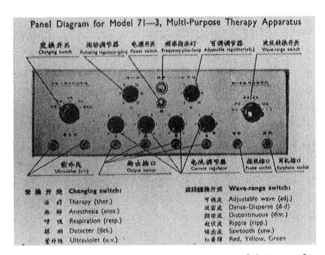

FIGURE 2–31. Panel diagram for Chinese model 71–3. This equipment is manufactured by the People's Republic of China; sole distributor, East Wind Medical Instruments Company, Ltd., 589 Nathan Road, Kowloon, Hong Kong. (Courtesy of East Wind Medical Instruments Co., Ltd.)

The sick animal will feel warmth and not burning pain. Moxibustion may last a few minutes to half an hour (Fig. 2–40). For a stronger stimulation, the burned moxa can touch the skin momentarily. For indirect moxibustion, the moxa is placed on a piece of ginger or green onion. The moxa is in the form of a round-bottomed pyramid

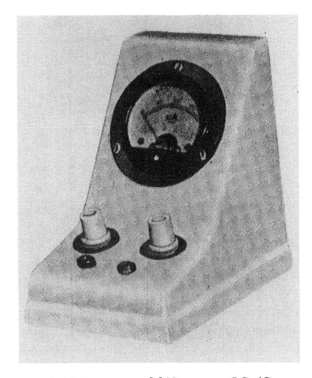

FIGURE 2–32. Japanese model Neurometer LC. (Courtesy of Nikka Overseas Agency Ltd., Vancouver, British Columbia, Canada.)

41 *Acupuncture Techniques and Equipment*

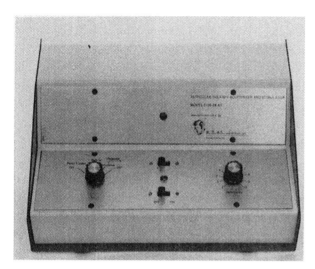

FIGURE 2–33. Auriculotherapy point finder and stimulator, model DHW 38–AT. (Courtesy of BX&L Industries, Irvine, California.)

and is placed and burned on the top of a thin layer of perforated ginger or green onion about 0.1 in. thick. When the thin piece of ginger or green onion becomes dried, a new piece should be used (Fig. 2–40). The duration of the treatment depends on the disease and the physical condition of the animal.

A modification of moxibustion is the use of moxa to heat an acupuncture needle that is in place. The burning moxa roll is brought near the handle of the needle or may touch it directly. The handle becomes very hot, but with reasonable application there is only a slight feeling of warmth in the tissue around the needle. Great care should be exercised when removing the needles so that the fingers are not burned. The only advantage that moxa has over tobacco such as cigarettes or cigars is that moxa probably burns at a cooler temperature.

The complications of moxibustion are obvious: injury to the patient (infection and pain), injury to the acupuncturist, and risk of starting a fire. Some of the points forbidden to moxa are understandable—for example, at the medial canthus of the eye.

Ryodoraku

Ryodoraku is a very specific form of acupuncture developed in Japan by Y. Nakatani.[4, 12–14, 16] His work began in 1950, and he soon founded the Ryodoraku Autonomic Nervous System Society of Japan.

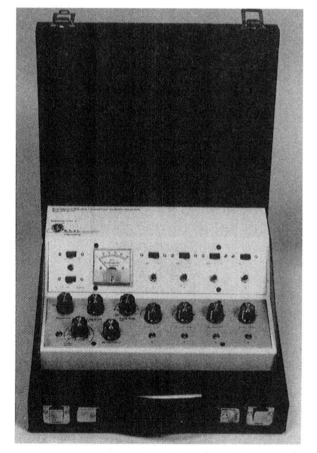

FIGURE 2–34. Multiwaveform stimulator, point finder, and meridian balance meter. Model DHW 38–4WF. (Courtesy of BX&L Industries, Irvine, California.)

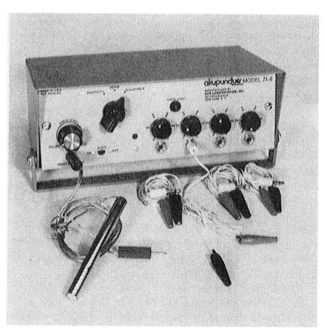

FIGURE 2–35. Acupuncture Model 71–6. (Courtesy of Ack Laboratories, New York, N.Y.)

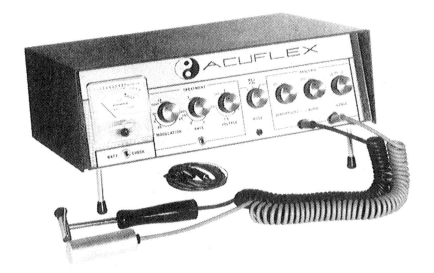

FIGURE 2–36. Acupuncture stimulator and point finder model CZ–110 Dual Neur-Metron. (Courtesy of Professional Medical Distributors, Wixom, Michigan.)

Nakatani's work and system involve measuring the electrical resistance of the skin, making certain conclusions from the measurements, and then treating according to these findings. When 21 volts dc is applied to the skin, many specific points of high current flow are found (described under "Point Find-ers", p. 37). These points are called "ryodo points" and are close to or exactly at the site of traditional Chinese acupuncture points. When 12 volts is applied only a few points are distinct. Ryodoraku are lines formed by linking ryodo points, and they correspond to traditional Chinese meridians. There are

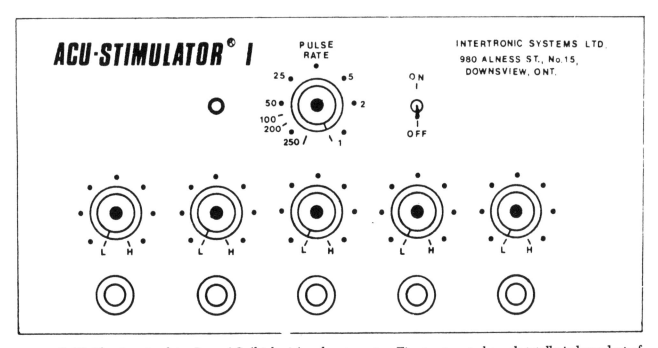

FIGURE 2–37. The Acustimulator I—an AC (biphasic) pulse generator. Five treatment channels totally independent of one another are provided through separate transformers. Each channel is controlled by its own output control. The output leads are color-coded for each pair. Polarity is indicated by the clips on the end. The pulse rate is continuously variable from 1 to 250 cycles/sec. (Courtesy of Intertronics Systems, Ltd., Ontario, Canada.)

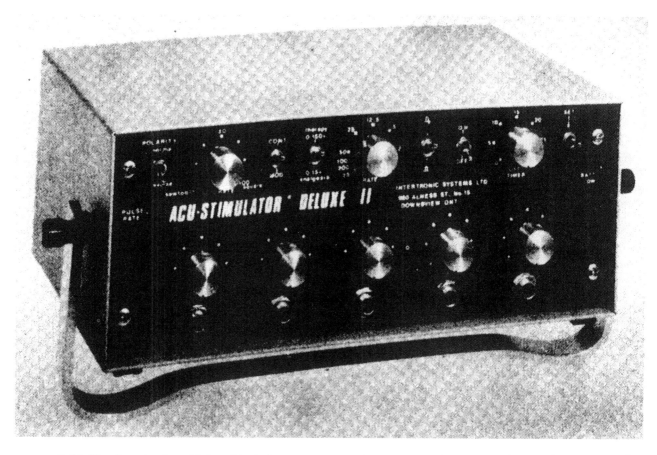

FIGURE 2–38. The Acustimulator Deluxe II–A therapeutic research instrument, the Acustimulator Deluxe II is similar to the Acustimulator I, but is a more sophisticated model. Two output waveforms are available by switch position—biphasic and pulsed square wave. The pulsed wave is used for treatment while the biphasic is generally used for analgesia. The pulse rate may be selected from 1 to 250 Hz, and each output is totally isolated from the others. If the unit is turned on with an output above zero, the unit warns of the condition by buzzer action (avoiding possible stimulation of the patient when not desired). Two output ranges are available, low 0–15 volts and high 0–150 volts. The latter is generally for less sensitive patients and for dorsal stimulation (bilateral transcutaneous dorsal stimulation). Polarity is changeable by flicking a switch. Another feature is the timer unit, which may be turned on at the beginning of treatment. When the time is reached, the unit shuts off. This is a completely solid-state timer of modern integrated-circuit construction, with no mechanical parts or clockwork to wear out. The battery provides about 100 hours of use, at which time the charger should be used. Recharging time is indicated by a battery-low light. Each output is color-coded. (Courtesy of Intertronics Systems Ltd., Ontario, Canada.)

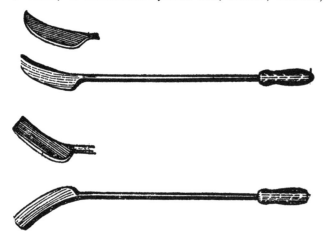

FIGURE 2–39. Cauterization irons. *Top,* Sharp-pointed iron for imprinting pattern. *Bottom,* Square-head iron for completion of the procedure.

six on each arm, H1-H6, six on each leg, F1-F6, and two on the midline, one anterior (VM) and one posterior (HM). The points are numbered starting at the distal end of the extremity.

The basic outline of ryodoraku measurement and therapy is as follows: Current flow is measured at a distal point of each ryodoraku on the limbs. The current flow is measured with 12 volts applied and with the device calibrated so that with the electrodes shorted together the current flow is 200 microamperes. The average of the current flow at the 24 points is calculated, and a line is drawn on a chart that has a range of readings for each ryodoraku (Fig. 2-41).

All the 24 measurements should fall within a specific range of the average line drawn. Any readings that do not fall into this range indicate that there is an abnormality of that ryodoraku. If the reading is higher than the average, the ryodoraku is hyperactive and needs to be sedated. If the reading is lower than the average, the ryodoraku needs to be tonified. Needles are placed in the appropriate points and stimulated with a direct current stimulator for 7 seconds. After successful treatment, the readings of the treated ryodorakus should fall within the average.

This technique has not yet been adapted to animals; however, some research is being conducted on this in Japan and in the United States on this.

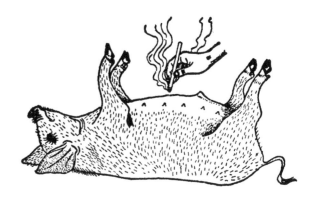

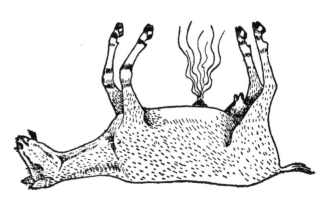

FIGURE 2-40. *Top,* Direct moxibustion with moxa roll. *Bottom,* Indirect moxibustion with moxa separated from the skin by a slice of ginger or green onion.

Regional Acupuncture Therapy

Several branches of acupuncture have developed that utilize only one small part of the body as the site for treating various diseases occurring throughout the body.

The most highly developed of these branches is auriculotherapy. In this system of diagnosis and treatment, the whole body is represented as an inverted fetus fitting within the ear (Figs. 2-42 and 2-43). The points at the various anatomic sites become sensitive and more electroconductive when there is disease of the anatomic site it represents (Fig. 2-44). The most well-known treatments involving this type of therapy are the placement of surgical staples in a specific region of the ear to treat obesity and to decrease the visceral effects of narcotic withdrawal in addicts. There has been relatively little work done in the area in animals. There are ear points in the horse for the production of acupuncture analgesia (see Chapter Six). There is a report of a study in which production of peritonitis in rabbits produced points in the ear with lower electrical resistance than normal.[11] Another report described the production of points in the ears of rabbits by the intramuscular injection of turpentine. These points had lower electrical resistance and also became stained blue when trypan blue was injected intravenously. The location of the points in the ear was specific for the anatomic location of the turpentine injection.[6]

Listed in Table 2-8 are the points in the ear of the human listed according to two systems of naming points. One is the translation of the Chinese name and the other is the numbering system created by E. C. Wong keyed to Fig. 2-45. After the list of points is a table of prescriptions (Table 2-9) for treating various disease conditions in the human as published by Wong.

Other regional treatment methods such as those utilizing the hand, foot, or nose are much less developed.

DR. YOSHIO NAKATANI'S CHART
for
RYODORAKU AUTONOMIC NERVE REGULATORY THERAPY

Name									Date of Exam.		
Address					Phone			Birth Date			

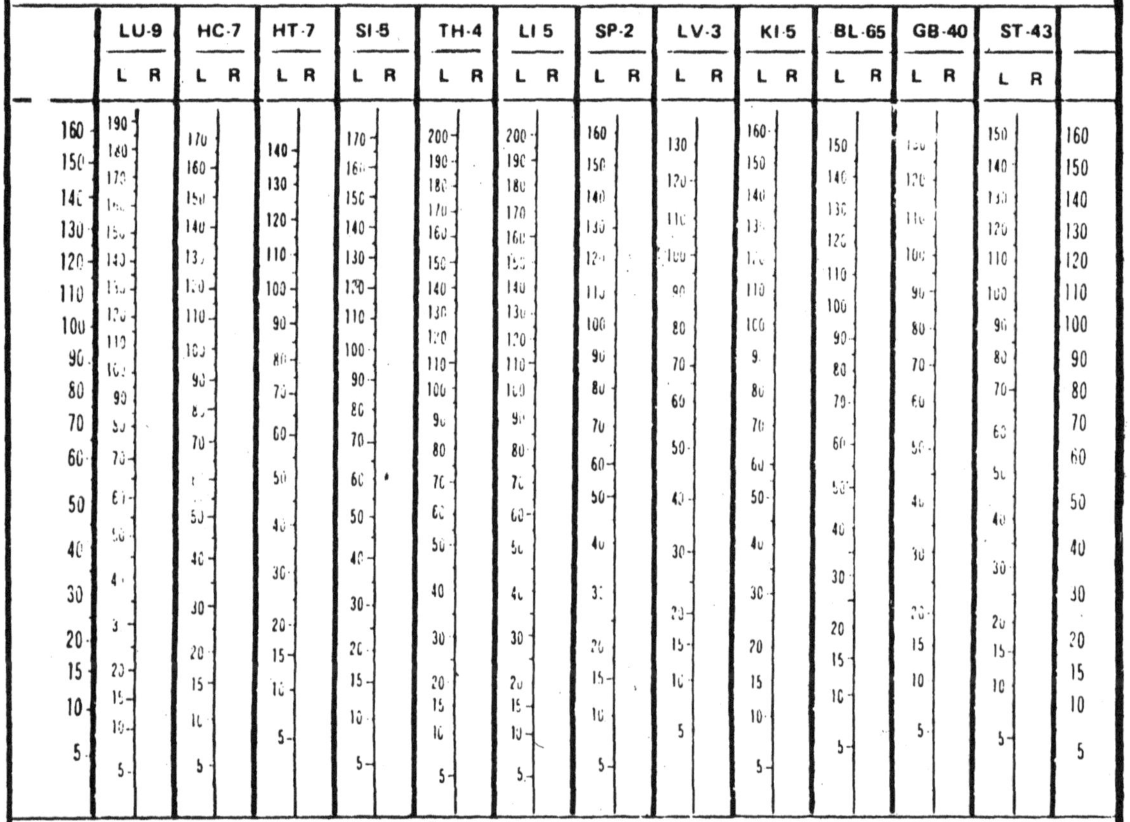

	LU-9	HC-7	HT-7	SI-5	TH-4	LI 5	SP-2	LV-3	KI-5	BL-65	GB-40	ST-43	
	L R	L R	L R	L R	L R	L R	L R	L R	L R	L R	L R	L R	

Meridian	LU	HC	HT	SI	TH	LI	SP	LV	KI	BL	GB	ST
Sed	LU-5	HC-7	HT-7	SI-8	TH-10	LI-2	SP-5	LV-2	KI-1	BL-65	GB-38	ST-45
Stim	LU-9	HC-9	HT-9	SI-3	TH-3	LI-11	SP-2	LV-8	KI-7	BL-67	GB-43	ST-41
Assoc.	BL-13	BL-14	BL-15	BL-27	BL-22	BL-25	BL-20	BL-18	BL-23	BL-28	BL-19	BL-21
Alarm	LU-1	CV-17	CV-14	CV-4	CV-5	ST-25	LV-13	LV-14	GB-25	CV-3	GB-24	CV-12
Source	LU-9	HC-7	HT-7	SI-4	TH-4	LI-4	SP-3	LV-3	KI-3	BL-64	GB-40	ST-42

APP Technique Seminars, inc.

FIGURE 2–41. Dr. Yoshio Nakatani's chart for ryodoraku autonomic nerve regulatory therapy. (Courtesy of Mr. E. C. Wong.)

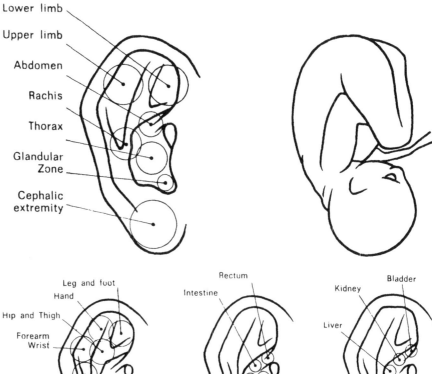

FIGURE 2–42. Relationship of fetal shape and position to location of auriculotherapy points. (Courtesy of Professional Medical Specialties, Inc., Orlando, Florida.)

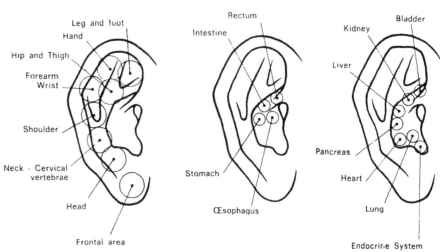

FIGURE 2–43. Areas of the ear related to various organs and structures. (Courtesy of Professional Medical Specialties, Inc., Orlando, Florida.)

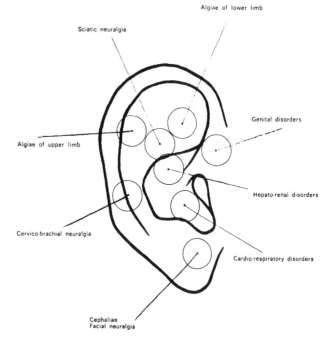

FIGURE 2–44. Treatment areas in the ear for certain conditions. (Courtesy of Professional Medical Specialties, Inc., Orlando, Florida.)

47 *Acupuncture Techniques and Equipment*

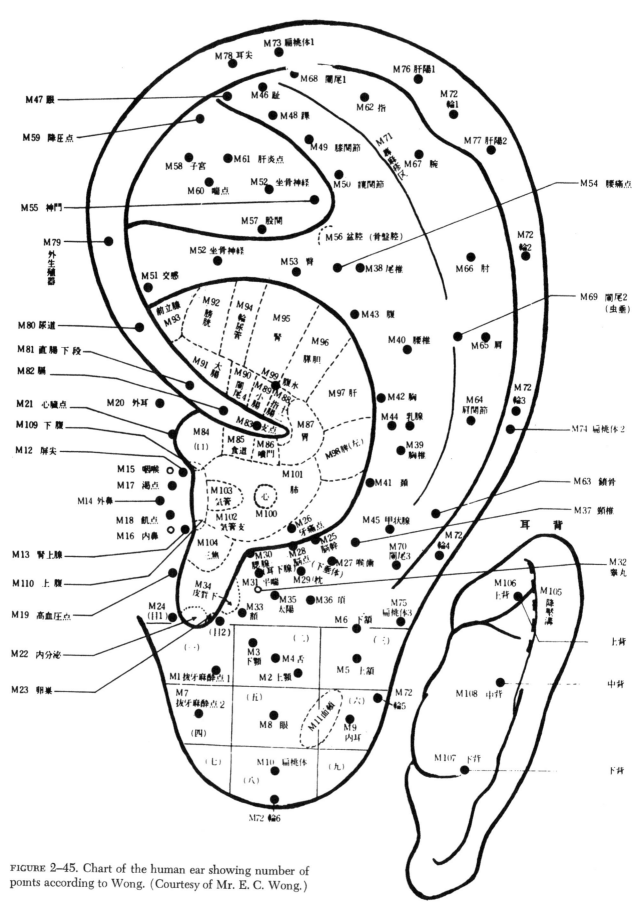

FIGURE 2–45. Chart of the human ear showing number of points according to Wong. (Courtesy of Mr. E. C. Wong.)

TABLE 2–8. *Chinese Auriculotherapy Points*

REGIONS	WONG'S EAR POINT NO.	EAR POINT	LOCATION
Auricular lobule	1	Anesthesia for extraction of teeth 1	At the posteroinferior part of the 1st area.*
	2	Upper jaw	At posteroinferior part of the 2nd area.
	3	Lower jaw	At anterosuperior part of the 2nd area.
	4	Tongue	At central point of the 2nd area.
	5	Shang-he (maxilla)	At central point of 3rd area.
	6	Hsia-he (mandible)	At central point of superior line of 3rd area.
	7	Anesthesia for extraction of teeth 2	At central point of 4th area.
	8	Eye	At central point of 5th area.
	9	Internal ear	At central point of 6th area.
	10	Tonsils 4	At central point of 8th area.
	11	Cheeks	Lying around borderline between 5th and 6th areas.
Tragus	12	Apex of tragus	The upper projection of tragus (at upper brim of projection if only one projection is found).
	13	Adrenal gland	The lower projection of tragus (at lower brim of projection if only one projection is found).
	14	External nose	At the central point of root region of the tragus.
	15	Pharynx and larynx	At inner surface of tragus opposing to orifice of external auditory meatus.
	16	Internal nose	At inner surface of tragus, slightly below acupuncture points of pharynx and larynx.
	17	Thirst Fluid removal therapy	The middle point between line connecting acupuncture points of apex of tragus and external nose.
	18	Hunger	The middle point between line connecting acupuncture points of adrenal gland and external nose.
	19	High blood pressure	The middle point between line connecting acupuncture of adrenal gland and eye.
Supratragic incisure	20	External ear	At depression in front of supratragic incisure.
	21	Heart point	The middle point of line connecting acupuncture points of apex of tragus, and external ear, slightly toward the posterior side.
Intertragic incisure	22	Internal secretion	The bottom part of intertragic incisure.
	23	Ovary	Lying between acupuncture points of subcortex and internal secretion.
	24	Eye 1, 2	At inferior part of intertragic incisure with acupuncture point of eye 1 in front and eye 2 behind.
Antitragus	25	Brain axis	At central point of supratragic incisure.
	26	Toothache	At inner surface of acupuncture point of brain axis and opposing to the Hou-ya.
	27	Hou-ya (Throat and teeth)	Lying between acupuncture points of cervical vertebrae and back of head.
	28	Brain (pituary body)	At central point of one-third of superior brim of the antitragus.
	29	Back of head	At posterosuperior part of the antitragus.
	30	Parotid	At central point of one-third of middle brim of antitragus.
	31	Ping-chuan (antihistamine)	At apex of antitragus (may locate at central point of brim of antitragus if apex of antitragus is not prominent).
	32	Testicle	About 0.2 mm inside the acupuncture point of parotid at medial side of the antitragus.

* The surface of the auricular lobule is divided into nine equal areas; they are the 1st area, the 2nd area and the 3rd area and so on.

TABLE 2–8. *Chinese Auriculotherapy Points* (continued)

REGIONS	WONG'S EAR POINT NO.	EAR POINT	LOCATION
	33	Forehead	At the anterointerior part of antitragus.
	34	Subcortex	At inner surface of antitragus.
	35	The sun (temple)	The middle point between line connecting acupuncture points of back of head and the forehead.
	36	Vertex	About 0.15 mm below acupuncture point of back of head.
Antihelix	37	Cervical vertebrae	A series of acupuncture points of vertebral column, lying along curved brim of cavum conchae on antihelix.
	38	Thoracic vertebrae	This line of acupuncture points could be separated by same level of acupuncture point of the lower segment of rectum and the same level of the acupuncture points of the shoulder joint into three segments.
	39	Lumbosacral vertebrae	The upper segment belonging to the field of lumbosacral vertebrae; the middle segment of the thoracic vertebrae; and the lower segment of the cervical vertebrae.
	40	Coccygeal vertebrae	At the lower projection of antihelix.
	41	Neck	At the notch between the borderline of antihelix and antitragus.
	42	Thorax	At the antihelix, at the same level of supratragic incisure.
	43	Abdomen	At the antihelix, with the same level of the lower border of the inferior crus of the antihelix.
	44	Mammary gland	At two sides of the upper part of the acupuncture point of the thoracic vertebrae with this point become an equilateral triangle.
	45	Thyroid gland	At the superior part of the acupuncture point of the cervical vertebrae near to the scapha.
Superior crus of the antihelix	46	Toes	At the posterosuperior part of superior crus of the antihelix.
	47	Heel	At the anterosuperior part of superior crus of antihelix.
	48	Ankle	At the anterosuperior part of the superior crus of the antihelix.
	49	Knee joint	At superior crus of antihelix, with same level of superior border of inferior crus of the antihelix.
	50	Hip joint	At superior crus of antihelix and the posteroinferior part of the acupuncture point of knee joint.
Inferior crus of the antihelix	51	Sympathetic	At the borderline between brim of inferior crus of antihelix and curved brim of the anterior portion of helix.
	52	Sciatica	At the middle point of superior border of the inferior crus of the antihelix (slightly toward the anterior side).
	53	Buttock	At the middle point of the superior border of the inferior crus of the antihelix (slightly toward the posterior side).
	54	Lumbago	At the lower projection of antihelix with same level of acupuncture point of coccygeal vertebrae.
Triangular fossa	55	Wonder point	At the bifurcation of crura of the antihelix.

TABLE 2–8. *Chinese Auriculotherapy Points* (continued)

REGIONS	WONG'S EAR POINT NO.	EAR POINT	LOCATION
	56	Pelvic cavity	At inner surface of the bifurcation of the crura of the antihelix.
	57	Buttock	At brim of the inferior crus of the antihelix with acupuncture point of ischium and buttock become an equilateral triangle.
	58	Uterus	At the middle point of the anterior portion of the triangular fossa just behind anterior portion of the helix.
	59	Depressing point Temp BP Tension	At the borderline between the superior crus of the helix and antihelix.
	60	Ping-chuan (Antihistamine)	About 0.2 mm from the posteroinferior part of the acupuncture point of the uterus.
	61	Hepatitis	About 0.2 mm lateral to the acupuncture point of the uterus.
Scapha	62	Fingers	At the scapha above the level of the auricular tubercle.
	63	Clavicle	At the scapha with the same level of the acupuncture point of the neck.
	64	Shoulder joint	At the scapha, lying between acupuncture point of the shoulder and clavicle.
	65	Shoulder	At the scapha with the same level of the supratragic notch (incisura anterior).
	66	Elbow	At the scapha, lying between the acupuncture points of the wrist and shoulder.
	67	Wrist	At the scapha with the same level of the auricular tubercle.
	68	Appendix	At the scapha, just above the acupuncture point of the fingers.
	69	Appendix[2]	At the scapha, at the same level of the acupuncture point of the shoulder (slightly toward the medial side of the antihelix).
	70	Appendix[3]	At the scapha, just below the acupuncture point of the clavicle.
	71	District of urticaria	Lying between the acupuncture points of the fingers and wrist (slightly toward the medial side of the antihelix).
Helix	72	Helix 1, 2, 3, 4, 5, 6	At equal intervals of six points beginning from the auricular tubercle of the helix downward to the middle point of the lower margin of auricular lobule.
	73	Tonsils[1]	Lying in the superior margin of the helix, vertically above the acupuncture point of the tonsils 4 on the auricular lobule.
	74	Tonsils[2]	At the helix with the acupuncture points of the tonsils 1 and tonsils 4 become an equilateral triangle.
	75	Tonsils[3]	The middle point between the line connecting the acupuncture point of tonsils 2 and tonsils 4.
	76	Kan-yang[1] (positive liver)	At the helix, above the level of the auricular tubercle.
	77	Kan-yang[2] (positive liver)	At the helix, on the lower margin of the auricular tubercle.
	78	Apex of the auricle	At the upper part of the helix and facing toward the terminal portion of the superior crus of the antihelix.

TABLE 2–8. *Chinese Auriculotherapy Points* (continued)

REGIONS	WONG'S EAR POINT NO.	EAR POINT	LOCATION
	79	External genital organs	At the anterior part of the helix with the same level of the inferior crus of antihelix.
	80	Urethra	At the anterior part of the helix with the same level of the acupuncture point of the urinary-bladder.
	81	Lower segment of the rectum	At the anterior portion of the helix with same level of acupuncture point of the large intestine.
Crus of the helix	82	Diaphragm	At the lower part of the crus of the helix.
	83	Point of support	At the end of the crus of the helix.
Cavum conchae	84	Mouth	At the posterior wall of the orifice of the external auditory meatus.
	85	Esophagus	At the upper portion of the cavum conchae just below the crus of the helix.
	86	Cardiac orifice	At the upper portion of the cavum conchae and just below the crus of the helix. Its acupuncture point lies behind that of the esophagus.
	87	Stomach	At the upper portion of the cavum conchae and just below the disappearance of the crus of the helix.
	88	Duodenum	Lying above the crus of the helix opposite to the acupuncture point of the cardiac orifice.
	89	Small intestine	At the lower portion of the cymba conchae and above the crus of the helix. It lies at point where slightly lateral to ½ of crus of helix.
	90	Appendix[4]	Just above the crus of the helix and lying among the acupuncture points of the large intestine and small intestine.
	91	Large intestine	At the anterointerior portion of cymba conchae and just above the crus of the helix.
Cymba conchae	92	Urinary bladder	At the anterosuperior part of the cymba conchae, just below the inferior crus of antihelix.
	93	Prostate	At the medial side of the acupuncture point of the urinary bladder.
	94	Ureter	In between the acupuncture point of the urinary bladder and kidney.
	95	Kidney	Lying in the upper part of the cymba conchae at the superior portion of the acupuncture point of the small intestine.
	96	Pancreas, gallbladder	At the posterior part of the cymba conchae, just anterior to the acupuncture point of the thoracic vertebrae. This point lies between the acupuncture points of the liver and kidney. On the left auricle, this point represents the pancreas, while on the right, the gallbladder.
	97	Liver	Lying immediately posterior to the acupuncture point of the stomach in the posteroinferior part of the cymba conchae.
	98	Spleen	The lower half of liver on the left auricle (on the right auricle the point of liver remains to be liver exclusively).
	99	Ascites	Lying among the acupuncture points of the kidney, pancreas, gallbladder, and small intestine.

TABLE 2–8. *Chinese Auriculotherapy Points* (continued)

REGIONS	WONG'S EAR POINT NO.	EAR POINT	LOCATION
Cavum conchae	100	Heart	The acupuncture point lying at the center of the deepest position of the cavum conchae.
	101	Lung	Lying around the circumference of the acupuncture point of the heart.
	102	Bronchi	At the acupuncture point of lung area.
	103	Windpipe	Lying between the acupuncture points of the heart and external auditory meatus.
	104	San-chiao (triple-burner)	In the cavum conchae and lying among the acupuncture points of the internal nose, lung, and internal secretion.
Back of the auricle	105	Depressing groove	A curved vertical groove on the back of the auricle.
	106	Upper back	At the upper cartilaginous eminence.
	107	Lower back	At the lower cartilaginous eminence.
	108	Middle back	Lying between the acupuncture points of the upper back and lower back.
Others	109	Lower Abdomen	At the superior wall of the orifice of the external auditory meatus.
	110	Upper abdomen	At the inferior wall of the orifice of the external auditory meatus.

TABLE 2–9. *Prescriptions for Auriculotherapy*

DISEASE	MAIN POINTS	SECONDARY POINTS
1. Infectious Diseases		
Common cold	16, 13, 33, 101	34, 29
Chicken pox	101, 22, 13, 29, 55	
Whooping cough	101, 102, 13	51, 29
Bacterial dysentery	91, 89, 81, 55, 22, 29	
Tuberculosis of lungs	101, 42, 13, 22	34, 104
Malaria	34, 22, 97, 13, 98	
2. Digestive System Diseases		
Acute and chronic gastritis	87, 51, 55	98, 43
Gastric ulcer	87, 51, 55	34, 88
Duodenal ulcer	88, 51, 55	34, 87
Gastroenteritis	87, 51, 55, 97	88
Spasm of the diaphragm	82, 55, 34	
Enteritis	91, 81, 51, 55	89, 98
Colitis	91, 22, 51	89, 55
Intestinal tuberculosis	91, 22, 51, 89, 55	29, 104,
Indigestion	89, 87, 51, 98, 96	91, 104
Nausea and vomiting	29, 87, 51, 55	34, 85
Diarrhea	91, 89, 51, 55	81, 98
Constipation	91, 89, 51, 87	43, 104
G-I Colic	55, 89, 51	110, 109
Functional disorder of the G-I system	91, 89, 51, 87	55, 104, 98
3. Respiratory Diseases		
Bronchitis	102, 55, 31, 13	51, 29

DISEASE	MAIN POINTS	SECONDARY POINTS
Acute lobar pneumonia	101, 42, 22, 13	55, 34
Bronchopneumonia	101, 102, 51, 55, 31	13, 29, 22
Asthma	55, 31, 51, 13	101, 29, 22, 60
Vesicular emphysema	101, 102, 51, 55, 31	13, 29
Pleurisy	101, 42, 22, 13	34, 104
Pleural adhesions	13, 42, 22	34, 55
Cough	55, 31, 13	29, 101
Pressure on chest	100, 51, 42	29, 101
Chest pain	55 C.P.*	
4. Cardiovascular Diseases		
Myocarditis	100, 51, 89, 55	29
Rheumatoid cardiopathy	100, 51, 22, 55	89, 37
Cardiac arrhythmia	100, 51, 55	34
Hypertension	100, 51, 55, 19	105
Hypotension	100, 51, 29, 13	
Peripheral circulatory disturbances	C.P.* 22, 13	
5. Diseases of the Blood System		
Leukopenia	97, 98, 22, 95, 100	29, 82, 51
Thrombopenic purpura	97, 98, 82, 51, 55, 22	29, 100
Jaundice	98, 89, 87, 22, 82	

* C.P. = Correspondence Part

53 *Acupuncture Techniques and Equipment*

TABLE 2–9. *Prescriptions for Auriculotherapy* (continued)

DISEASE	MAIN POINTS	SECONDARY POINTS
6. Genitourinary Diseases		
Acute nephritis	95, 92, 51, 55, 97	13, 98, 22
Pyelonephritis	95, 92, 51, 55, 97	13, 98, 22
Renal dysfunction	95, 92, 51, 55	13, 29
Hematuria	95, 92, 97, 82, 13	
Urine retention	95, 92, 51, 79	34
Incontinence of urine	28, 92, 83	29, 95
Impotence, frigidity in male, female	58, 79, 32, 22, 95	
Prostatitis	93, 92, 95, 22	29
7. Endocrine Diseases		
Hypothyroidism	45, 22, 28, 55	
Hyperthyroidism	45, 22, 28, 55	37
Diabetes insipidus	98(L), 95, 55, 96(L), 28, 22	
8. Diseases of the Locomotion System		
Neck pain	37, 41, 55	
Hypertrophic spondylopathy	C.P.* 22, 13, 34	95, 55
Periarthritis of shoulder	55, 64, 65 (C.P.*)	13, 63
Rheumatoid arthritis	22, 29, 95, 55 (C.P.*)	34, 55
9. Neurologic Disorders		
Trigeminal neuralgia	11, 5, 6, 55, 29	20
Facial paralysis	11, 8, 84, 29	2, 3, 97
Facial spasm	11, 55, 34, 35	
Meniere's disease	95, 55, 29, 9	34, 87
Intercostal neuralgia	42, 29	
Sciatica	52, 55, 29, 53	13
Multiple neuritis	C.P.* 55, 13, 22	
Amyotrophic lateral sclerosis	95, 22, 25, 29, 104	
Cerebellar ataxia	25, 29, 37	95, 55
Epilepsy	95, 55, 29, 100, 87	34
Migraine	35, 55, 95, 34	
Excessive sweating	51, 101, 13, 22, 29	
Neurasthenia	100, 95, 55, 29, 87	34
Aftereffects of meningitis	95, 25, 29, 55, 100	87, 34
10. Other Diseases		
Furuncle, carbuncle, and paronychia	C.P.* 55, 13, 29	
Cellulitis	C.P.* 55, 13	
Erysipelas	C.P.* 55, 13, 101, 29, 22	
Mastitis	44, 22, 13, 29	
Mammary abscess	44, 22, 13, 29	
Appendicitis	68, 91, 51, 55	
Gallstone	96, 51, 55	97, 88
Chronic pancreatitis	96, 22, 51, 55	

DISEASE	MAIN POINTS	SECONDARY POINTS
Paralytic intestinal obstruction	91, 89, 51, **34, 43**	
Ureteral calculus	94, 95, 51, 55	
Hernia	110, 34, 22	
Anal fissure and prolapse	55, 81, 91, 34	98
Chrinc cholecystitis	96, 97, 51, 55	22
Internal and external piles	81, 91	34, 98, 13
Cystitis	92, 95, 51, **55**	13, 29
Prostatis	93, 92, 95, 22	29
Orchitis and epididymitis	32, 55, 13, 22	79, 57
Fracture, contusion, sprain, and injuries	C.P.* 55, 34, 95	13
Renal calculus	95, 94, 55	34
11. Gynecologic Disorders		
Dysmenorrhea	58, 22, 51, 55	
Amenorrhea	58, 22, 23, 13, 95	
Functional uterine hemorrhage	58, 22, 97, 98, 95, 28	13
Endometritis	58, 23, 22, 13	79
Uterine prolapse	58, 34	79
Vulvar prutitus	59, 29, 13, 55, 101, 22	
12. Ophthalmologic Disorders		
Hordeolum and chalazion	8, 97, 98	
Acute conjunctivitis	8, 97	
Follicular conjunctivitis	8, 97	
Glaucoma	8, 97, 95, 24	
Optic atrophy	8, 97, 95	
Night blindness	8, 97, 24	
Myopia	8, 97, 95, 24	
Diplopia	8, 97, 95, 24	
13. Otorhinolaryngologic (ENT) Disorders		
Tinnitus	95, 9, 20, 29	
Loss of hearing	95, 9, 20, 29	
Furunculosis of the external meatus	95, 9, 22	20
Otitis media	95, 9, 22	20
Rhinitis	16, 13, 33	101
Epistaxis	16, 13, 33, 22	
Chronic laryngitis	16, 13, 33	
Chronic pharyngitis	15, 55, 100, 22	
Chronic tonsillitis	15, 55, 100, 22	101, 27
Hoarseness	15, 55, 100, 101	22
Acute tonsillitis	15, 10, 73, 74, 75	72
Uvular edema	15, 55, 13	
14. Stomatologic Disorders		
Toothache	5, 6, 55, 26	27
Periodontitis	5, 6, 84, 13	95

* C.P. = Correspondence Part

* C.P. = Correspondence Part

TABLE 2–9. *Prescriptions for Auriculotherapy* (continued)

DISEASE	MAIN POINTS	SECONDARY POINTS
Mycotic stomatitis	84, 22, 13, 98, 29	
Glossitis	4, 84, 22, 100	

15. Dermatologic Disorders

Folliculitis and herpes zoster	C.P.* 101, 29, 22, 13	
Dermatitis solaris	101, 22, 13, 29	
Urticaria	101, 55, 13, 29, 22	
Cutaneous pruritus	101, 22, 13, 29, 55	
Neurodermatitis	C.P.* 101, 22, 29, 13	
Acne	101, 22, 32, 11	
Sunburn	55, 101, 22, 13	

16. Other Disorders

Heat stroke	29, 100, 34, 13	
Shock	13, 100, 29	28
Alcoholism	33, 34, 29	
Seasickness	29, 87	9, 55

* C.P. = Correspondence Part

Ancillary Drug Administration

The effect of concomitant drug administration on acupuncture therapy or analgesia is not well-known. The use of many types of drugs before and during surgery under acupuncture analgesia is reasonably well-documented in the Chinese literature. Drugs such as phenothiazine tranquilizers (chlorpromazine, promethazine), narcotics (meperidine), barbiturates (phenobarbital sodium), anticholinergics (atropine, scopolamine), and local anesthetics (procaine, lidocaine) have all been used extensively during acupuncture analgesia.[2]

Limited clinical experience has shown that drugs such as diphenylhydantoin, phenylbutazone, and corticosteroids have not prevented a response from acupuncture therapy.[5] Some experimental studies have measured cardiovascular responses to acupuncture stimulation in dogs under general anesthesia. These dogs had been given thiopental and were under halothane anesthesia at a level of about 1 MAC, receiving a continuous intravenous succinycholine drip.[7-10]

It is often taught, however, in human and veterinary acupuncture courses that the administration of some drugs, especially corticosteroids, inhibits the response to acupuncture therapy.

The problem of drug influences is especially important in veterinary medicine, where it is often difficult to treat an animal adequately without the administration of some drug for chemical restraint such as phenothiazine tranquilizers, narcotics, xylazine, or occasionally general anesthesia.

Importation of Foreign Equipment

Equipment has been manufactured and sold in the United States for a few years; however, much equipment is made in many other countries, especially China and Japan. This equipment is imported and sold in the United States. Such importation is controlled by very specific regulations enforced by the federal Food and Drug Administration in the Department of Health, Education and Welfare. The major reason for the detention of equipment at ports of entry is inadequate labeling of the items. The following example occurred during an attempt to bring several sets of veterinary acupuncture needles into the United States from China.[5] The package, which was being hand-carried, was detained at the port of entry (Anchorage, Alaska). The form "Notice of Detention and Hearing" was issued along with a copy of a page of the Federal Register and a sheet titled "Warning".

The text from the Federal Register is as follows:

From the Federal Register of March 9, 1973; 38 F.R. 6419
DEPARTMENT OF HEALTH, EDUCATION AND WELFARE
Food and Drug Administration

Acupuncture Devices Labeling–Notice to Manufacturers, Packers and Distributors

The Commissioner of Food and Drugs is aware of the current interest in the United States surrounding the use of acupuncture needles, stimulators, and other accessories for medical purposes. Acupuncture paraphernalia are being imported into this country and are also being manufactured domestically for various medical uses, including the treatment and diagnosis of serious diseases, anesthesia, and pain relief. These products are devices and must comply with all applicable provisions of the Federal Food, Drug, and Cosmetic Act.

It is the position of the Food and Drug Administration that the safety and effectiveness of acupuncture devices have not yet been established by adequate scientific studies to support the many and varied uses for which such devices are being promoted, including uses for analgesia and anesthesia. Although various theories have been advanced as to how medical results can be obtained through the use of acupuncture, none has been proved or generally accepted, and there is a body of scientific opinion which questions the safety and effectiveness of acupuncture in many of the uses for which it is now being applied.

Under the Federal Food, Drug, and Cosmetic Act, all devices must be properly labeled to be in compliance with the law. Devices which are not safe for use by the laity, or for which adequate directions cannot be written for safe use by the laity, must be labeled as prescription devices and must be accompanied by labeling which provides the prescribing practitioner with adequate directions for their safe and effective use. Because the safety and effectiveness of acupuncture devices have not yet been adequately demonstrated, and labeling therefore cannot be devised, which would provide adequate directions for safe and effective use, they may not be labeled in accordance with the requirements for prescription devices as stated in 21 CFR 1.106(d). Until evidence is obtained demonstrating that acupuncture is a safe and effective medical technique, acupuncture devices must be limited to investigational or research use.

Current Food and Drug Administration regulations do not contain specific provisions governing the shipment of investigational devices in interstate commerce for clinical research or experimental use. The Commissioner of Food and Drugs is aware of the need for such regulations to provide adequate guidance as to the labeling for experimental devices to be used on human beings. Therefore, the Commissioner intends to publish at a later date proposed regulations which would govern all investigational devices. In the interim, this notice will apply to all acupuncture devices.

In order to establish guidelines under which manufacturers, packers, and distributors can properly label acupuncture devices for investigational use, the Food and Drug Administration met on September 22, 1972, with individuals concerned with the use of acupuncture in the United States. These included representatives of the States of California and New York, the city of New York, the American Society of Anesthesiologists, the National Institutes of Health, the Federation of State Medical Boards, the American Medical Association, medical practitioners, and the Food and Drug Administration Medical Device Advisory Committee. It was the consensus of this group that acupuncture devices should be restricted to investigational use by licensed practitioners and that the labeling for these devices should include this restriction in addition to other information.

Accordingly, the Commissioner of Food and Drugs concludes that until substantial scientific evidence is obtained by valid research studies supporting the safety and therapeutic usefulness of acupuncture devices, the Food and Drug Administration will regard as misbranded any acupuncture device shipped in interstate commerce if the following information does not appear in the labeling:

(a) The name of the device.

(b) The name and place of business of the manufacturer, packer, or distributor.

(c) An accurate statement of the quantity of the contents.

(d) The composition of the device and whether it is sterile, nonsterile, reusable, or disposable.

(e) The dimension or other pertinent physical characteristics of the device.

(f) The following statement: "Caution: Experimental device limited to investigational use by or under the direct supervision of a licensed medical or dental practitioner. This device is to be used only with informed consent under conditions designed to protect the patient as a research subject, where the scientific protocol for investigation has been reviewed and approved by an appropriate institutional review committee, and where conditions for such use are in accordance with State law."

Instructions for the use of the device for the purpose for which it is being investigated and, to the extent such information is known, any human hazards, contraindications, precautions, or side effects associated with its use, should be provided to researchers and investigators. The Food and Drug Administration, however, will regard as misbranded any acupuncture device shipped in interstate commerce if accompanied by claims of diagnostic or therapeutic effectiveness.

Pending promulgation of separate regulations for conducting clinical investigations of investigational devices, researchers and investigators shall assure adequate informed consent and institutional committee review for such investigations, utilizing as a guideline the standards established for investigational drugs in 21 CFR 136.37 and in Division 10, unit C of form FD-1571, in 21 CFR 130.3(a)(2).

Dated: February 21, 1973.

SHERWIN GARDNER,
Deputy Commissioner of Food and Drugs

The text of the sheet titled "Warning" is as follows:

Warning Please read enclosed notices carefully. If submitted labels are not in strict accord with sections "a" through "f" of the Federal Register notice of March 9, 1973, they will not be acceptable. You will be requested to re-submit the labels. This might cause a delay of several months in your receiving the shipment. A large number of acupuncture entries and the failure of consignees to provide proper labels have resulted in a heavy backlog in our work.

Your cooperation in this matter will enable us to serve you more efficiently. Thank you.

After sending the labels as proscribed in the Federal Register, the material was immediately released; however, arrangements then must be made with commercial custom house bookers to pick up the materials, pack them, and then ship them. This is at the importer's expense. The importation of these materials should be greatly expedited if the appropriate labels are prepared beforehand and attached to the items before the time of entry.

REFERENCES

1. Anon. 1972. *Chinese Veterinary Handbook* (in Chinese). Lan Chou Veterinary Research Institute. Gan shu, China: The Peoples Publishing Co.
2. Anon. 1974. *The Principles and Practical Use of Acupuncture Analgesia.* Hong Kong: Medicine and Health Publishing Co.
3. Babich, A. M. 1973. An analysis of a portable electronic stimulator manufactured in the Peoples Republic of China. *Amer. J. Chinese Med.* 1:341–50.
4. Gunji, R. 1973. *Electric Acupuncture (Introduction to Simple Ryodoraku Treatment).* Tokyo: Bunkodo Co.
5. Klide, A. M. 1974–76. Unpublished observations.
6. Kvirchishvilli, VI. 1974. Projections of different parts of the body on the surface of the concha auriculae in humans and animals. *Amer. J. Acupuncture* 2:208.
7. Lee, D. C. 1976. Inhibition of the cardiovascular effects of acupuncture (moxibustion) by propanolol in dogs during halothane anesthesia. *Canad. Anaesth. Soc. J.* 23:307–18.
8. Lee, D. C. *et al.* 1974. Cardiovascular effects of acupuncture in anesthetized dogs. *Amer. J. Chinese Med.* 2:271–82.
9. Lee, D. C. *et al.* 1975. Cardiovascular effects of moxibustion at jin chung (GV 26) during halothane anesthesia in dogs. *Amer. J. Chinese Med.* 3:245–61.
10. Lee, M. O., *et al.* 1975. Cardiovascular effects of acupuncture at tsu san li (ST 36) in dogs. *J. Surg. Res.* 18:51–63.
11. Li, C., *et al.* 1973. Survey of electrical resistance of rabbit penna during experimental peritonitis. *Chinese Med. J.* No. 7, July:94.
12. Nakatani, Y. 1961. *Actual Ryodoraku Clinic.* (in Japanese). Japan: Ryodoraku Research Institute.
13. Nakatani, Y. 1961. *Detailed Explanation of Ryodo Points and Ryodoraku Treatment* (in Japanese). Japan: Ryodoraku Research Institute.
14. Nakatani, Y. 1966. *Outline of Ryodoraku Medical Science.* (in Japanese). Japan: Ryodoraku Research Institute.
15. Nogier, P. 1972. *Treatise of Auriculotherapy.* Lyon, France.
16. Sato, T, and Nakatani, Y. 1974. Acupuncture for chronic pain in Japan. In *Advances in Neurology,* 4: 813–18. New York: Raven Press.

APPENDIX: *Instruction Guides for Electrical Acupuncture Stimulators*

Chinese Model 626–1, Multipurpose Electrotherapeutic Apparatus (FIG 2–29)

DESCRIPTION

This model is a portable type of transistorized, multipurpose electrotherapeutic apparatus that has a wide application with high therapeutic effects, and it can be used for treatment, acupunctural anesthesia, artificial respiration, and diagnostic purposes.

It is small, lightweight, portable, and convenient to use. The power is supplied by a 9V dry battery, and this apparatus is therefore extremely suitable for the medical unit and the electroacupunctural therapy.

METHOD OF USE:

Method of operation for the treatment:

1. The position of the patient, either in sitting or sleeping posture, should be to the utmost kept comfortably.
2. After selecting the points for stimulation with the electrodes, first insert the needles well into these points as directed by the new method of general acupuncture or the electric conduction method.
3. Connect the needles to the electrodes of the output. Generally, the positive electrode bears the auxiliary point, whereas the negative bears the principal point, and as a rule, the principal point must be coupled with the auxiliary, just as the up with the down, but this can be modified according to the conditions when required.
4. Turn the power switch, adjust the desired mode of current and frequency, then turn the output control, and adjust to the appropriate current of stimulative intensity where the patient has a marked feeling of stimulation without any intolerable pain. Before the operation starts, the output control should be turned to the left back on the "O" position, and when the operation starts, the output control is then turned slowly to the right so that the output can be gradually increased.
5. At the end of the treatment, first turn off the output control, then the power, and then take away the output terminals (the clips) before removing the needles.
6. This apparatus is separated into three output leads, which can be applied simultaneously to six points or to several patterns for the treatment and/or the acupunctural anesthesia.

Method of operation for the acupunctural anesthesia:

Operate the same way as above. All three modes of current can be chosen for the acupunctural anesthesia, but in general, the adjustable mode is more preferable.

Method of operation for the artificial respiration:

1. First select the points for stimulation from the bilateral phrenic nerves of the neck, and then plunge the needles.

2. Connect the needles to the electrodes of the output.

3. Turn the operation mode knob to the ripple (sawtoothed) mode position.

4. Adjust the frequency and the stimulative intensity suitable for the required times per minute of the artificial respiration.

Method of operation for detecting the Auricular Point:

1. Turn the operation mode knob to the adjustable mode position, and plug the jack socket of the probe into the point detector. While the patient is grasping the metal tube with one hand, use the probe to touch the ear lightly and uniformly in order to find out the auricular point. When the site of the point is touched, a sound of high frequency will occur immediately. If the sound is too small, first try to make a short circuit between the metal tube and the probe, and then read-

just the frequency regulator for a greater sound.

2. The place to be detected should be clean and dry; otherwise the finding will become inaccurate.

Method of operation for detecting the sites of the Meridian Points:

1. Turn the operation mode knob to the adjustable mode position.

2. Plug the jack socket of the probe into the point detector and while the metal tube is grasped in the hand of the patient, use the probe to touch the skin where the meridian point is to be detected. If the site of the point is touched, a sound of high frequency will occur immediately. According to individual sensitivity, fitly readjust the frequency regulator so as to control the current of the stimulative intensity.

3. The place to be detected should be clean and dry.

Chinese Model 71–1, Acupuncture Anesthesia Apparatus (FIGS. 2–30, 2–31)

This is a new type fully transistorized electrical acupuncture anesthesia apparatus, and also can be used as an electrotherapeutic apparatus. It sends pulsating currents of adjustable intensities and frequencies transmits through the acupuncture needles to human body. For therapeutic or anesthesia purposes, the nervous or muscular system is excited or inhibited by means of stimulation. This apparatus is suitable for use in acupuncture anesthesia of various kinds of surgery and may also be used in association with acupuncture treatment for many kinds of diseases. It is an ideal tool in modern medical science.

As the circuit is transistorized, the average power consumption is very small, yet the instantaneous output is high. In addition to the above mentioned features, this apparatus is simple in manipulation, compact, lightweight, and easy to carry.

RANGE OF APPLICATIONS

Anesthesia: This apparatus is suitable for use in acupuncture anesthesia of various kinds of surgery.

Therapeutic: It can improve the peripheral circulation and adjust the tonicity on the nervous and muscular systems. It is to be used in association with acupuncture treatment in various diseases such as contusion, sprain, strain, lumbago, sore legs, and tenosynovitis.

DIRECTIONS FOR OPERATION

1. Turn the changing switch to the required wave. The illumination of the frequency pilot light indicates that the apparatus starts to output pulse current.
This apparatus is provided with a range of three waveforms:

   a. Turn the changing switch to ⊓ position:

No. 1, 2, 3, & 4 output sockets are all in the wave of ⊓

   b. Turn the changing switch to ⊓⊓ position: No. 1 & 2 output sockets are in the wave of ⊓ which stimulating effect is comparatively strong. No. 3 & 4 output sockets are in the wave of ⊓ of which stimulating effect is comparatively weak.

   c. Turn the changing switch to ⊓ position: No. 1, 2, 3, & 4 output sockets are all in the wave of ⊓

2. Connect the output electrode wire plug to the output sockets (No. 1 to 4) by plugging. On each electrode wire, there are two clips that can be held firmly on the acupuncture needles. The four sets of output sockets can afford eight points, of which current strength can be adjusted by turning the current regulators.

POWER SUPPLY

DC 9 Volts. Insert six No. 1 batteries.

NOTES

1. When the apparatus is not in use, turn the changing switch to "off" position.

2. For the purpose of checking the power consumption, you may turn the changing switch to "battery" position. The pilot-lamp situated at the left underside corner will light and according to its brightness you can judge whether the batteries should be changed or not.

3. This apparatus has been put in clinical practice but its efficiency is closely related with a good grasp of the exact location of the major points, as well as the clinical experience of a physician.

Chinese Model 71–3 Multi-purpose Therapy Apparatus (FIGS. 2–32, 2–33)

This is a fully transistorized multipurpose therapy apparatus, which transmits pulsating currents of different intensities and frequencies through the acupuncture needles to human body. For therapeutic or anesthesia purposes, the nervous or muscular system is excited or inhibited by means of stimulation. This apparatus is used in the treatment of various diseases, in clinical operations using acupuncture anesthesia and in the rescue of patients from the failure of respiration. It is also suitable for use in finding the exact location of point in order to promote the efficacy of acupuncture treatment or acupuncture anesthesia. This apparatus is equipped with an ultraviolet lamp, which gives the action of radiation therapy. It is an ideal tool in modern medical science.

As the circuit is transistorized, the average power consumption is very small, yet the instantaneous output is high. In addition to the above mentioned advantages, this apparatus is small, lightweight, of robust construction, and easy to carry.

RANGE OF APPLICATIONS
1. Therapeutic: It can improve the peripheral circulation and adjust the tonicity on the nervous and muscular systems. It is suitable for all kinds of diseases that can be treated by acupuncture, such as contusion, sprain, strain, lumbago, sore legs, and tenosynovitis.
2. Anesthesia: For acupuncture anesthesia in various kinds of clinical operations.
3. Respiration: For patients with failure or sudden stop of respiration.
4. Detection: To find the exact location of points, in order to enhance the efficacy of acupuncture treatment or acupuncture anesthesia.
5. Ultraviolet: It gives a sterilization effect and is indicated for the treatment of various skin diseases and the promotion of healing.

DIRECTIONS FOR OPERATION
1. For therapeutic or anesthesia:
    a. Turn the changing switch to "therapeutic" or "anesthesia" as required.
    b. Turn the wave-range switch to the required wave. This apparatus is provided with a range of five waveforms:
    Adjustable wave (range of frequency: 2–50 cycles/sec, and can be controlled by an adjustable regulator). Dense-disperse wave, discontinuous wave, ripple wave, sawtooth wave (range of modulation frequencies: 15–25 cycles/min, and can be controlled by a pulsating regulator)
    c. Connect the electrode wire plug (accessories A) to the output socket (No. 1–4) by plugging. On each output electrode wire there are two clips which can be held firmly on the acupuncture

needles. These four sets of output current can afford eight points, whose output current strength can be regulated by "Current Regulator" individually. Therefore, it can be used for treatment or anesthesia of one to four patients at the same time without any mutual interference on output strength.
    d. Turn the power switch to "on". The illumination of the frequency pilot light indicates that the apparatus starts to output pulse current.
2. For respiration:
    a. Turn the Changing Switch to "respiration".
    b. Turn the Wave-range Switch to "red, yellow, green" three color points.
    c. Regulate the pulsating regulator to the required frequency. Range of frequency for respiration: 15–25 cycles/min. It is suitable for different frequencies required by adults and children.
    d. Connect the electrode wire plug (accessories A) to anyone of the output socket. The electrode wire is fitted with two clips capable of holding firmly on the acupuncture needles used on the patient's phrenic nerve points. Adjust the output current strength by turning the current regulator, which is above the output socket.
    e. Turn the power switch to "on". The illumination of the frequency pilot light indicates that the apparatus starts transmitting pulse current.

Remarks:
The phrenic nerve point is at the location 1–2 cm above the middle of each collar bone. There are two points, one is on the left and the other is on the right.

When the patient is under an acupuncture treatment with pulsating current and rhythmical abdominal respiration appears, it means that he has obtained the therapeutic effect.
3. For detection:
    a. Turn the changing switch to "detector".
    b. Turn the wave-range switch to "red, yellow, green" three color points:
    c. Connect the detector wire plug (accessories B) to the probe socket by plugging. The test probe is used for tracing points, an earphone is used by a doctor and the electrode, made of brass with chromium plating, is to be held tightly by patient.
    d. Turn the power switch to "on". The illumination of the frequency pilot light indicates that the apparatus starts transmitting pulse current. Because the frequency and output are fixed, all the regulators lose their function.
    e. When the test probe touches the point, you may hear immediately such a noise "po, po, po, . . ." from the earphone.

Remarks:

1. When the sensitivity of detection is affected due to the difference of temperature, humidity, and the skin resistance, you may remove the back cover plate of this apparatus and take out the battery, then use a screw driver to adjust the potential metre on the left side hole, clockwise for increasing sensitivity: counter-clockwise for decreasing sensitivity.

2. For detection, the frequency pilot lamp is in light only when the point is found. But the exact point is subjected to such a noise "Po, Po, Po, . . ." heard from the earphone.

4. For Ultraviolet:

 a. Turn the changing switch to "Ultraviolet".

 b. Turn the wave-range switch to "red, yellow, green" three color points.

 c. Connect the ultraviolet lamp wire plug (accessories C) into ultraviolet socket by plugging. Remove the cover from the ultraviolet lamp. The ultraviolet therapy is to be directed by a physician. In general, the patient can obtain satisfactory therapy by using one erythema dose in clinic when the affected area is exposed to the ultraviolet not exceeding 1 min at a distance of 1 cm.

 d. Turn the power switch to "on". The ultraviolet lamp is in light and the time for stability takes about 1–2 min. Because the ultraviolet frequency and output are fixed, all regulators lose their function.

Remarks:

If the room temperature is comparatively low, the working current of ultraviolet may drop and the lamp tube may probably not light. Then, you may remove the back cover plate of this apparatus, take out the battery and use a screw driver to adjust the potential meter on the right side hole, clockwise for increasing current, counterclockwise for decreasing current.

POWER SUPPLY

D.C. 9 Volts. Insert six No. 1 batteries.

NOTES

1. Do not touch the ultraviolet lamp tube. If it is dirty, you may clean it with a piece of alcohol cotton.

2. You should pay attention to the battery consumption frequently. When the frequency pilot lamp is dim, it shows that the battery should be changed.

3. This apparatus has been put in clinical practice but its efficiency is closely related with a good grasp of the exact location of the major points as well as the clinical experience of a physician.

ACCESSORIES

a. Output electrode wires with plugs and clips (4 sets).

b. Detection wire with plug, test probe, earphone and chromium-plated brass electrode (1 set).

c. Ultraviolet lamp (with an extra spare ultraviolet tube) (1 set).

Technical Data—Acuflex Model CZ-110 Dual Neur-Metron (FIG. 2–38)

PHYSICAL DATA

15″ Wide × 4⅛″ High × 9¾″ Deep

Unit Weight: 11 lbs.

Portable with 2½-inch removable steel legs, rubber protectors on legs and case.

FINISH

Steel case and cover, beige and brown baked enamel.

POWER REQUIREMENTS

Self-contained: Battery (rechargeable) 1–9V Battery 2U6

CONTROLS AND INDICATORS

Meter: 300 amp with nomenclature.

Battery Condition Pushbutton: Push to test.

Calibrate Procedure: With sensitivity on, adjust to 200 microamps, calibrate position on meter.

Solid-State Lamp: Indicates when unit is on. If not on when unit is turned on recharge battery.

Treatment (silver) Jack: Harness connection.

Negative (black) Jack: Probe connection.

Positive (red) Jack: Grip connection.

Modulation Knob*: Detent Position—continuous (steady rate) and adjustable from 15–100 groups of pulses/min. In "cont." position, the output pulses are continuous at the rate set on the rate knob. At other than the "cont." position, the train of pulses is interrupted so that the pulses are on for a specific ime and then off for the same length of time. This modulation is adjustable from 15 to 100 times/min.

Rate Knob*: Adjustable frequency from 1–100 pulses/ sec.

* With modulation in continuous detent, rate knob controls output frequency. With modulation in adjustable section the frequency is still controlled by rate knob, but groups of pulses are created according to setting on modulation knob.

Voltage: Adjusts the output voltage from "0" to a maximum of 250 volts peak to peak (not calibrated).

Mode Knob: Controls whether the treatment side or the analytical side is operable. Waveform on treatment side is bipolar with slightly more energy in one direction. The pulse is of very short duration (less than 1 msec) in each direction and decays with a short RC constant. The mode switch has two positions, which internally interchange the output leads. When the mode is at the 10 o'clock position, more energy eminates (higher pulse) through the black lead. When the mode is set in "rev pol." more energy eminates from the red lead. When using the analytical side, the range sets voltage available at the probe and grip (red, positive potential; black, negative). This is a direct current (dc) and its maximum can be set by turning on the sensitivity knob, shortening the probe and grip together, and reading resultant microamps (300 maximum). When the range is in X, the voltage is 12 volts, but the meter is shunted to produce a 450 microamp, full-scale reading (used with needle injection). The audio signal is synchronized with the output of the meter and increases in frequency as the current increases.

Sensitivity Knob: Rotate clockwise to turn machine on, adjust to 200 microamps by shorting probe and grip together.

Audio Knob: Rotate clockwise to turn audio on, adjust to acceptable level (turn off after use, so not to deplete battery).

Range: 12–12 volt position
  21–21 volt position
  × –12 volt position with damped meter (= 450 microamp max.) capacity.

STANDARD ACCESSORIES
1–Treatment harness.
1–Probe with color-coded retractable cord.
1–Grip with color-coded retractable cord.
Rechargeable 12-volt battery system—includes recharger. Unit is inoperative when charger is plugged into rear panel.

ELECTRONIC CONSTRUCTION
All solid-state, mounted on two quality printed circuit boards.

CONTRAINDICATIONS
Use standard electrical precautions when analyzing and treating patients with pacemakers.

Instruction Guide Sheet for the Acuflex Dual—C2 110 Neur. Metron

This instruction sheet is to be used as an added guide for the use of the Acuflex CZ-110 Dual and is not to be construed as the only way of use.

ANALYSIS

Step One:
Turn the mode switch to "Analysis."
Step Two:
Turn on the sensitivity switch and the audio switch, with the range switch either in 12-volt or 21-volt position. Now you must place the probe and grip together by placing metal to metal. This will short the two, enabling you to tune the sensitivity switch to the 200 microamp arrow on the meter. At this point, you are ready to analyze. You must recalibrate if you change from 12 to 21 on the range switch.
Note:
The X position on the range switch is for use with a needle gun, which would replace the probe and you would then select the output by turning the sensitivity to the output desired.

TREATMENT

Turn the mode switch to the left, pointing to "treatment."
Step Two:

Turn the voltage switch on and set the pulse rate to the desired setting. The rate is 60 times whatever is shown on the rate scale.
Step Three:
Modulation is as follows: In the "cont." position, you can do pain control or anesthesia. From 15 to 35 is the stimulation range and from 35 to 100 is the sedation range depending on the method of treatment.

BATTERY

To check the battery level, turn the mode switch to "analysis" position. With all knobs in the "off" position, push the battery-check button, which puts the needle on the meter in the battery-good range. If the battery reads "low," charge the system with the battery charger supplied with the instrument. When you plug in the battery charger, the instrument will not operate, thus eliminating line hazard to patient.
Note:
You cannot overcharge this system, so do not worry about leaving it charging over a weekend.

PROBE

The probe has many uses but one is to place cotton in the cup end and dampen it with a conductive material, saline solution for example.

User's Manual for the Multiwaveform Stimulator/Acu Point Finder and Meridian Balance Meter Model DHW 3B–4WF (FIG. 2–36)

CONTENTS

1. IMPORTANT STATEMENT TO ALL USERS

Until substantial scientific evidence is obtained in the U.S. by valid research studies supporting the therapeutic usefulness of acupuncture, the Food and Drug Administration requires the following statement to be included in all acupuncture devices: "This experimental device is limited to investigational use by or under the direct supervision of licensed medical or dental practitioners. It is to be used only under conditions designed to protect the patient as a research subject and where the scientific protocol for investigation has been reviewed and approved by an appropriate institutional review or where conditions for such use are in accordance with state law." Users are also urged to read this operational manual carefully before using this instrument.

2. INTRODUCTION

This model combined in one instrument the three functions most often performed in acupuncture treatment, acupoint location, meridian diagnosis, and electrical stimulation. The range of different waveforms and output levels available cover those required for therapeutic treatment, anesthesia, and artificial respiration, etc. In fact, the ranges are wider than those available in instruments imported from China and Japan. This is intentional because it is believed that further experimentation is probably required in order to determine the optimum conditions (parameters) for each application.

2.1 Summary of the Working Principles of the Instrument

In the 1950's, Japanese researchers headed by Dr. Kyugo

Sasagawa studied the physiologic basis of acupuncture and arrived at two main conclusions: First, there exists on the human body points of low electrical resistance that the traditional Chinese medical literature refers to as acupuncture points. Second, they reported pathways with good electrical conductivity (low electrical resistance), which they termed "ryodoraku." These pathways again agree very well with those of the meridians. Finally, in about the same period, it has been discovered by acupuncture practitioners in China that the delicate needle manipulation techniques can be replaced by the application of electrical stimuli. They have found by experimentation the waveforms and pulse rates most likely to produce results.

This instrument is designed on these principles. It is a sophisticated electronic instrument that, when used as an acupoint finder, can sense sudden reduction in electrical resistance; when used as a meridian balance meter, it can monitor the current through the meridian for a fixed voltage; when used as a stimulator, it delivers a train of pulses of adjustable pulse rates and is modulated by a variety of waveforms.

3. SPECIFICATIONS

A. On-Off Switch

Always switch off the instrument if it is not being used to avoid draining the batteries.

B. Point Finder and Normal Switch

If the instrument is being used as an acupuncture point finder, slide the switch to the left, as marked. This activates the sonic circuit. For any other applications of this instrument, slide this switch to the right, marked "normal."

C. Waveform Control Switch

This switch controls the waveform, or shape, of the electric stimulus. In the "off" position, all electrical outputs are switched off.

C.1 In the uniform pulse-amplitude position, the stimulus is a train of pulses a fraction of a millisecond in duration, having uniform amplitude and pulse rate. The pulse rate can be adjusted by the pulse-rate switch from a low rate of 1 pulse every 2 sec to a high rate of 200 pulses/sec. Every step of the switch approximately doubles the pulse rate. At the position marked "DC", the pulse rate is so high that the stimulation can be considered continuous. At this position, the light should blink at the pulse rate controlled by the pulse-rate switch marked.

C.2 In the dense-disperse position, the stimulus is a train of pulses having uniform amplitude but changing automatically from a high pulse rate of 200 pulses/sec (dense) to a low rate of 0.5 pulses/sec (disperse). The period the high rate persists is typically 1, 2, or 0.5 sec, and the period the low rate persists is typically 4, 2, 1, or 0.5 sec. The exact periods are controlled by the frequency switch.

C.3 In the square-wave position, the envelope or the modulating waveform is rectangular. This means that the train of uniform-amplitude pulses is turned on (typically for about 1, 2, or 0.5 sec) and then off (typically for about 4, 2, 1, or 0.5 sec). The exact on period and off period are controlled by the frequency switch.

C.4 In the triangular-wave position, the envelope or the modulating waveform is triangular. This means that the train of pulses has uniform pulse rate, but their amplitudes fluctuate, rising steadily from zero amplitude to a peak wave (which is adjustable by output-level switches) and then falls gradually to zero. The entire sequence takes typically 1–6 sec. The pulse train remains off for typically 0.5–4 sec before its amplitude rises steadily gain. Again, the on period and off period are controlled by the frequency switch.

D. *The Frequency Switch*

The switch controls the waveform of the envelope or the modulating wave. Its application has been referred to in paragraph 3. The meaning of each switch position is detailed as follows:

Position	On-Time or dense period	Off-Time or disperse period
1	1 sec	4 sec
2	2 sec	2 sec
3	1 sec	2 sec
4	2 sec	1 sec
5	1 sec	1 sec
6	0–5 sec	0–5 sec

E. *Pulse-rate Switch*

This switch controls the pulse rate or frequency, as referred to in section C.2 above. The pulse rate for each position is typically as follows:

Position	Pulse-Rate
0.5 pps (1)	1 pulse /2 sec
2	3 pulses/2 sec
3	2 pulses/sec
4	3 pulses/sec
5	5 pulses/sec
6	10 pulses/sec
7	20 pulses/sec
8	40 pulses/sec
DC (9)	200 pulses/sec

F. *The Multifunction Switch*

When the instrument is used as a point finder, the switch should be set at one of the sensitivity positions (9, 12, 21, or 30). Each number indicates the number of volts (DC) being applied across the exploring and holding electrodes. The 12-volt position is more sensitive than the 9-volt position, and so on.

When the instrument is used as a meridian-balance meter, using the exploring electrode and the cup electrode, turn this switch to the "meridian-balance" position, (and, of course, the point finder/normal switch—see paragraph 2 above—should be in normal position). *When the instrument is used as a stimulator,* this switch is turned to one of the four positions under "monitor." For example, at position 3, the microammeter is monitoring the current in microamperes being delivered through the leads plugged into output jack numbered "3". When the push-button switch is pushed down the pointer of the microammeter will move to give the appropriate reading. Therefore, by turning this switch to any of the four positions (marked "1", "2", "3", "4" under "monitor"), the four output currents can be measured.

G. *"MB-S" Slide Switches*
(MB ± Meridian Balance, S = Stimulator)

Each of these four slide switches is related to the output-level control and output jack directly under it. Thus, *if the switch above output 1 is slided to the "MB" position,* the voltage across the output clips from jack 1 is a constant DC voltage. The microammeter will read (push push-button 1 down) the DC current through the meridian. (It is assumed that the clips are attached to two needles inserted into the same meridian). This reading will tell the cognizant practitioner about the state of the meridian (hyper- or hypoactive). *If the slide switch above output 1 is on the "S" position,* the voltage across the clips from jack 1 would be the stimulating voltage with a waveform, frequency, and pulse-rate determined by switchs 3, 4, and 5, respectively. The microammeter then reads (push push-button 1 down) the stimulating current.

H. *Output-Level Control*

Each of these 4 controls, control the output voltages coming out of the jack immediately below it. The output voltage is maximum when the control is at the most clock-wise position (zero output voltages) before the instrument is switched on.

I. *Push-Button Switches*

This set of 4 push-button switches are "normally closed" switches. They are connected across the microammeter, and as such, will normally allow the stimulating current to bypass the microammeter.

However, when, for example, one of the switches is pushed down (and the multifunction switch is turned to the appropriate position), the push-button switch is opened and the microammeter will measure the current through output 1.

J. Stimulator-Output Jacks

This set of 4 output jacks deliver a constant DC voltage if slide switches marked "Meridian Balance/Stimulator" are in position MB and deliver the stimulating waveforms if it is in position S. These jacks are used if the meridian balance function is performed in conjunction with needles.

K. Point-Finder and Meridian Balance Jack

This jack is used for acupuncture point location and if the meridian balance is performed in conjunction with the cup electrodes.

L. Indicator Light

If the instrument is used as a stimulator, this light will blink at the pulse rate and frequency used. It gives a rough indication of the waveform being used. If excessive current is drawn from any one of the output jacks, this light may become rather dim. This may also be because one or more batteries is dead.

M. Microammeter

This microammeter can monitor the meridian balance or stimulator current through any one of the 4 stimulator outputs, and the meridian balance or point-finder current through the point-finder and meridian balance jacks by appropriate positioning of the multifunction switch.

To obtain the correct current reading, multiply the meter reading by a factor of 2. Thus, the full-scale reading for the meter is 200 microamperes.

N. Sensitivity Control

This control is used for the meridian balance meter setup. Whenever meridian balance diagnosis is performed, it should be used to adjust the reading of the meter to read 200 (100 $\times$ 2). Both electrodes must be shorted while adjusting this meter reading. *For any other monitoring purposes, this control must be turned up to the maximum (all the way to the right) so that the meter will give an accurate reading in microamps of the stimulator output.*

4. OPERATIONAL PROCEDURES

A. Important Basic Procedure

Before turning the instrument on,

a. Check that all 4 output level controls are in the most anticlockwise positions. IMPORTANT: This must be done in order to avoid administering dangerous and unpleasant shocks to the patients.
b. Check that the multifunction switch is in the 9-volt position.
c. Check that the waveform switch is in the off position.
d. Read and refresh your mind by re-reading this user's manual until you are sure of the function of all the controls.

Before putting this instrument away,

e. Check that the power on-off switch is in off position.

This is to avoid the unpleasant experience of finding all the batteries drained and dead.

f. Go through steps a, b, and c above.
g. Check that the indicator light is not blinking.

B. As an Acupuncture Point-Finder

B.1 Preliminary Checking
Check that the multifunction switch is in the 9-volt position. Insert the plug (with the two leads provided) into the socket located in the left-most position.

B.2 Turn the multifunction switch to the 12-volt position, and the slide-switch to the point-finder position. Avoid contacting the electrodes because this would send in a current of a magnitude sufficient to damage the meter.

B.3 The instrument is now ready to be used. Ask the subject to hold cylindrical electrode with one hand. The exploring probe is then applied with moderate pressure to the vicinity of the acupuncture point to be located. The exact location of this point is a low-resistance point and is indicated by a rapid increase in current-meter reading, accompanied by a correspondingly high-pitched audio note. This instrument is uniquely designed so that the frequency of the audio note increases as the exploring probe gets nearer to the exact point location.

B.4 Precaution
Some points have area in the order of only 1 sq mm, and hence careful searching is necessary before they can be located accurately. The skin should be kept dry; otherwise, the point location may not be found easily.

B.5 Sensitivity Switch
In the point-finding process, if the meter reading remains low and the audio-note low-pitched, it may be necessary to turn the sensitivity switch to the 21-volt or 30-volt position. In general, points on the chest, shoulder, and the face require less voltage, and points on the limbs require higher voltages.

B.6 Criterion
The presence of a point is not indicated by low resistance alone, but by a sudden drop in resistance, as evidenced by a jump in the current meter reading and a higher-pitched note. In other words, it is the change in these quantities that is important not their absolute values. In some cases, in order to observe these changes, proper selection of the sensitivity switch is necessary. For some subjects, the drop in electrical resistance at the acupuncture point relative to that of the surrounding tissue is not marked, and one has to be content with a not-so-precise indication. Erroneous acupoint location may be caused by moisture and by scratching the surface of the skin. To avoid the former, the part of the body being studied should be kept dry.

C. As a Meridian Balance Meter in Conjunction with Cup Electrodes

C.1 Preliminary Checking

Turn the multifunction switch to the meridian balance position and the slide switch to the "normal" position.

C.2 Setting Up

Insert the plug into the socket in the left-most position.

C.3 Fill the cup in the exploring electrode with cotton soaked in saline solution.

C.4 Ask the subject to hold the cylindrical electrode in one hand. The practitioner will place the cup electrode over the yuan, or source, point of each of the 12 meridians, left side first, then right side. The cup electrode should make uniform, firm contact with the point, and as the meter needles rises to a steady final reading, this then is taken to be the measured value.

C.5 The 24 measured values are plotted on graph paper and each value is compared with the average of the 24 readings. One can draw general conclusions as follows:

a. For the same meridian, marked difference between readings for the left and right sides implies unbalance.

b. A higher-than-average reading indicates that the meridian is hyperactive; a lower-than-average value implies hypoactivity.

D. *Electrical Stimulation in Conjunction with Acupuncture Needles*

D.1 Preliminary Checking.

Before turning the instrument on, check that all the output level controls are in the most anticlockwise positions.

D.2 Select the appropriate waveforms. If the first waveform is selected, also select a pulse rate (ranging from 0–5pps to DC). If one of the other three waveforms is selected, turn the pulse-rate switch to a high pulse-rate position (for example, the last position next to that marked "DC"). Now select a frequency. The first frequency switch position has a stimulation period of 1 sec. followed by a relaxation period (absence of stimulation) of 4 sec. (see Sect. 3.4).

D.3 *Making Sure That the Output-Level Control Is in the Most Anticlockwise Position.*

Now insert the plug into one of the four output jacks and attach the clips to the acupuncture needles, which we assume have been inserted into the appropriate acupuncture points. Slowly turn the output level control clockwise

until the subject can feel the electric impulses. At this stage, proceed very gradually until the subject experiences a numbing and pulsating feeling and yet without feeling unduly uncomfortable and painful. This then is the appropriate voltage setting.

D.4 *Measuring the Output Currents.*

If the output current is to be measured, turn the multifunction switch to the appropriate position (1, 2, 3, or 4, depending on which output current is to be measured) under "monitor" and press the corresponding push-button down. The reading obtained, when multiplied by a factor of 2, is the output current delivered to the patient in microamperes.

D.5 *Four Independent Outputs.*

The four outputs deliver the same waveform, frequency, and pulse rate, but the output level can be controlled independently. The interaction between outputs is minimal. *As a safety precaution, if more than one output is being used, and then one output is to be turned off completely, always do this gradually, and reduce the other outputs whenever necessary.*

E. *Electrical Stimulation in Conjunction with Cup Electrodes*

For this application, proceed as described in the previous section, except that attach the clips onto the pair of cup electrodes provided. The cups are filled with a ball of cotton soaked in a saline solution. Apply the electrodes to the acupuncture points selected for the particular treatment.

F. *Meridian Diagnosis prior to Application of Stimulation (with Needles in Position)*

Before or in the procedures described in Sections 4.5 and 4.6, if it is desired to determine the condition the meridian being used (for example, to find whether it is hyperactive or hypoactive or to see if the electrical stimulation has resulted in any change) just slide the "MB-S" switch to the "MB" position, press the push-button down and note the current reading (of course, the multifunction switch should monitor the appropriate output jacks).

G. *How to Use the Microammeter*

Please refer to Sect. 3.13 for a detailed explanation.

Acu-Stimulator I Portable Electronic Pulse Generator (FIG. 2–39)

PLEASE READ THESE PAGES BEFORE YOU PLACE THE INSTRUMENT IN USE

The basic action of the Acu-Stimulator is simple. Controls on the device allow tailoring of the output for specific treatment effects.

The frequency and amplitude of the output may be individually adjusted. There are five outputs, which are

all isolated from each other. The use of separate output transformers for each output achieves this and provides greater flexibility.

OPERATION

Frequency Control

This control adjusts the output pulse rate and is adjustable from 1 to 250 pulses/sec. There is a visual monitor of the output frequency beside this control.

Output Controls

These should be left to their extreme counterclockwise position when not connected to the patient. Thus, if the output wires are being connected to the patient, there is no possibility of shock. This is very important as *failure to do so could startle the patient.* The control may then be adjusted from the low position to the desired level of stimulation.

Note

The output wires should be plugged into the jack under the appropriate output control. The alligator clips on the ends of these wires should be connected to the electrode in such a manner that they do not put unnecessary leverage on the skin. The red clip is positive and the black is negative.

Wires that are not in use should be stored neatly to avoid wire tangling.

Adequate precautions should be taken to ensure the patient's safety when the region extending between the electrodes passes near the vicinity of the heart. Although the current from the stimulator is well below levels that could induce cardiac fibrillation, the fact that some people may be unusually sensitive should be considered.

No tests have thus far been made that would predict the effect of electrostimulation on the operation of cardiac pacemakers. Caution should be exercised if the patient has any implanted electrical or electronics devices within the body.

Intertronic Systems Limited assumes no consequential damages for use or misuse of this device.

TECHNICAL INFORMATION

Frequency range: 1–250 Hz
Peak current at maximum O/P into 500 ohms load: 100 ma
Peak power at maximum O/P into a 500 ohms load: 5W
Maximum RMS current into a 500 ohms load: 8 ma
Maximum duty cycle (positive half cycle only): 10%
DC level on output: not measurable at 5mv/division
$Z_{In} = 10$ Meg.
Battery voltage: 9V

MAX output voltages at various loads

Voltage P-P	Load Resistance (ohms)
163	
152	20K
140	10K
115	5K
95	2K
79	1K
55	500

Waveform: Positive cycle 0.5 m.s.
Negative cycle 0.4 m.s.

ELECTRICAL STIMULATION CONTRAINDICTIONS

Direct and Alternating Stimulation

a. A stinging sensation may result from poor contact between the electrode and the skin.
b. A burning sensation may result if the stimulating electrodes are in close proximity.
c. In certain cases of patients with sensitive skin, there may be an unfavorable skin reaction or infection.
d. Acupuncture ear stapling is not recommended because an extremely high infection rate has been reported. This could result in serious inner ear infection with consequent hearing loss.
e. Electric burns may result from a high intensity stimulation or prolonged DC stimulation. These may cause unforseen nerve damage.
f. Electrolytic burns may be caused by polarization effects.
g. Unforeseen muscle paralysis or spasms may result from improper stimulation.
h. DC stimulation has a very strong effect and is commonly used for skin problems, neuralgia, and mental illness. It may, however, cause electrolysis, which has a corrosive effect on the skin. It is advisable to switch the polarity or turn the current off every 1–3 min. Treatment times should not exceed 15 min. Pulsed DC decreases the risk of electrolysis.
i. In stimulation, the positive and negative electrodes must be connected to the right points. The positive electrode can relieve pain syndromes, inflammation, and swelling; the negative electrode can stimulate peripheral circulation.
j. Never put two electrodes across from each other, on the sides of the spine above the third lumbar vertebra.
k. Nervous or hypertension patients, cardiac patients, and pregnant women are not good candidates for electroacupuncture.

3

Animal

Acupuncture Points

In ancient China, practitioners of veterinary acupuncture relied on Chinese veterinary classics and the experience of the family or master. With the advent of government support for research and development of veterinary acupuncture, the veterinary classics were edited, and the experiences of practitioners were documented. In modern Chinese publications, the location, names, and functions of acupuncture points in large animals is, in general, consistent (see Chapter Eight).

As clinical studies progressed, only those acupuncture points that showed good therapeutic efficacy were taught to students of veterinary medicine. Therefore, in Chinese books of the 1950s and '60s, one may find differences from books published since 1970. The latest standard text in China is the *Chinese Veterinary Handbook*, compiled by the Lanchow Veterinary Research Institute in 1972.

Large animal acupuncture points used in, or derived from, Oriental countries are essentially based on *Yuen Heng Liao Ma Chi* (1608).* Veterinary acupuncture, as it has developed in Europe, appears to have as its base human acupuncture information and anatomical transposition of human points onto animals. As it developed in the United States, veterinary acupuncture utilized both Oriental and European information. Several different charts of the horse, cow, dog, and cat have been produced in the United States (Figs. 3–73 to 3–99; 3–101 to 3–117), and are based on one or several of the methods for locating points, as described below.

The nomenclature for acupuncture points in the West is in a confused state—a situation attributable to several causes. The rapid acquisition and translation into English of Oriental information by many individuals and groups has resulted in the use of dif-

ferent English systems for naming points. There are two parts to the problem, the first concerning the transliteration of the sounds produced by spoken Chinese. This technique, called Romanizing, converts the sounds of the spoken Chinese language into Roman alphabet letters and words. There are several recognized systems for performing this conversion. The system used by the authors is Wade-Giles; the system used in the Sobin horse model booklet (see page 69) is Pin Yin. When standardized systems such as Wade-Giles or Pin Yin are used, words can be recognized by individuals familiar with the system. But to those not familiar with either system, the Romanized words for a particular Chinese character would appear to be different. Although this causes some confusion, the use of recognized systems of Romanizing is the correct method for converting Chinese words to the Roman alphabet. Unfortunately, many people have Romanized the names of acupuncture points using various dialects and unrecognized conversion systems; this is further compounded by the admixture of other Oriental languages.

We have included material that has been Romanized by others in various ways. This material is included as it was provided by the various sources in order to provide as much as possible the available information on veterinary acupuncture. No attempt was made to change the material into the Wade-Giles system of Romanizing.

The second part of the problem is that as veterinary acupuncture charts and texts were brought into the United States, the points were given Roman letters and Arabic numerals rather than, and in addition to, the Chinese names. As each person or group acquired charts, they labelled them differently; consequently the Roman letter and Arabic numeral designation for any specific point varies from chart to

---

* There is no information on small animal acupuncture from ancient China.

chart. For example, the point we call FL7 (ch'ang feng) from other sources is called 42, FL9, or small intestine 6, and is missing from two other charts.

Another existing problem concerns the question of whether there are meridians in the animals comparable to those of the human. In an ancient Chinese chart with 12 points (Fig. 3–12, and Fig. 1–4), each of these points represents a whole meridian as described in man (see p. 16).[4] None of the Chinese horse charts, or other Chinese animal charts, have meridian lines composed of many points. One chart of the horse, showing meridian lines, was produced by the Japanese acupuncturist Dr. Meiyu Okada (Figs. 3–13 to 3–18). It reportedly has as its source an ancient Chinese text, *Ba Ryo Taizen*, probably written about 50–150 B.C.[13] In this chart, the names given to the meridians are the same as those in the human. However, the number of points on each meridian shown for the horse is different than in the human. The names of the points would be confusing if one were communicating with someone who was using anatomic transposition (see below) for location and names of points—for example, the human point stomach 36 (tsu-san-li) is called stomach 21 (tsu-san-li). Another set of horse charts were produced by Dr. H. Grady Young[18]; these were based on Okada's chart (Figs. 3–19 to 3–26).

Determining the Location of Acupuncture Points

At present, there are several ways of determining the location of acupuncture points. There are two practical methods (anatomic transposition and published charts) and two investigational methods (electric point finders and provocation).

ANATOMIC TRANSPOSITION

The method used initially and still in use in the western world is anatomic transposition of the human acupuncture points. Oriental investigators are also using this method in small animals. The human points are located anatomically, and then the same anatomic location is found in the animal species of interest, and that point in the animal is given the human name and function. Some points are very easy to transpose—for example, conception vessel 8 is located in the umbilicus. However, other points are more difficult to transpose. The very important association points of the bladder meridian are located on the back, lateral to the vertebral column at a level between various spinous processes. For example, bladder 23 is located between the spinous process of

the 2nd and 3rd lumbar vertebrae. This site can be found in the various animal species, but the total number of preceding vertebrae varies in the different species: for example, in the human the 2nd lumbar vertebra is the 21st vertebra (counting from the head). In the horse, it is the 27th vertebra; in the dog it is the 22nd; and in the pig, it is the 23rd or 24th. Therefore, the question is whether one can use the 2nd lumbar vertebra as a landmark in different species.

A problem of even more complexity is the location of points in the area of the phalanges: for example, the extremely important point, large intestine 4, is located in the human between metacarpals 1 and 2. In the horse, metacarpal 1 is missing, and metacarpal 2 is very small and tightly attached to metacarpal 3. The cow has the 3rd and 4th metacarpal bones fused, and the 1st and 2nd metacarpal bones are missing altogether. Metacarpal 1 is missing in the pig.

The only published work describing anatomic transposition in animals is relatively old and has been modified extensively by the author since that publication.[12]

Acupuncture Units of Measurement

In the human, distances between acupuncture points are measured in acupuncture "inches" (also called *chun, tsun,* or *pouce*) and fen, which are 0.1 inch. These inches are different for each individual and are measured using anatomic relationships. The classic definition of an inch is the length of the second phalanx of digit 3 of the hand. Other larger numbers of inches are defined anatomically also—for example, the distance between the wrist and the elbow is 12 inches, and the distance between the nipples is 8 inches (Fig. 3–100).

In animals, no system exists. The only reference to an inch found is in the booklet accompanying an acupuncture model for the horse (p. 70 below), which states that an inch in the horse is the width of the 16th rib at the level of the tuber coxae. Whether the relationships described for the human apply to the dog or any other animal is not known at present.

PUBLISHED CHARTS

The various published charts can be used to locate points. These charts vary considerably, and the available Chinese charts are only for farm animals (Figs. 3–1 to 3–7 and 3–27 to 3–72). Charts are now available in English for small animals, but these are based on anatomic transposition and vary with the individual's opinion of the precise way to do the transposition (Figs. 3–73 to 3–99). One can attempt to verify the locations utilizing electric point finders. However, even though points can be found at approximate anatomic locations, one cannot be sure they are, in fact, the same in name and function as the human points. Many extra points can be found, and several points may be found in an area supposed to anatomically contain a certain human point. Because of the large number of charts in this chapter, they are all placed together at the end of the chapter (pp. 120–210).

ELECTRIC POINT FINDING

One can find points, with an instrument, as areas of low electrical resistance (see chapter 2). Many points are found in animals in locations similar to those in man. Whether these points serve the same functions as in man is not yet known.

The electrical locating of points in animals adds some information; however, there are more questions. The number of low-resistance points found on any one individual, animal or human, is quite variable. It varies in the same individual, from day to day, with the voltage of the seeking instrument, and with the duration of seeking in two ways. If the point-finder electrode is held in one position for more than a few seconds, it will damage the skin, producing a false low-resistance point. If one seeks points on dogs, the longer the process continues during any one session, the more points will begin to appear.

PROVOCATION

Points can be studied by provocation—that is, causing a lesion in an organ and finding points on the body that become painful and/or have altered conductivity. This has been done in cattle by Dr. O.

Kothbauer.[7-10] He injected an iodine solution into various organs and located points on the skin that were painful and had altered electrical conductivity. His work has slowly progressed over a period of 20 years. Most of his provocation work has been related to the reproductive organs of the cow.

Kothbauer has also tried to relate naturally occurring diseases in an organ to the appearance of painful spots with altered electrical conductivity. The verification of the condition was by clinical examination and/or postmortem examination. Through this work, Kothbauer has been able to map many points in cows (Figs. 3–8 to 3–11). The finding of these painful points is another piece of useful information in diagnosis.

A provocation study has also been done in the rabbit, involving auriculotherapy.[11] According to this branch of acupuncture, the entire body is represented inside the ear, disease of an organ produces a painful altered electrical resistance point at a consistent location, and the condition may be treated by stimulating that point. In a rabbit study, turpentine was injected intramuscularly, and points were looked for in the ear. Very small zones of decreased electrical resistance appeared in the ear in specific locations that varied with the site of the turpentine injection. Thus, specific projection zones seem to exist in the ear for various parts of the body. Not only did electrical resistance of the points change, but sweating, hyperemia, and ulceration or intensive desquamation of the skin also occurred. In another study to visualize these points, the rabbits were given trypan blue IV, after the turpentine injection. Within a short time, only the corresponding projection zone in the ear was colored.

Acupuncture Points in Large Animals

The following descriptions of the acupuncture points of large animals, their locations, method of stimulation, and indications for their use are from Sobin, Ottaviano,[15] Shin,[16] and a Chinese veterinary handbook.[3]

HORSE

Sobin Horse Model (Fig. 3–27)*

This acupuncture model of a horse and its accompanying booklet are imported from China. The book-

let includes: names of the points, anatomic locations, methods of needling, and conditions the point should be used to treat. The numbers accompanying the names of points refer to the numbers in the horse model. The English text of the booklet is reproduced on pages 70–81.

* This model of the horse was imported into the United States by Julian M. Sobin, president of Sobin Chemicals, Inc., Boston, Massachusetts 02210. Mr. Sobin is very interested in,

and has been a leader in, trade arrangements with China. He was the first American businessman invited to Peking,[14] and he attended the 31st Canton Trade Fair (Chinese Export Commodities Fair at Kwangchow) in 1972 and every trade fair since then. Mr. Sobin negotiated the first sale of U.S. goods ever made at a Canton Trade Fair,[1] where it is estimated that 50% of China's trade is negotiated. Mr. Sobin agreed to allow us to completely reproduce the booklet distributed with the horse model, with no restrictions, so that we could produce as complete a book on the subject as possible.

Localization	Name of the Point	Location of the Point	Method of Acupuncture or Cauterization	Animal response to Acupuncture	Indication
Head and Neck	1 Ta-feng-men	On the top of the head, middle of the natural line of the root of mane, namely at the crosspoint of the external parietal crest of the parietal bone.	Puncture with a new needle 2-3 tsun* downwards under the skin.	The two ears standing upright and backwards.	Tetanus, encephalitis, encephalomyelitis, encephaledema.
	2 Tung-tien	At the centre of the forehead. At the midpoint in between the two eyes.	Cauterize with mugwort or iron.		Pus accumulation in frontal sinus, cerebral hyperemia.
	3 Lung-hui	At the midpoint on the line in between the two lateral canthi of eyes.	,,		Cerebral hyperemia, cerebral anemia, rheumatism of the neck
	4 Tung-tang	At the midpoint in between the two medial canthi.	,,		Same as Lung-hui.
	5 Shang-kuan	Above the mandibular articulation, in the depression below the zygomatic arch. Bilateral.	Puncture with a round sharp needle obliquely downward from 8 fen to 1 tsun deep.	Shaking head, twitching of the nose and lips.	Tetanus, paralysis of the facial nerve.
	6 Hsia-kuan	Below the mandibular articulation, 1 tsun below and in front of Shang-kuan. Bilateral.	Puncture with a round sharp needle obliquely upward 1.5-2 tsun deep.	Same as Shang-kuan.	Same as Shang-kuan.
	7 Yan-mo	On the blood vessel about 5 fen behind Tai-yang. Bilateral.	Same as Tai-yang.		Same as Tai-yang.
	8 Tai-yang	On the transverse facial vein about 1 tsun below and behind the lateral canthus. Bilateral.	Puncture with the small broad needle along the blood vessel 2-3 fen deep. Bleeding.		Conjunctivitis, Keratitis, periodical ophthalmia, heat stroke.
	9 Chuan-nao	Above the lateral canthus, on the fold of the eye lid, at the rim of the supraorbital process. One on each eye.	Press the eyeball downwards. Puncture with the round sharp needle along the rim of the supraorbital process 2-2.5 tsun deep.	Same as Ching-ming.	Same as Ching-ming.
	10 Ching-shu	At the midpoint of the superior palpebra, on the lower rim of the supra-orbital process. One in each eye.	Press the eyeball downwards. Puncture with the round sharp needle along the lower rim of the supra-orbital process 2-2.5 tsun deep.	Same as Ching-ming.	Same as Ching-ming.

*Tsun 寸 is a measure of length in acupuncture to indicate the depth of needle insertion or the location of sites. One tsun is divided into ten fen 分. The width of rib on the point inter-crossed by the level of Tuber coxae and the 16th rib is one tsun. (Hold the rib with thumb and forefinger and measure the width between the two fingers).

Localization	Name of the Point	Location of the Point	Method of Acupuncture or Cauterization	Animal response to Acupuncture	Indication
Head and Neck	11 Kai-tien	At the midpoint of the lower border of the cornea, on its line of demarcation with the sclera. One on each eye-ball.	Use local anaethsia when the worm is in the anterior chamber of the eye. Open the eye lids and fix the eye-ball. Puncture quickly and skillfully with the thin triangular needle or ophthalmia needle 1 fen deep, quickly withdraw, let the worm flow out together with the aqueous humor.		Microfilaria of Setaria equi
	12 Ching-ming	In the lower eyelid 1/3 point of the upper border of the lacrimal bone. One point in each eye.	Press the eyeball upward, puncture with a round sharp needle along the upper border of the lacrimal bone 2-2.5 tsun deep.	Close and open of the eye intermittently, and lacrimation.	Conjunctivitis, keratitis, periodical ophthalmia, pannus.
	13 San-chiang	About 1 tsun below the medial canthus on the angular vein. Bilateral.	Puncture with a triangular needle along the blood vessel upwards for 2-3 fen deep until bleeding.		Spasm of the bowel, inflation of bowel, constipation, indigestion, conjunctivitis, keratitis, periodical ophthalmia.
	14 Ta-mo	On the vein about 7 fen below and behind San-chiang. Bilateral.	Same as San-chiang.		Same as San-chiang.
	15 Hsueh-tang	At the two sides of the nose, 2 tsun from the upper rim of the nostrils. Bilateral.	Puncture with a triangular needle transversely through the septum nasi. Bleeding.		Rhinitis, over-exertion, cerebral hyperaemia, congestion of the lung.
	16 Pi-shu	1 tsun below Hsueh-tang. Bilateral.	Same as Hsueh-tang.		Same as Hsueh-tang.
	17 Cho-chin	In the fossa between the two nostrils. One point only.	Make a cut in the fossa about 4-5 fen long, hook out the tendon of leavator labii superioris proprius, drag forcefully and repeatedly.		Rheumatism of the neck.
	18 Fen-shui	In the centre of the vortices pilorum of the upper lip. One point only.	Puncture with a round sharp needle 1-1.5 tsun deep.	Obvious contraction and swinging of the upper lip.	Spasm of the bowel, inflation of the bowel, constiption, dilatation of the stomach, indigestion.
	19 Chiang-wen	On the outer surface of the upper lip, on the line along the lower border of the two nostrils, 3 fen beside the medial wing of nostril. Bilateral.	Puncture with a round sharp needle perpendicularly 3-5 fen deep.	Obvious contraction of the upper lip.	Common cold, high fever, heat stroke, over exertion.
	20 Wai-chuen-yin	On the outer surface of the upper lip, just in between the lower border of the two nostrils. One point only.	Puncture with a Middle broad needle perpendicularly 3 fen deep.		Stomatitis, indigestion, pharyngolaryngitis.

Localization	Name of the Point	Location of the Point	Method of Acupuncture or Cauterization	Animal response to Acupuncture	Indication
Head and Neck	21 Nei-chuen-yin	On the inner surface of the upper lip, 1 tsun from the gum of teeth, 5-8 fen beside the fraenula labii superioris. Bilateral.	Puncture with a triangular needle 3 fen deep.		Stomatitis, indigestion, pharyngolaryngitis.
	22 Chiang-ya	On the top of the cartilage of the alae nasi. Bilateral.	Puncture with a triangular needle 3 fen deep.		Spasm of the bowel, constipation, dilatation of stomach.
	23 Suo-kou	On the outer rim of the orbicularis oris, 7 fen above and posterior to the Anguli oris. Bilateral.	Puncture with a round sharp needle upward and backward 2-3 tsun deep.	Contraction of the lip and mouth muscles.	Tetanus, paralysis of the facial nerve.
	24 Kai-kuan	At the cross point of the prolonged line of the commisurae labiorum and the anterior border of the masseter. Bilateral.	Puncture with a round sharp needle upward and backwards 3 tsun deep or downwards and forewards through to Suo-kou.	Obvious fibrillation of masseter and brachiocephalicus, fibrillation of lips, mouth, and buccinator, when puncture through to Suo-kou.	Same as Suo-kou.
	25 Bao-sai	2.5 tsun below the facial crest, and about 2 tsun behind the anterior border of the masseter. Bilateral.	Puncture with a round sharp needle or a fire needle obliquely upwards 6-8 fen deep.		Swelling of the face, osteomalacia, spasm of the masseter.
	26 Cheng-chiang	In the centre of the lower lip, about 1 tsun from the rim. One point only.	Puncture with a round sharp needle about 3 fen deep.		Paralysis of the facial nerve, stomatitis.
	27 Yu-tang	5 fen beside the median line of the hard palate on the 3rd ruga palatina inside the mouth.	Puncture with a triangular needle upward and forward 3 fen deep. Rub with salt after bleeding.		Stomatitis, indigestion, heat stroke, overexertion, common cold.
	28 Erh-chien	On the posterior auricular vein at the dorsal side of the ear or at the tip of the ear. Bilateral.	Puncture with a small broad needle into the blood vessel to bleed or puncture with a triangular needle at the tip of the ear 3-4 fen deep until bleeding.		Spasm of the bowel, common cold.
	29 Ting-erh	At the medial side of the root of the ear, in the fossa in front of the occipital crest. Bilateral.	Puncture with a round sharp needle or a fine needle 1 tsun under the skin.		Paralysis of an ear, dullness, exhaustion.
	30 Feng-men	1 tsun behind the ear, 2 tsun from the natural line of the mane, in the fossa in front of the wing of the atlas. Bilateral.	Puncture with a round sharp needle obliquely upwards 2 tsun deep.	Standing upright of the ear of the same side.	Encephalitis, common cold, tetanus.
	31 Fu-tu	2 tsun behind the ear, 1.5 tsun from the natural line of the mane, in the fossa behind the wing of the atlas. Bilateral.	Same as Feng-men.	Same as Feng-men.	Same as Feng-men.

Localization	Name of the Point	Location of the Point	Method of Acupuncture or Cauterization	Animal response to Acupuncture	Indication
Head and Neck	32 Chiu-wei	There are nine points on each side of the neck. The 1st point (Yi-wei) is 2 tsun below and posterior to Feng-men, 1.2 tsun from the lower natural line of the mane; The 9th (Chiu-wei) is 1.5 tsun in front of the anterior angle of the scapula (Bo-chien), 1.8 tsun below the lower natural line of the mane. The total length between the 1st and 9th points is divided into 8 equal parts. The 8 points from the front backwards are named Erh-wei (2nd), San-wei (3rd), Sze-wei (4th), Wu-wei (5th), Liu-wei (6th), Chi-wei (7th), and Ba-wei (8th). All the points are distributed alone the lower margin of the rhomboid-eus forming an arc.	Puncture with a round sharp needle perpendicularly 1.5-3 tsun deep.	Contraction of the neck and shoulder muscles. Fibrillation of the muscles of the withers.	Rheumatism of the neck, tetanus.
	33 Ching-mo	At between the upper and middle 1/3 of the jugular vein. Bilateral.	Make the vein congested at first, then puncture with a large broad needle or a bleeding needle along the blood vessel to bleed.		Overexertion, heat stroke, toxication, cerebral hyperemia, congestion of the lung, laminitis, stomatitis.
Fore Limb	34 Bo-chien	In the fossa beside the junction of scapular cartilage and the anterior angle of the scapula. Bilateral.	Puncture with a round sharp needle along the medial border of the scapula slightly downward 3-4 tsun deep.	Fibrillation of the muscles of the withers.	Paralysis of the suprascapular nerve, arthritis of the shoulder joint, rheumatism of the fore limb.
	35 Fei-men	On the anterior border of the scapula, in the middle of the neck, 4 tsun below and in front of Bo-chien. Bilateral.	Puncture with a round sharp needle along the medial border of the scapula backward and downward 3-4 tsun deep.	Fibrillation of the shoulder muscle.	Same as Bo-chien.
	36 Bo-chung	On the anterior border of the scapula, 2 tsun below Fei-men. Bilateral.	Puncture with a round sharp needle along the medial border of the scapula backward and inward obliquely 2.5-3 tsun deep.	Fibrillation of the shoulder and elbow muscles.	Rheumatism of the fore limb, arthritis of shoulder and elbow joints, paralysis of suprascapular nerve, myositis of sterno-brachio cephalicus.
	37 Chien-chin	On top of the shoulder, in the fossa of the lateral upper border of the lateral tuberosity of the humerus. Bilateral.	Puncture with a round sharp needle backward and downward 2-2.5 tsun deep.	Lifting of the fore limb.	Rheumatism of the fore limb, arthritis of the shoulder joint, myositis of sterno-brachiocephalicus, paralysis of the suprascapular nerve.
	38 Kung-tzu	3 tsun below the midpoint of the upper border of the sca-pular cartilage. Bilateral.	Puncture with a round sharp needle downwards obliquely 4-5 tsun deep.	Fibrillation of the shoulder muscles.	Paralysis of the suprascapular nerve, atrophy of the shoulder and brachial muscles, chronic shoulder lameness.

Localization	Name of the Point	Location of the Point	Method of Acupuncture or Cauterization	Animal response to Acupuncture	Indication
Fore Limb	39 Bo-lan	In the fossa at the junction of scapular cartilage and the posterior angle of the scapula. Bilateral.	Puncture with a round sharp needle along the medial border of the scapula foreward and downward 3-4 tsun deep.	Same as Bo-chien	Same as Bo-chien.
	40 Fei-pan	On the posterior border of the scapula, 4 tsun in front of and below Bo-lan. Bilateral.	Puncture with a round sharp needle towards the shoulder of the same side, along the medial border of the scapula 2.5-3 tsun deep.	Fibrillation of the shoulder muscles.	Paralysis of the suprascapular nerve, myositis of the sternobrachiocephalicus, rheumatism of the fore limb.
	41 Chung-tien	In the sulcus muscularis 3 tsun above and posterior to Chiang-feng. Bilateral.	Puncture with a round sharp needle perpendicularly 3-3.5 tsun deep.	Lifting of fore limb, contraction of shoulder muscles.	Same as Chiang-feng.
	42 Chiang-feng	In the fossa behind the humerus, on the posterior border of the deltoideus and in between the long head and the lateral head of the triceps brachii. Bilateral.	Puncture with a round sharp needle perpendicularly 2.5-3 tsun deep.	Obvious contraction of the muscles of the same area and lifting of that limb.	Arthritis of all joints of the fore limb, myositis of sternobrachiocephalicus, paralysis of radial nerve, rheumatism of the fore limb.
	43 Chien-wai-yu	In the depression of the posterior border of the lateral tuberosity of humerus. Bilateral.	Puncture with a round sharp needle along the posterior border of humerus perpendicularly 2.5-3 tsun deep.	Same as Chien-yu.	Same as Chien-yu.
	44 Chien-yu	On top of the shoulder, in the depression of the lower-border of the lateral tuberosity of the humerus. Bilateral.	Puncture with a round sharp needle along the anterior border of humerus inward and upward 1 tsun deep.	Contraction of muscles around the shoulder.	Arthritis of the shoulder joint, myositis of sternobrachiocephalicus, paralysis of radial nerve.
	45 Yan-chou	On the elbow line in the depression 1.5 tsun above and posterior to the Processus anconaeus of the ulna. Bilateral.	Puncture with a round sharp needle forward and slightly obliquely downward 8 fen — 1 tsun deep.	Fibrillation of the muscles around the elbow.	Rheumatism of the muscles of the elbow area.
	46 Cheng-deng	In the depression about 1.3 tsun below and posterior to the Processus anconaeus on the medial surface. Bilateral.	Puncture with a round sharp needle obliquely forward and upward 8 fen — 1 tsun deep.	Same as Yan-chou.	Same as Yan-chou.
	47 Chou-shu	In the depression just in front of the tip of the elbow. Bilateral.	Puncture with a round sharp needle perpendicularly 1.5 tsun deep.	Fibrillation of muscles of the elbow.	Arthritis of the elbow joint.
	48 Cheng-chung	On the outer surface of the fore arm, in the depression below the lateral tuberosity of radius, in the groove of common extensor tendon. Bilateral.	Puncture with a round sharp needle slightly obliquely forward 1.5-2 tsun deep.	Lifting of the limb.	Rheumatism of the fore limb, arthritis of the elbow and carpal joints, paralysis of radial nerve, myositis and tenositis, tenovaginitis.

Localization	Name of the Point	Location of the Point	Method of Acupuncture or Cauterization	Animal response to Acupuncture	Indication
	49 Chien-san-li	2 tsun below and in front of Cheng-chung, in the groove between anteroir carpal extensor and common digital extensor muscles. Bilateral.	Puncture with a round sharp needle perpendicularly 1-1.5 tsun deep.	,,	Besides the same as Cheng-chung, also for arthritis of the fetlock joint, and tetanus.
	50 Kuo-liang	1 tsun above the lateral side of the carpal joint, in the depression between the posterior border of radius and the lateral carpal flexor. Bilateral.	Puncture through with a round sharp needle inward from outside.	Contraction of the elbow muscles and elevation of the limb.	Arthritis of the carpal joint.
	51 Hsiung-tang	On the brachial subcutaneous vein in the lower part of the thoracic lateral groove near to the upper part of the forearm. Bilateral.	Puncture quickly with a large broad needle 3 fen deep to bleed.		Acute arthritis of the shoulder and elbow joints, myositis of sterno-brachiocephalicus, laminitis, rheumatism of the shoulder and arm.
Fore Limb	52 Chia-chi	In the axilla, or in the muscular groove of the upper part of the forearm, at the centre of the medial surface and the trunk. Bilateral.	Lift up the sick limb, drag it forward and outward. Cut along the point, puncture with Chia-chi needle backward and upward towards Chiang-feng 7-8 tsun deep. Withdraw and then sway the limb several times. Strict disinfection during operation is needed.		Chronic shoulder lameness, paralysis of scapular nerves.
	53 Tung-chin	On the subcutaneous vein of the forearm, 2 tsun below Chia-chi. Bilateral.	Puncture with a small broad needle 3 fen deep to bleed.		Same as Hsiung-tang.
	54 Tsan-chin	On the lateral superficial volar vein at the lateral anterior border of the deep flexor digital tendon, 2 tsun below the lower border of the carpal joint, at the lateral upper end of the volar portion. Bilateral.	Puncture with a small broad needle 3 fen deep to bleed.		Arthritis of the carpal joint, osteoma of the volar bone (early stage), tenositis, tenovaginitis, arthritis of fetlock joint.
	55 Chien-chan-wan	On the medial and lateral digital veins on the upper border of the fetlock joint. Two points on each fore limb.	Puncture with a small broad needle 2-3 fen deep to bleed.		Contusion of the fetlock joint, arthritis of fetlock joint, acute arthritis of carpal joint, tenositis, tenovaginitis.
	56 Ming-tang	In the depression inferior to the sesamoid bone at the lateral posterior lower part of the fetlock joint. Bilateral.	Puncture with a small broad needle upwards 3-4 fen deep.		Contusion of the fetlock joint, arthritis of fetlock joint, flexor tenositis, tenovaginitis.
	57 Chien-chiu	In the depression above the bulb, in the middle of the posterior surface of the hoof. Bilateral.	Lift the limb and hold it. Puncture with a round sharp needle 1-1.5 tsun deep towards the tip of the hoof.	Lifting up of the limb.	Arthritis of the fetlock joint, laminitis, tenositis, arthritis of carpal joint, rheumatism of forelimb.

Localization	Name of the Point	Location of the Point	Method of Acupuncture or Cauterization	Animal response to Acupuncture	Indication
Fore Limb	58 Chien-ti-men	In the depression behind the cartilage of the hoof, on the upper border of the bulb. One point on each side of the hoof.	Puncture with a small broad needle 3 fen deep.		Inflammation of the bulb of the hoof.
	59 Chien-ti-tou	7-8 fen lateral to the median point of the coronary border of the hoof. Bilateral.	Puncture with a large broad needle quickly 3 fen deep to bleed.		Laminitis, colic pain, inflammation of the bulbs of the hoof.
Lateral side of the thorax and abdomen	60 Tu-shu	In the last but 9 intercostal space in the musculus iliocostalis groove. Bilateral.	Puncture with a round sharp needle obliquely inward and downward 1-1.3 tsun deep.	Fibrillation of the intercostal muscles.	Spasm of the bowel, overexertion.
	61 Fei-shu	In the last but 8 intercostal space in the musculus iliocostalis groove. Bilateral.	Same as Tu-shu.	Same as Tu-shu	Pleuritis, bronchitis, pneumonia.
	62 Ke-shu	In the last but 7 intercostal space in the musculus iliocostalis groove. Bilateral.	,,	,,	Gastroenteritis constipation, trachitis.
	63 Tan-shu	In the last but 6 intercostal space in the musculus iliocostalis groove. Bilateral.	,,	,,	Intestinal constipation, fever, icterus, chill, laryngopharyngitis.
	64 Wei-shu	In the last but 5 intercostal space in the musculus iliocostalis groove. Bilateral.	,,	,,	Indigestion, spasm of the bowel, inflation of the bowel, dilatation of the stomach.
	65 Kan-shu	In the last but 4 intercostal space in the musculus iliocostalis groove. Bilateral.	Same as Tu-shu.	Same as Tu-shu	Conjunctivitis, keratitis, indigestion.
	66 San-chiao-shu	In the last but 3 intercostal space in the musculus iliocostalis groove. Bilateral.	,,	,,	Indigestion, spasm of bowel.
	67 Pi-shu	In the last but 2 intercostal space in the musculus iliocostalis groove. Bilateral.	,,	,,	Indigestion, spasm of bowel, inflation of bowel. dilatation of stomach.
	68 Chi-hai-shu	In the last but one intercostal space in the musculus iliocostalis groove. Bilateral.	,,	,,	Dilatation of the stomach.
	69 Ta-chang-shu	In the last intercostal space of the musculus iliocostalis groove. Bilateral.	Puncture with a round sharp needle obliquely inward and downward 1.2-1.5 tsun deep.	,,	Indigestion, spasm of bowel, inflation of bowel, enteritis, constipation.
	70 Kuan-yuan-shu	In the musculus iliocostalis groove behind the 18th rib. Bilateral.	Puncture with a round sharp needle perpendicularly 2-2.5 tsun deep. It would be better to use an electric needle.	Contraction of abdominal muscles, increase of intestinal peristalsis, winding and defecation when use an electric needle.	Intestinal constipation, indigestion, spasm of bowel, inflation of bowel, dilatation of stomach.
	71 Hsiao-chang-shu	About 1 tsun behind Kuan-yuan-shu in the musculus iliocostalis groove. Bilateral.	Puncture with a round sharp needle obliquely inward and downward 1.2-1.5 tsun deep.	Contraction of intestinal muscle.	Same as Kuan-yuan-shu.

Localization	Name of the Point	Location of the Point	Method of Acupuncture or Cauterization	Animal response to Acupuncture	Indication
Lateral side of the thorax and abdomen	72 Tuan-hsueh	On the dorsal median line, in the depression in between the Proc. spinosis of the 17th-18th Thoracic vertebrae, 18th thoracic-1st lumbar vertebrae, and 1st-2nd lumbar vertebrae. There are three points altogether.	Puncture with a round sharp needle perpendicularly 8 fen to 1 tsun deep.	Fibrillation of the intercostal muscles.	Bleeding after castration, epistaxis, haematuria, hemofecia.
	73 Chueh-yin-shu	In the last but 11 intercostal space, in the depression at the lateral border of the M. iliocostalis, about 6.3 tsun from the dorsal median line. Bilateral.	Puncture with a round sharp needle obliquely inward and downward 1 tsun deep.	Fibrillation of the intercostal muscles.	Heat stroke, spasm of bowel, polyhidrosis
	74 Tai-mo	About 2 tsun behind processus anconaeus, on the lateral thoracic vein. Bilateral.	Puncture with a large broad needle 3 fen to bleed.		Enteritis, spasm of bowel, heat stroke.
Loin and Buttock	75 Yao-chien	2 tsun in front of Yao-chung. Bilateral.	Puncture with a round sharp needle inward and downward 2-2.5 tsun deep.	Same as Shen-shu.	Rheumatism of the loin, paralysis of the loin.
	76 Yao-chung	2 tsun in front of Yao-hou. Bilateral.	,,	,,	,,
	77 Yao-hou	2 tsun in front of the Shen-peng. Bilateral.	,,	,,	,,
	78 Shen-peng	2 tsun in front of the Shen-shu. Bilateral.	Same as Shen-shu.	,,	Same as Shen-shu.
	79 Shen-shu	2 tsun lateral to Pai-hui. Bilateral.	Puncture with a round sharp needle perpendicularly 1.5-2 tsun deep.	Contraction of the loin and buttock muscles.	Rheumatism of the hind quarter, paralysis of hind quarter, paralysis of the loin.
	80 Shen-chueh	2 tsun behind Shen-shu. Bilateral.	,,	,,	,,
	81 Pai-hui	In the depression in between the Processus spinosus of the last lumbar vertebra and the Processus spinosus of the 1st sacral vertebra. One point only.	Puncture with a round sharp needle perpendicularly 3-3.5 tsun deep.	Arching of the loin, fibrillation of the loin and buttock muscles	Rheumatism of the hind quarter, arthritis of hip joint, paralysis of the hind quarter, common cold, heat stroke, overexertion, tetanus, colic.
	82 Pa-chiao	1.5 tsun beside the dorsal median line, in between the Processi spinosi of the sacrum. There are four points on each side from cranial to caudal: Yi-chiao, Erh-chiao, San-chiao, Szu-chiao.	Puncture with a round sharp needle perpendicularly 1-1.5 tsun deep.	Fibrillation of the buttock muscles.	Rheumatism of the hind quarter, paralysis of the loin, paralysis of the penis.
	83 Tung-chang	Make a horizontal line from tuber coxae to the posterior border of the last rib. Then make vertical lines from the tuber coxae and the posterior border of the last rib towards the dorsal median line. The midpoints of the two lines are the points. The anterior point is Tung-chang 1. The posterior point is Tung-chang 2. Bilateral.	Puncture with a round sharp needle perpendicularly 2-2.5 tsun deep.	Fibrillation of the loin and intercostal muscles.	Intestinal constipation, inflation of bowel, spasm of bowel.

Localization	Name of the Point	Location of the Point	Method of Acupuncture or Cauterization	Animal response to Acupuncture	Indication
Hind Limb	84 Yan-chih	Make a perpendicular line from the Tuber coxae towards the dorsal median line. The point is at the lateral 1/3 of the line. Bilateral.	Puncture with a round sharp needle posteriorly downward and inward 2.5 tsun deep.	Fibrillation of the loin and buttock muscles.	Rheumatism of the hind quarters' muscles, arthritis of the hip and knee joints.
	85 Tan-tien	In the depression behind and below the Tuber coxae. Bilateral.	Puncture with a round sharp needle perpendicularly 2.5-3.5 tsun deep.	Same as Yan-chih.	Same as Yan-chih.
	86 Pa-shan	At the midpoint between Pai-hui and the anterior convexity of the trochanter major femoris. Bilateral.	Puncture with a round sharp needle perpendicularly 3-3.5 tsun deep.	Contraction of the buttock muscles.	Rheumatism of the hind quarters' muscles, arthritis of hip joint, myositis of M. biceps femoris, paralysis of sciatic nerve.
	87 Lu-ku	At the lateral 1/3 between the Pai-hui and the anterior convexity of the trochanter major femoris. Bilateral.	Same as Pa-shan.	Same as Pa-shan	Same as Pa-shan.
	88 Huan-tiao	In the depression at the anterior border of the hip joint. Bilateral.	Puncture with a round sharp needle obliquely downward inward, and backward 3.5-4 tsun deep.	Contraction of buttock muscles, lifting up of hind limb.	Paralysis of sciatic nerve, paralysis of femoral nerve, rheumatism of hind quarters, arthritis of hip joint, myositis of semitendinosus and semimembranosus, and biceps femoris.
	89 Ta-kua	In the depression below and in front of the anterior convexity of the trochanter major femoris. Bilateral.	Puncture with a round sharp needle along the anterior border of the femur forward, inward and obliquely 2-3.5 tsun deep.	Contraction of the thigh and hip muscles.	Arthritis of the hip joint, rheumatism of the posterior limb, paralysis of the femoral nerve, paralysis of the tibial and fibular nerves.
	90 Hsiao-kua	In the depression below and behind the trochanter tertius of the femur. Bilateral.	Puncture with a round sharp needle along the posterior border of the femur slightly downward 2-3 tsun deep.	Same as Ta-kua.	Rheumatism of the posterior limb, paralysis of the femoral, tibial and fibular nerves, myositis of biceps femoris.
	91 Hsie-chi	Beside the root of the tail about 2 tsun in the groove of the biceps femoris. Bilateral.	Puncture with a round sharp needle perpendicularly 2.5-3 tsun deep.	Fibrillation of the hip and thigh muscles swinging of the tail.	Rheumatism of femoral and rump muscles, arthritis of hip joint, myositis of biceps femoris, myositis of semitendinosus and semimenbranosus, paralysis of sciatic nerve, paralysis of femoral nerve.
	92 Han-kou	In the same muscle groove and 3 tsun below Hsie-chi. Bilateral.	Same as Hsie-chi.	Same as Hsie-chi.	Same as Hsie-chi.
	93 Yang-wa	In the same muscle groove and 3 tsun below Han-kou. Bilateral.	Same as Hsie-chi.	Same as Hsie-chi.	Same as Hsie-chi.
	94 Chien-shen	In the same muscle groove and 3 tsun below Yang-wa. Bilateral.	,,	,,	,,

Localization	Name of the Point	Location of the Point	Method of Acupuncture or Cauterization	Animal response to Acupuncture	Indication
Hind Limb	95 Hou-fu-tu	At the midpoint between the anterior convexity of the trochanter major femoris and the patella. Bilateral.	Puncture with a round sharp needle 1.5-2 tsun deep.	Contraction of the thigh muscles.	Rheumatism of the posterior limb, arthritis of the hip and stifle joints.
	96 Yin-shi	In the depression above the upper border of the patella. Bilateral.	Puncture with a round sharp needle inward and downward 1-1.2 tsun deep.	Contraction of the surrounding muscles, lifting up of the hind limb.	Arthritis of the stifle joint, rheumatism of the hind limb.
	97 Lue-tsiao	Below the patella, in the depression between the lateral and middle patellar ligaments. Bilateral.	Puncture with a round sharp needle obliquely backward and upward 1.5-2 tsun deep.	Fibrillation of the muscles around the stifle joint.	Arthritis of the stifle joint, rheumatism of hind limb, paralysis of femoral nerve, paralysis of tibial and fibular nerves, tenositis.
	98 Yang-ling	Behind the stifle joint in the depression above the posterior upper border of the lateral condyle of the tibia. Bilateral.	Puncture with a round sharp needle forward and inward 2.5-3 tsun deep.	Lifting up of the limb, fibrillation of muscles.	Arthritis of stifle joint, indigestion, rheumatism of the hind limb.
	99 Feng-lung	Behind the stifle joint, in the depression of the posterior lower border of the lateral condyle of the tibia. Bilateral.	Puncture with a round sharp needle perpendicularly 2-3 tsun deep.	Lifting up of the limb, fibrillation of the leg muscles.	Indigestion, rheumatism of hind limb, paralysis of the tibial and fibular nerves.
	100 Hou-san-li	Obliquely below and behind Lue-tsiao about 3 tsun, in the muscular groove of long digital extensor and lateral digital extensor muscles, in the depression below the head of fibula. Bilateral.	Puncture with a round sharp needle perpendicularly 1.5-2 tsun deep.	Same as Feng-lung.	Indigestion, arthritis of stifle joint, arthritis of tarsal joint, paralysis of tibial and fibular nerves.
	101 Chiao-dang	On the same saphenous vein 2 tsun above Shen-tang. Bilateral.	Same as Shen-tang.		Same as Shen-tang.
	102 Shen-tang	On the saphenous vein about 4 tsun below the midpoint of the root of the inner surface of the thigh. Bilateral.	Puncture with a small broad needle 3 fen deep to bleed.		Arthritis of hip joint, arthritis of stifle joint, myositis of Semitendinosus and Semimembranosus, myositis of biceps femoris, orchitis, laminitis, edema of hind limb and scrotum.
	103 Tu-hsüeh	On the same vein 2 tsun below Shen-tang. Bilateral.	Same as Shen-tang		Same as Shen-tang.
	104 Chu-shang	In the depression 1 tsun above Chu-chih. Bilateral.	Puncture with a round sharp needle obliquely inward and upward 1-1.2 tsun deep.	Lifting up of that limb.	Arthritis of metatarsal joint, paralysis of tibial and fibular nerves.

Localization	Name of the Point	Location of the Point	Method of Acupuncture or Cauterization	Animal response to Acupuncture	Indication
Hind Limb	105 Chu-chih	On the medial dorsal metatarsal vein in the depression lateral to the metatarsal joint. Bilateral.	Puncture quickly with a small broad needle 2-3 fen deep to bleed.		Acute arthritis of the metatarsal joint.
	106 Hou-chan-wan	On the medial and lateral digital veins above the upper border of the fetlock joint. One point on each side on both hind limbs.	Puncture with a small broad needle 2-3 fen deep to bleed.		Contusion of the fetlock joint, arthritis of fetlock joint, acute arthritis of metatarsal joint, tenositis, tendovaginitis.
	107 Lao-tang	Same as Ming-tang on the fore limb.	Same as Ming-tang on the fore limb.		Contusion of the fetlock joint, arthritis of fetlock joint, tenositis, tendovaginitis.
	108 Hou-chiu	In the depression above the bulb, in the middle of the posterior surface of the hoof. Bilateral.	Lift the limb and hold it. Puncture with a round sharp needle 1-1.5 tsun deep towards the tip of the hoof.	Lifting up of the limb.	Laminitis, rheumatism of the hind limb, paralysis of the tibial and fibular nerves, arthritis of fetlock joint, tenositis, tendovaginitis.
	109 Hou-ti-men	On the upper border of the bulb, in the depression behind the cartilage of the hoof. One point on each side of the hoof.	Puncture with a small broad needle 3 fen deep.		Inflammation of the bulb of the hoof.
	110 Hou-ti-tou	At the midpoint of the coronary border of the hind hoof. Bilateral.	Puncture with a large broad needle quickly 3 fen deep to bleed.		Laminitis, colic pain, inflammation of the bulbs of the hoof.
Tail	111 Chui-feng	In the depression between the 1st and 2nd coccygeal vertebrae, on the dorsal side of the root of the tail. One point only.	Lift up the tail a little, puncture with a round sharp needle perpendicularly 5 fen to 1 tsun deep.	Fibrillation of the hip muscles and swinging of the tail.	Rheumatism of the loin, paralysis of the loin.
	112 Hou-hai	In the depression between the anus and the root of tail. One point only.	Puncture with a round sharp needle upward and forward 4-6 tsun deep.	Lifting up of the tail, contraction of the anus.	Indigestion, diarrhoea, constipation, inflation of the bowel, paralysis of rectum.

Localization	Name of the Point	Location of the Point	Method of Acupuncture or Cauterization	Animal response to Acupuncture	Indication
Tail	113 Wei-pen	On the blood vessel in the middle of the lower surface of the tail 2 tsun from the root. One point only.	Lift the tail straight upward, puncture with a large broad needle upward 3 fen deep to bleed.		Acute arthritis of hip joint, constipation, rheumatism of the loin.
	114 Wei-chien	On the tip of the tail. One point only.	Puncture with a triangular needle or broad needle perpendicularly 4-5 fen deep to bleed.		Overexertion, heat stroke, common cold, spasm of bowel.

Ottaviano[15] (Fig. 3–108)

Foreleg

FL1 (Lateral side point above coronary band) Laminitis, ringbone, sidebone, navicular disease, all hoof afflictions.

FL2 (Center point above coronary band) Same as above (FL1) plus convulsions and colic.

FL3 (Medial point above coronary band) Same as FL1.

FL4 Arthritis of fetlock, bowed tendons, secondary point for laminitis and sidebones.

FL5 Arthritis of fetlock, bowed tendons, inability to flex fetlock, secondary point for laminitis.

FL6. Bowed tendons, inflammation in area.

FL7. Knee joint inflammations, bowed tendons.

FL8 All metacarpal problems.

FL9 *Guo-liang.* Important point for all afflictions of the knee joint, bowed tendons, arthritis of knee, fetlock, navicular bone, laminitis. Reflex point to fetlock, hoof, and shoulder area.

FL10 Local point for joint, muscle.

FL11 Energy point, arthritis or pain of shoulder, scapular region. Knee pain. Use with FL21 for analgesia of knee.

FL12 Paralysis of nerve, local joint and muscle inflammation.

FL13 Paralysis of nerve, local joint. (Same as above FL12.)

FL14 Shoulder and scapular pain, muscular pain, nerve paralysis, local analgesia.

FL15 Shoulder and muscle pain in region.

FL16 Main point for shoulder pain of all types.

FL17 Same as above.

FL18 Shoulder and scapular pain, reflex point for scapula.

FL19 Same as above.

Head

H20 Emergency point. Convulsions, colic, abdominal problems, syncope.

H21 Nasal problems, lung hemorrhage.

H22 Nasal problems, facial paralysis.

H23 All eye afflictions.

H24 Eye afflictions, excessive tearing, facial paralysis.

H25 Tranquilizer, facial paralysis, maxilla and mandible afflictions, tetanus, facial swelling from insect bite, mastication problems.

H26 Tip of Ear (*Er-Jian*). Facial paralysis special point, eye problems, epilepsy, convulsions, common cold, fevers.

H27 Hemorrhage of lungs, eye afflictions, tetanus.

H28 Cervical problems, wobblers, cerebral problems, torticollis.

H29 Same as above.

H30 through H37 *Jiu-Wei.* Cervical afflictions, cerebral problems, wobblers, torticollis, tetanus, arthritis in area.

Trunk

T38 Arthritis of any joint of forelimb. Scapular pain. Reflex point to pain in front limb.

T39 Scapular pain—reflex to shoulder pain, similar but secondary to T38.

T40 Same as T39.

T41 Important point. Convulsions, fever, lungs, stomach laminitis, shoulder pain, appetite.

T42 Important point. Organic afflictions, reflex point to shoulder and scapular area. Whenever sensitive, treat with needle.

T43 Convulsions, fever, lungs.

T44 Lungs, edema of chest, emphysema, not enough wind, convulsions, local point.

T45 Lungs, pulmonary hemorrhage, local point.

T46 Intestinal influence, lumbar pain, colic secondary point, local influence.

T47 Throat area, fevers, jaundice, liver, wind and breathing, lower lungs, local.

T48 Stomach swelling, intestinal influence, local.

T49 Same as T48.

T50 Same as T48, colic.

T51 Colic, convulsions, inflammation of stomach.

T52 Same as T48.

T53 Lumbar pain and arthritis, tying up, intestines, diarrhea, colic, stomach.

T54 Lumbar pain, kidney afflictions, tying up syndrome.

T55 Lumbar pain and arthritis, kidney inflamation, hind limb paralysis.

T56 100 Meeting Places (*Bai Hui*)—Important point. All balance problems, cerebral-cervical problems, lumbar pain and arthritis, colic, energy, hip problems, paralysis, tying up, etc.

T57 Lumbar arthritis and pain, vertebra inflammation, reproductive organ influence, urinary difficulties, bladder.

T58 Lumbar pain, hind limb paralysis, rectal problems.

T59 End of Tail (*Nei Jien*). Emergency, fever, convulsions, common cold, low back pain, urinary incontinence.

T87 Lumbar pain, arthritis, and tying up. Similar uses as RL86 but secondary. Deals more with lumbar pain.

T88 Kidney and liver influence. Reflex point. If painful, puncture point. Has minor influence over lungs.

T89 Controls liver, reflex point for organic dysfunctions, circulation and energy. Key point, also used for laminitis.

T90 Point of the Lungs—all problems with lungs. If tender, treat reflex point.

T91 Lung problems, fever, convulsions.

T92 Tri-heater function/lower-upper-middle. Organic problems, fevers, lungs, hemorrhage from lungs, reflex to mouth, tendon and hoof problems.

T93 Lung, upper heater and middle heater, heart problems, wind, pain of front limbs due to arthritis.

T94 Shoulder pains reflex point—skin problems, scapular pain, arthritis of any part of front limbs.

Rear Leg

RL60 Local point, arthritis and pain in area, including area down to stifle.

RL61 Same as RL60.

RL62 Same as RL60.

RL63 All problems with hip and stifle area.

RL64 Same as RL60.

RL65 Same as RL60.

RL66 Same as RL60.

RL67 Same as RL60.

RL68 Stifle pain and arthritis, weakness in the entire leg, stomach, large intestine.

RL69 Same as RL68.

RL70 Same as RL68.

RL71 Tibia and fibula pain, stifle pain, patella pain, tarsal joint, stomach influence, energy, appetite, strength.

RL72 Hock problems (capped, spavin) (can use heat—moxa stick).

RL73 Local pain (can use heat).

RL74 Same as RL72 (can use heat).

RL75 Local joint pain.

RL76 Local pain, arthritis, flexor tendons.

RL77 Same as FL2.

RL78 Same as FL1.

RL79 Same as FL3.

RL80 Same as FL4.

RL81 Local joint afflictions. (Heat can be used.)

RL82 Bilateral. Same as RL76.

RL83 Point exists medial and lateral to tendons. Point is used for tendon problems.

RL84 Tendon, muscular, and bone problems of area.

RL85 Uses are similar to RL72.

RL86 Local joint problems, arthritis of rear quarters, lameness and paralysis of real quarters. Excellent local point when tender.

Shin[16] *(Fig. 3–109)*

1. Inside of Comb *Nae Ra*

Location. Mid-line—below the tendon of lavator labii superioris proprius muscle.

Method. 1 cm perpendicular insertion.

Indication. Facial paralysis, syncope, pay attention at races.

2. House of the Blood *Hyul Dang*

Location. Under the tendon of the muscularis labii superioris proprius muscle.

Method. 5 mm perpendicular insertion.

Indication. Facial surgery, facial paralysis.

3. Three Red *Sam Hong*

Location. Junction of the V-shaped tendon of the muscles on the mid-line on the dorsal part of the nose.

Method. 2.5 mm perpendicular insertion.

Indication. Stroke, facial paralysis.

4. Chewing Sound *Soi Jin*

Location. Between the nose and the upper lip, ventral to the nares.

Method. 5 mm perpendicular insertion on the obicularis oris muscle.

Indication. Chewing problems.

5. Pearl House *Ok Dang*

Location. Caudal to the nose, lateral side, on the dilatator naris lateralis.

Method. 5 mm perpendicular insertion.

Indication. Coughing and the common cold.

6. Go to Heaven *Tong Chun*

Location. Mid-line on same level as the eyes.

Method. 3 mm perpendicular insertion.

Indication. Colds, cough.

7. Door of the Wind *Aung Moon*

Location. Mid-line, one half the distance between level of the eyes and the top of the head.

Method. 3 mm perpendicular insertion.

Indication. Cough, cold, syncope, dizziness, facial paralysis.

8. Closing Mouth *Shoe Ku*

Location. On the V-junction of the levator naso-labialis and the zygomaticus.

Method. 5 mm perpendicular insertion.

Indication. Chewing problems.

9. Small Eye *So Ahn*

Location. Lateral border of dorsal orbital depression.

Method. 3 mm perpendicular insertion.

Indication. Syncope, facial paralysis.

10. Point of Ear *Ei Chim*

Location. Medial convex side of the ear, lateral side of the medial spine, midway in a dorso-ventral plane.

Method. Prick 2 mm.

Indication. Cranial nerve disorders, syncope, facial paralysis.

11. The Sun *Tai Yang*

Location. Sub-zygmoatic fossa, ventral to the zygomatic arch, right above the facial nerve.

Method. 5 mm perpendicular insertion.

Indication. Wobblers (Fredrick's ataxia of the spine), cervical ataxia.

12. Lung Point *Tie Yiu*

Location. Above the intermediate tendon of the masseter muscle, rostral to the angle of the jaw.

Method. 5 mm perpendicular insertion.

Indication. Controls lung disorders.

13. Point of Cloud *Un Chim*

Location. Cranial to the first thoracic vertebra, between the 7th cervical and the 1st thoracic vertebrae.

Method. 5 cm perpendicular insertion.

Indication. Paralysis of the shoulder, chest pains, arthritis of the forelegs, pneumonia.

13–1. First Step *Il Wui*

Location. On the mid-line between the first and second cervical vertebrae (C_1 and C_2).

Method. Perpendicular insertion.

Indication. Neck muscle spasm, cough, facial nerve paralysis.

13–2. Second Step *Yi Wui*

Location. On the mid-line between C_2–C_3.

Method. Perpendicular insertion.

Indication. Back (lumbar) pain, cervical arthritis, conjunctivitis.

13–3. Third Step *Sam Wui*

Location. On the mid-line between C_3–C_4.

Method. Perpendicular insertion.

Indication. Dermatitis on foreleg, carpal arthritis, cervical spine subluxation, syncope from trauma.

13–4. 4th Step *Sa Wui*

Location. On the mid-line between C_4–C_5.

Method. Perpendicular insertion.

Indication. Indigestion, (from stomach lazy condition) diarrhea.

13–5. 5th Step *O Wui*

Location. On the mid-line between C_5–C_6.

Method. Perpendicular insertion.

Indication. Shoulder joint arthritis, cervical myalgia, foreleg lameness, laminitis, ring bone.

14. Very Thin Point *Bak Chim*

Location. Cranial and ventral to the first thoracic vertebra on the brachiocephalicus muscle.

Method. 3–4 cm perpendicular insertion.

Indication. Pneumonia and shoulder arthritis.

15. House of the Chest *Hyung Dang*

Location. Ventral end of scapula, near the insertion of the deltoid muscles.

Method. 4 cm perpendicular insertion.

Indication. Stomach disorders, scapular pain, relaxation after racing.

16. Very Thin Lily *Bak Rahn*

Location. On the scapula, above the 5th rib.

Method. 3 cm perpendicular insertion.

Indication. Arthritis of the forelegs, chest pain, shoulder pain.

17. Tree Wing *Chang Poong*

Location. Caudal to the spine of the scapula and dorsal to the 3rd intercostal space.
Method. 3–4 cm perpendicular insertion.
Indication. Wobblers, cervical disorders, shoulder pain.

17–1. Reaching Heaven *Chung Cheun*

Location. Cranial to the spine of scapula, at the level of C₆–C₇.
Method. 3 cm perpendicular insertion.
Indication. Pain in scapula, shoulder joint arthritis, cervical ataxia, cough.

18. Muscle of Chest *Dong Keun*

Location. Cranial and ventral to the humerus where at the attachment of the biceps brachii.
Method. 2 cm perpendicular insertion.
Indication. Colic, indigestion (gas forming conditions), pain in the foreleg, laminitis.

19. Welcome Wind *Young Poong*

Location. 9th intercostal space, One Horse Inch (9 cm, 3½ inches) lateral to the tip of the spinous process.
Method. 2 cm perpendicular insertion.
Indication. Emphysema, cough, fever, cold (Viral infections of respiratory tract), pneumonia.

19–1. Thin Hole *Park Kong*

Location. Mid-shaft lateral humerus, at the level of the 2nd costal attachment to the sternum.
Method. 2 cm perpendicular insertion.
Indication. Stomach disorders, diarrhoea.

20. Heart Point *Sim Yu*

Location. Middle of the 2nd intercostal space at the level of the scapulo-humeral joint.
Method. 2 cm perpendicular insertion.
Indication. Circulatory disorders, blood pressure, arterial problems.

20–1. Stomach Point *Wui Yu*

Location. In the 3rd intercostal space, ⅓ of distance from dorsal part of space.
Method. 3 cm perpendicular insertion.
Indication. Stomach disorder, diarrhea, constipation, colic, enteritis, gastritis, (This functional point is same as human ST 36).

21. Night Eye *Ya Ahn*

Location. In the chet nut, in the medial side of ulna, originally this is forbidden point.
Method. 3 cm Diagonal (ventral) insertion.
Indication. Insommnia, hypnotic purpose [sedation?]

21–1. Energy Coming from Inside *Nai Nae Ki*

Location. Dorsal cranial to the olecrenon, on the lateral side, at the head of the biceps brachii.
Method. 1 cm perpendicular insertion.
Indication. General weakness, lameness of foreleg, Wobbler syndrome.

21–2. Front Ulna *Jeon Chuk*

Location. Lateral side of the mid-shaft of radius where the muscle of lateral extensor attaches.
Method. 1 cm diagonal (caudal) insertion.
Indication. Laminitis, leg pain, sore muscle of fore leg.

21–3. Center of Arm *Chung Wan*

Location. Dorsal to accessory carpal bone, medial side of foreleg, caudal to ulna, at the insertion of flexor carpi ulnaris.
Method. 7 mm perpendicular insertion.
Indication. Carpal arthritis, laminitis, ring bone, side bone.

21–4. Front Knee *Jeon Kae*

Location. Ventral to accessory carpal bone, medial side of foreleg.
Method. 7 mm perpendicular insertion.
Indication. Carpal arthritis, lameness of lateral side of foreleg.

21–5. Front of Arm *Jeon Wan*

Location. Cranial and ventral to carpal bones, on the tendon of extensor carpi obliquus.
Method. 5 mm perpendicular insertion.
Indication. Knee joint arthritis, edema of foreleg.

21–6. Gate of Knee *Seul Moon*

Location. Cranial medial distal side of Ulna, on the extensor carpi radialis.
Method. 5 mm perpendicular insertion.
Indication. Knee joint arthritis, lameness of foreleg.

22. Cap of Knee *Seul Kae*

Location. Lateral epicodyle of radius, in the depression.
Method. 1 cm horizontal insertion (caudal).
Indication. Carpal arthritis, dysuria, enuresis, cystitis.

22–1. Out side of knee *Oe Wan*

Location. Cranial to and between the third and fourth carpal bone.
Method. 1 cm horizontal insertion (caudal).

Indication. Knee joint arthritis, edema on foreleg.

22–2. Inside of Knee *Nae Seul*
Location. Ventral to lateral side of accessory carpal bone, caudal lateral side of carpal bones.
Method. 1 cm horizontal (caudal) insertion.
Indication. Tendonitis, fetlock joint arthritis.

22–3. Point of Knee *Jeong Seul*
Location. Dorsal to knee joint, where common extensor tendon is attached.
Method. 1 cm transverse horizontal insertion.
Indication. Sprain, strain of knee joint.

23. Energizing the Blood *Whal Hyul*
Location. Lateral, caudal to the distal end of metacarpal bone.
Method. 1 cm perpendicular insertion.
Indication. Anemia, bucked shin, tendonitis, arthritis of fetlock joint.

23–1. Tie of Bright *Kyul Myung*
Location. Lateral, caudal to the proximal side of metacarpal bone.
Method. 1 cm perpendicular insertion.
Indication. Tendonitis, bucked shin.

23–2. Circle of Joint *Whan Jeol*
Location. Lateral, caudal to the middle of metacarpal bone.
Method. 1 cm perpendicular insertion.
Indication. Tendonitis, arthritis of fetlock joint, bursitis.

24. House of Labor *No Dang*
Location. Lateral, ventral to lateral sesamoid bone.
Method. 1 cm perpendicular insertion.
Indication. Periostitis, edema on fetlock joint, arthritis, laminitis.

25. Side Door *Pyon Moon*
Location. Cranial, lateral to distal end of 1st phalanx (P_1) in the space between P_1 and P_2 of front leg.
Method. 1 cm horizontal caudal insertion.
Indication. Edema of ankle joint, tendonitis, sprain, strain, pain in the leg.

26. Nail of the Foot *Je chim*
Location. Cranial, medial to the space between P_2 and P_3.
Method. 1 cm horizontal, caudal insertion.
Indication. Laminitis, ring bone, side bone.

27. Door of the Foot *Je Moon*

Location. Medial, ventral to medial sesamoid bone.
Method. 1 cm perpendicular insertion.
Indication. Periostitis, edema of ankle joint, arthritis, laminitis.

28. White Heaven *Cheon Bak*
Location. Medial, ventral to distal P_1.
Method. 1 cm perpendicular insertion.
Indication. Tendonitis, periostitis, general weakness of forelegs.

28–1. Bright Well *Myung Jung*
Location. Caudal, mid line of forefoot, distal P_1.
Method. 7 mm perpendicular insertion, usually bleed with triangle needle.
Indication. Laminitis, tendonitis, navicular disease.

28–2. Side door *Cheuk Mun* (same as point 25, this is medial)
Location. Cranial, medial distal end of P_1 in the space between P_1 and P_2 of foreleg.
Method. 1 cm perpendicular insertion.
Indication. Ring bone, side bone.

29. Arm of Knee *Seul Wan*
Location. Medial side of the carpus, ventral to the accessory carpal bone.
Method. 1 cm perpendicular insertion.
Indication. Tendonitis, metacarpal arthritis, periositis, laminitis.

29–1. Inside of Bright-Tie *Nae Kyul Myung*
Location. Medial, caudal to the proximal side of third metacarpal bone (MCIII).
Method. 1 cm perpendicular insertion.
Indication. Tendonitis, bucked shins.

29–2. Inside Circle *Nae Whan*
Location. Medial, caudal to distal MCIII.
Method. 1 cm perpendicular insertion.
Indication. Tendonitis, arthritis of fetlock joint.

29–3. Inside of Energizer *Nae Whal*
Location. Cranial to the distal end of MCIII.
Method. 7 mm perpendicular insertion.
Indication. Arthritis of fetlock joint, strain of ankle joint.

29–4. Inside of Circle of Joint *Nae Whan Jeol*
Location. Medial, cranial to mid MCIII.
Method. 1 cm perpendicular insertion.
Indication. Tendonitis, arthritis of fetlock joint, bursitis.

30. Armor of the Hair *Bal Kap*

Location. 10th intercostal space, one Shin horse inch lateral to the midline.
Method. 1 cm perpendicular insertion.
Indication. Shoulder pain, backache, cervical ataxia.

31 through 40. Spinal Bridge Holes *Chunk Yang Hyul*

Location. 11th intercostal space.
Method. 1 cm perpendicular insertion.
Indication. Liver disorders, skin disease, back aches.

32. At 12th intercostal space.

Method. 1 cm perpendicular insertion.
Indication. Lung disorders, emphysema, common cold, fever.

33. At 13th intercostal space. (also known as a liver point)

Method. 1 cm perpendicular insertion.
Indication. Colic, intestinal disorders.

34. At 14th intercostal space.

Method. 1 cm perpendicular insertion.
Indication. Thoracic vertebral arthritis.

35. At the 15th intercostal space.

Method. 1 cm perpendicular insertion.
Indication. Colic, intestinal disorders, indigestion.

36. At the 16th intercostal space.

Method. 1 cm perpendicular insertion.
Indication. Backache, laminitis, front leg lameness.

37. At the 17th intercostal space.

Method. 1 cm perpendicular insertion.
Indication. Backache, foreleg lameness.

38. Between T_{17} and L_1.

Method. 1 cm perpendicular insertion.
Indication. Lumbago, lumbar arthritis, colic, emphysema, laminitis.

39. Between L_1 and L_2.

Method. 1.5 cm perpendicular insertion.
Indication. Pain in lumbar vertebrae, foreleg lameness, laminitis.

40. Between L_2 and L_3.

Method. 1.5 cm perpendicular insertion.
Indication. Back pain, tendonitis, arthritis in forefoot.

41. One Hundred Meeting *Baek Hoe*

Location. On the mid line between L_6 and S_1. Same functional point as GV20 in human (Pai Hui).
Method. 5 mm perpendicular insertion.

Indication. Mental disorders, any lameness, lung disorders, liver disorders, intestinal disorders, connecting point for any combination of acupuncture formulae.

42. Lung Point *Pei Yu*

Location. 4th intercostal space at the level of scapulo-humeral joint.
Method. 1 cm perpendicular insertion.
Indication. Emphysema, dermatitis, lung disorder.

42–1. Lung Point *Pei Yu*

Location. 7th intercostal space at the level of scapulo-humeral joint.
Method. 1 cm perpendicular insertion.
Indication. Emphysema, cough, colic, dermatitis.

43. Lung Point *Pei Yu*

Location. 5th intercostal space at the level of the middle of the scapula.
Method. 1 cm perpendicular insertion.
Indication. Cough, emphysema, dermatitis, colic, fever.

44. Liver Point *Kan Yu*

Location. 12th intercostal space at the level of the middle of the humerus.
Method. 1.5 cm perpendicular insertion, for 25 mins.
Indication. Backache, emphysema, laminitis, toxemia, fever.

45. Spleen Point *Bi Yu*

Location. 15th intercostal space at the level of the middle of the scapula.
Method. 1 cm perpendicular insertion.
Indication. Indigestion, gas forming syndromes, liver disorders.

46. Kidney Point *Shin Yu*

Location. Caudal to ilium, 3rd sacral space, 1″ lateral to the spine.
Method. Laminitis, reproductive problems, kidney and bladder disorders.
Indication. 1.5 cm perpendicular insertion, for 25 mins.

47. Great Mountain *Pa San*

Location. Dorsal to coxa-femoral joint and greater trochanter.
Method. 3 cm perpendicular insertion.
Indication. Hip lameness, hip joint arthritis.

48. Root of Tail *Mi Keun*

Location. Lateral to the 4th coccegeal vertebra.

Method.   2 cm perpendicular insertion.
Indication.   Dysuria, cystitis, spinal ataxia, hindleg lameness.

49. Proper Swap *Kyo Dang*
Location.   Middle of the lateral shaft of femur.
Method.   3 cm perpendicular insertion.
Indication.   Stifle joint arthritis, hindleg lameness.

50. Umbrella of Kidney *U Shin*
Location.   Ventral to the lateral side of patella.
Method.   2 cm perpendicular insertion.
Indication.   Luxation of patella, locked stifle.

51. Eight Point *Pal Hyul*
Location.   Between medial condyle of tibia and tuber calcus.
Method.   2 cm diagonal insertion (upward).
Indication.   Arthritis of hock joints, local swelling.

51–1. Same name
Location.   Cranial to distal end of tibia.
Method.   2 cm horizontal insertion, (laterally).
Indication.   Pain in the hock.

51–2. Same name
Location.   Cranial to tibial tarsal bone.
Method.   2 cm perpendicular insertion.
Indication.   Same as 51–1.

51–3. Same name
Location.   Caudal, medial to tibial tarsal bone.
Method.   2 cm perpendicular insertion.
Indication.   Tendonitis, ankle sprain, arthritis of tarsal bones.

52. Small Joint *So Jeol*
Location.   Between lateral condyle of tibia and tuber calcus.
Method.   2 cm diagonal insertion (upward).
Indication.   Arthritis of hock joint, hip lameness.

53. Bird's Joint *Jo Jeol*
Location.   Caudal, lateral to the proximal end of the third metatarsal bone (MTIII) and ventral to tuber calcis.
Method.   1 cm perpendicular insertion.
Indication.   Tendonitis, muscle pain (Hamstring, gastrocnemius, superficial digital flexor,) arthritis of tarsal bones.

53–1. Same name
Location.   Caudal posterior, middle of MTIII.
Method.   1 cm perpendicular insertion.
Indication.   Inflammation of achilles tendon, (30 min-utes insertion and five minutes moxibustion, three times in a week).

54. Curved Scale *Gok Chuck*
Location.   Cranial, ventral to the distal ends of MTIII.
Method.   1 cm perpendicular insertion.
Indication.   Ankle joint arthritis, ankle strain.

54–1. Same name
Location.   Lateral, ventral to lateral sesamoid bone of hind foot.
Method.   1 cm perpendicular insertion.
Indication.   Laminitis, joint arthritis, tendonitis.

54–2. Same name
Location.   Cranial, medial to distal end of first phalanx P_1 in the space between P_1 and P_2 of hind foot.
Method.   1 cm horizontal insertion (downward).
Indication.   Laminitis, ring bone, side bone.

55. Rear Foot *Hu Je*
Location.   Cranial midline of hind foot between P_2 and P_3.
Method.   1 cm horizontal insertion, (downward).
Indication.   Laminitis, cervical ataxia, ring bone, side bone.

56. Side Door *Pyon Moon*
Location.   Cranial midline of the hind foot between P_1 and P_2.
Method.   1 cm perpendicular insertion.
Indication.   Laminitis, ring bone, side bone.

56–1. Same name
Location.   Medial, caudal to the proximal side of MTIII.
Method.   1 cm perpendicular insertion.
Indication.   Tendonitis, bucked shins.

56–2. Same name
Location.   Medial, caudal to the middle of MTIII.
Method.   1 cm perpendicular insertion.
Indication.   Tendonitis, arthritis of ankle joint.

56–3. Same name
Location.   Medial, caudal to the distal end of MTIII.
Method.   1 cm perpendicular insertion.
Indication.   Tendonitis, arthritis of ankle joint, ring bone.

56–4. Same name
Location.   Medial, ventral to medial sesamoid bone hindleg.
Method.   1 cm perpendicular insertion.

Indication. Laminitis, edema on ankle joint.

56–5. Same name

Location. Caudal, mid line of distal portion of hind P₁.

Method. 7 mm perpendicular insertion, usually needs bleeding with triangle needle.

Indication. Laminitis, tendonitis, navicular disease.

57. Thousand Gold *Cheun Geum*

Location. Medial, ventral to the patella.

Method. 2 cm perpendicular insertion.

Indication. Patella luxation, locked stifle.

58. Great Wing *Dae Ik*. Human ST36 *Hu Sam Li*.

Location. Lateral, ventral to the lateral condyle of tibia.

Method. 2 cm perpendicular insertion.

Indication. Stifle joint arthritis, luxation of stifle.

59. House of Chicken *Ge Ok*

Location. Ventral to the greater trochanter of femur.

Method. 3 cm perpendicular insertion.

Indication. Hip joint arthritis, muscle pain, (after racing).

60. Sweat Well *Han Jeong*

Location. Lateral, caudal to the distal portion of femur.

Method. 2 cm perpendicular insertion.

Indication. Stifle joint problems.

Chinese Veterinary Handbook[3] *(Figs. 3–28 to 3–43)*

The asterisks next to some of the points indicate those points that produce a strong needle feeling (te ch'i; see pp. 249–251). Some of these points have been used for the production of acupuncture analgesia.

Head and Neck

HN1. Upper Gate *Shang Kuan* (Figs. 3–28, 3–30).

Location. In the depression caudal and dorsal to the mandibular joint and ventral to the zygomatic arch.

Method. Hot needle, 5 fen to 1 tsun.†

Indication. Facial paralysis, tetanus.

HN2. Lower Gate *Hsia Kuan* (Fig. 3–28).

Location. In the depression rostral and ventral to the mandibular joint, one tsun rostral to HN1.

Method. Hot needle, 5 fen to 1 tsun, at an angle.

Indication. Same as HN1.

HN3. Open Heaven *K'ai T'ien* (Figs. 3–28, 3–33C).

Location. Immediately below the midpoint of the ventral margin of the pupil, at the line of demarcation between the lower border of the cornea with the sclera.

Method. Cold water is splashed onto the eye and the parasite swims to the anterior chamber of the eyeball. Apply 2–3% procaine to constrict the pupil. Use a curved needle to pierce the cornea, and the parasite will flow out with the aqueous humor.

Indication. Microfilariae of *Setaria equi*.

HN4. Three Rivers *San Chiang* (Figs. 3–28, 3–32).

Location. One tsun rostral to the medial canthus on the angular vein.

Method. Small, wide needle or prism needle inserted at an angle into the blood vessel about 3 fen. Bleed 50–100 cc.

Indication. Spasm of the bowel, gaseous distension of the bowel, constipation, indigestion, conjunctivitis, keratitis, periodic ophthalmia.

*HN5. The Great Yang *T'ai Yang* (Fig. 3–32).

Location. On the transverse facial vein, one tsun caudal to the lateral canthus.

Method. The medium, wide needle, about 3 fen; bleed.

Indication. Conjunctivitis, keratitis, periodic ophthalmia (bleed 100–200 cc), sunstroke, encephalitis (bleed 400–800 cc).

*HN6. Vessels of Eyes *Yan Mai* (Figs. 3–28, 3–32).

Location. On the transverse facial vein 1.5 tsun caudal to the lateral canthus or about 5 fen behind T'ai Yang (HN5).

Method. Same as HN5.

Indication. Same as HN5.

*HN7. God of Nose *Pi Shu* (Figs. 3–28, 3–32).

Location. The middle point between the dorsal margin of the nasal orifice and the rostral tip of the nasal bone.

Method. One hand is used to grasp the two sides of the nasal bridge. A small, wide needle or prism needle is inserted through the

† The tsun is a measure of length used in acupuncture to indicate the depth of needle insertion and anatomic distances. One tsun is divided into ten fen. The width of the 16th rib at the level of tuber coxae equals 1 tsun. (Hold the rib with thumb and the index finger and measure the width between the two fingers.)

nasal orifices and septum nasi; bleed 100–300 cc.

Indication. Unconsciousness, rhinitis, overexertion, cerebral hyperemia, congestion of the lung.

*HN8. Hall of Blood *Hsueh T'ang* (Figs. 3–28, 3–32).

Location. Two tsun caudal to the dorsal margin of the nasal orifice. One on each side of the nasal bridge.

Method. Same as HN7.

Indication. Same as HN7.

*HN9. Ginger Tooth *Chiang Ya* (Figs. 3–28, 3–32).

Location. At the cartilage of the ala nasi, 5 fen lateral to the midpoint of the outer margin of the nasal orifice.

Method. Small, wide needle inserted until it reaches the cartilage, about 3 fen.

Indication. Spasm of the bowel, constipation, dilatation of the stomach.

HN10. Pulling Tendon *Ch'ou Chin* (Figs. 3–28, 3–34B).

Location. At the midpoint of the line joining the corner of the nasal orifices. Single point.

Method. The upper lip is pulled up with one hand. The large, wide needle is used to cut the skin to expose the tendon of the levator labii superioris proprius muscle. The tendon is then cleaned from the underlying connective tissue and pulled several times, forcefully but without inducing physical damage.

Indication. Stiff neck and back.

*HN11. Dividing Water *Fen Shui* (Figs. 3–28, 3–34B).

Location. At the middle of the spirally arranged hair (vortex pilorum) of the outer surface of the upper lip. Single point.

Method. The prism needle or small, wide needle is inserted 0.3 fen until there is slight bleeding.

Indication. Spasm of the bowel, gaseous distension of the bowel, constipation, dilatation of the stomach, indigestion.

HN12. Holding Chin *So K'ou* (Figs. 3–28, 3–32).

Location. Seven fen caudal and dorsal to the corner of the mouth, at the outer margin of orbicularis oris muscle.

Method. The hot needle is inserted from the corner of the mouth caudal 2.5–3 tsun in the same direction.

Indication. Facial paralysis and trismus.

HN13. Gate Switch *K'ai Kuan* (Figs. 3–28, 3–29).

Location. The cranial margin of the masseter muscle at the level of the table surface of the molars and on a line from the corner of the mouth.

Method. The hot needle; caudal-dorsal direction, 8 fen to 1 tsun, or insert the hao chen for 2.5–3 tsun in the same direction.

Indication. Same as HN12.

HN14. Inner Lip Ying *Nei Ch'un Ying* (Fig. 3–33B).

Location. At the blood vessel 5 fen to 1 tsun lateral to the midpoint on the dental surface of the upper lip, 1 tsun from the gum of the tooth, 5–8 fen beside the frenulum labii superioris; or the needle may be inserted at the papillae of the swollen area.

Method. The prism needle is inserted 2–3 fen until bleeding occurs or it pierces through a swollen area.

Indication. Swollen lip, stomatitis, indigestion, pharyngolaryngitis.

*HN15. Jade Mansion *Yu T'ang* (Fig. 3–33A).

Location. Inside the third ridge of the hard palate in the mouth, approximately 5 fen from the midline.

Method. After the mouth is opened, pull out the tongue; insert a small, wide needle or prism needle, slanting up 3 fen deep from the corner of the mouth and bleed (do not insert straight upward, to prevent severe bleeding).

Indication. Gastric discomfort, ulcer of the tongue and stomach, indigestion, stomatitis, heat stroke, overexertion, common cold.

HN16. Passing Gate (Lip Ying) *T'ung Kuan* (She Yin) (Fig. 3–34A).

Location. The blood vessels at both sides of the ventral surface of the tongue.

Method. The tongue is pulled outside the mouth and turned upside down. A small, wide needle or prism needle is inserted 2–3 fen until bleeding occurs.

Indication. Swelling of the tongue, ulcer of the tongue, gastric discomfort, loss of appetite.

HN17. Tip of Ear *Erh Chien* (Figs. 3–28, 3–35A).

Location. The bifurcation of posterior auricular vein at the dorsal tip of the ear.

Method. Puncture with a small, wide needle to

rupture the blood vessel and cause bleeding.

Indication. Spasm of bowel, common cold.

*HN18. Vein of Neck (Vein of Bird, Great Blood) *Ching Mai, (Ku Mai or Ta Hsueh)* (Figs. 3–28, 3–32).

Location. The jugular vein at the cranial and middle third of the jugular vein.

Method. The vein is held off (as in venipuncture). The large, wide needle is inserted 3–4 fen into the blood vessel to bleed 500–1500 cc.

Indication. Sunstroke, encephalitis, lung congestion, acute pneumonia, urticaria, intoxication, laminitis, stomatitis.

HN19. Throat Door *Hou Men* (Figs. 3–28, 3–32).

Location. One tsun caudal and ventral to the larynx, at the external maxillary vein.

Method. Same as HN18. Bleed 300–500 cc.

Indication. Laryngitis, pharyngitis.

HN20. Nine Divisions *Chiu Wei* (Figs. 3–28, 3–29).

Location. There are nine points on each side of the neck. The first of the nine points is 3 tsun caudal and ventral to the ear. The ninth point is 1.5 tsun cranial to the anterior angle of the scapula. The distance between these two points is divided into eight equal parts. All the points are distributed along the lower margin of the rhomboideus muscle forming an arc.

Method. Hot needle, 8 fen to 1 tsun; or hao chen, 1.5–3 tsun.

Indication. Rheumatism of the cervical region, tetanus.

Forelimb (FL)

FL1. Small Row *Kung Tsu* (Figs. 3–28, 3–30).

Location. Caudal to the tuber spinae of the scapula and 3 tsun below the midpoint of the upper border of the scapular cartilage.

Method. Air is injected subcutaneously and is pushed downward with the fingers so that the subcutaneous tissue of the shoulder is filled with air. As an alternative, a hot needle is inserted 4–5 tsun downward at an angle.

Indication. Paralysis of the nerves of the scapular region, muscle atrophy of the shoulder, chronic shoulder lameness.

FL2. Tip of Shoulder *Po Chien* (Figs. 3–28, 3–30).

Location. In the depression between the anterior angle of the scapula and the scapular cartilage.

Method. The hao chen is inserted in a caudal and ventral direction 2–3 tsun or the hot needle is inserted 8 fen to 1 tsun.

Indication. Paralysis of the nerves of the scapular region, arthritis of the shoulder joint, rheumatism of the forelimb.

FL3. Middle of Shoulder *Po Chung* (Figs. 3–28, 3–29).

Location. At the intersection of the cranial margin of the scapular muscle and the dorsal margin of the brachiocephalicus muscle.

Method. The hao chen is inserted in a caudal and ventral direction 3 tsun, or a hot needle is inserted 1 to 1.5 tsun.

Indication. Paralysis of the nerves of the scapular region, arthritis of shoulder and elbow, rheumatism of the upper portion of the forelimb, myositis of the sternobrachio-cephalicus muscle.

FL4. Shoulder Fence *Po Lan* (Figs. 3–28, 3–30).

Location. At the anterior margin of the scapula, midway between FL2 and FL3.

Method. The hao chen is inserted 3–4 tsun in a caudal and ventral direction, or a hot needle is inserted 1 tsun.

Indication. Same as FL2.

Note: In other sources (see p. 74), this point is said to be located where FL5 is.

FL5. Door of Lung *Fei Men* (Figs. 3–28, 3–30).

Location. The depression at the caudal border of the scapular cartilage in the middle of the neck.

Method. Hao chen is inserted 1–1.5 tsun or a hot needle is inserted 8 fen to 1 tsun.

Indication. Bronchitis, paralysis of the suprascapular nerve, arthritis of the shoulder, rheumatism of the forelimb.

Note: In other sources (see p. 73), this point is said to be located where FL4 is.

FL6. Lung Approach *Fei P'an* (Figs. 3–28, 3–30, 3–37, 3–38).

Location. The cleft between the caudal margin of the scapula and the underlying rib. The distance between FL5 and FL6 is the same as between FL2 and FL4.

Method. Hao chen is inserted 2 tsun or a hot needle 1 tsun.

Indication. Same as FL5.

°FL7. Wind Chase *Ch'ang Feng* (Figs. 3–28, 3–29, 3–37, 3–38, 3–39).

Location. Five tsun caudal and ventral to the shoulder joint in the deepest area, at the intersection of the plane between the long head and the lateral head of the triceps muscle and the deltoid muscle. This is an important point in the fore-limb.

Method. Hao chen is inserted 2–3 tsun, or a hot needle 1.8–2.3 tsun.

Indication. Twisted shoulder joint, rheumatism of forelimb, arthritis of forelimb, strained elbow muscle, paralysis of the ulnar nerve, paralysis of the nerves in the scapular region, strained biceps muscle, twisted elbow joint. Acupuncture analgesia (see pp. 260–263).

°FL8. Celestial Rush *Ch'ung T'ien* (Figs. 3–28, 3–29, 3–37, 3–38).

Location. The depression caudal and dorsal to FL7. The distance between FL7 and FL8 is equal to the distance between FL8 and FL10.

Method. Hao chen is inserted 2–2.5 tsun or a hot needle 1.2–1.5 tsun.

Indication. Same as FL7.

°FL9. Shoulder Chastity *Chien Cheng* (Figs. 3–28, 3–29).

Location. Cranial to FL8 in the muscle cleft at the caudal margin of the scapula.

Method. Hao chen is inserted 2–2.5 tsun.

Indication. Same as FL7.

FL10. Celestial Ancestry *T'ien Ts'ung* (Figs. 3–28, 3–29).

Location. The point between the middle third and the ventral third segments of a line joining the middle of the upper margin of the scapular cartilage and FL7. It is located in the muscle cleft at the caudal margin of the scapula.

Method. Hao chen is inserted 2 tsun.

Indication. Same as FL7.

°FL11. Shoulder Well *Chien Ching* (Figs. 3–28 to 3–30, 3–37, 3–38).

Location. In the depression of the lateral dorsal border of the shoulder joint at the ventral extension line of the scapular spine.

Method. A hot needle is inserted in a caudal and ventral direction 1–1.5 tsun, or hao chen 2–2.5 tsun.

Indication. Twisted shoulder joint, strained biceps muscle, rheumatism of the forelimb, arthritis of the shoulder, myositis of the sternobrachiocephalicus muscle, paralysis of the suprascapular nerve.

FL12. Shoulder Solemnity *Chien Yu* (Figs. 3–28, 3–30, 3–37, 3–38).

Location. The depression cranial and ventral to the shoulder joint.

Method. A hot needle is inserted in a caudal and ventral direction 5–8 fen, along the cranial border of humerus.

Indication. Same as FL11.

FL13. Outside Shoulder God *Chien Wai Yu* (Figs. 3–28, 3–30, 3–37, 3–38).

Location. Cranial and ventral to FL9 in the depression at the caudal margin of the shoulder joint.

Method. Hao chen is inserted 2–2.5 tsun, or a hot needle 1–1.2 tsun.

Indication. Same as FL11.

FL14. Elbow God *Chou Shu* (Figs. 3–28 to 3–30, 3–34, 3–37, 3–38).

Location. Cranial and dorsal to the tip of the elbow, in the depression at the junction of middle third and caudal third of the straight line joining FL7 and the tip of the elbow.

Method. Hao chen is inserted 2–2.5 tsun, or a hot needle 1–1.5 tsun.

Indication. Twisted elbow joint, rheumatism of the forelimb, arthritis of the elbow.

FL15. Gas Releasing *Chia Ch'i* (Fig. 3–34B).

Location. The middle of the axilla or the muscular groove of the upper part of the forearm at the center of the medial surface and the trunk.

Method. The affected limb is lifted forward and outward. The skin along the point is cut and the chia ch'i needle is directed backward and upward 7–8 tsun. The needle is then withdrawn and the limb is swayed several times.

Indication. Chronic shoulder lameness, paralysis of scapular nerves.

FL16. Pectoral Hall *Hsiung T'ang* (Fig. 3–34B).

Location. The subcutaneous median vein located

ventral to the biceps muscle tendon on the medial side of the forelimb.

Method. Use the middle, wide needle; quickly pierce the vein 3 fen deep. Bleed 300–500 cc.

Indication. Acute shoulder joint twist, acute elbow muscle sprain, acute biceps tendon sprain, intercostal and shoulder pain, indigestion, edematous inflammation of the forelimb, acute rheumatism of the shoulder and arm.

FL17. Eye of Knee *Hsi Yen* (Figs. 3–28, 3–34B).

Location. In the depression slightly lateral to the middle of the lower margin of the cranial surface of the carpal joint.

Method. The medium, wide needle is used with a quick insertion 2–3 fen to release edematous fluid.

Indication. Carpal synovitis, arthritis of the carpal joint.

FL18. Knee vein *Hsi Mai* (Figs. 3–28, 3–35B).

Location. The blood vessel cranial to the tendon of the 4th carpal bone and behind the bone 2 tsun below the ventral to the carpal point.

Method. The medium, wide needle is inserted 3 fen; bleed 100–300 cc.

Indication. Flexor tendonitis, acute arthritis of the carpal joint, carpal synovitis.

*FL19. Wrist Entangled *Ch'an Wan* (Figs. 3–28, 3–35B).

Location. On the medial and lateral digital veins, dorsal and caudal to fetlock joint. There are eight points on four limbs.

Method. The medium, wide needle is inserted 3 fen to bleed 100–300 cc.

Indication. Twisted fetlock joint.

*FL20. Hoof Head *T'i T'ou* (Figs. 3–28, 3–34B, 3–37).

Location. On the blood vessel 3 fen dorsal to the hairline of the hoof, about 4–8 fen lateral to the midline. The blood vessels in this area are relatively large and pulsate on palpation. The points on the front feet are more lateral than those on the hind feet.

Method. The medium, wide needle is inserted quickly 3 fen to bleed 300–500 cc.

Indication. Inflammation of coronary corium, in-

flammation of laminar corium, twisted fetlock joint, compression injury of hoof, colic pain.

FL21. Hoof Door *T'i Men* (Figs. 3–28, 3–35A).

Location. At the midpoint of the cartilages of the hoof, one on the medial and one on lateral side of the hoof.

Method. A small, wide needle is used in a straight insertion for 3 fen. Bleed 100–300 cc.

Indication. Pain in the hollow of the heel, inflammation of coronary corium; inflammation of laminar corium.

FL22. Front Depression (Celestial Balance) *Ch'ien Chiu (T'ien P'ing)* (Figs. 3–35A, 3–37).

Location. The pit in the hollow depression at the middle of the caudal surface of the hoof.

Method. A medium, wide needle is inserted 3 fen to slightly bleed.

Indication. Pain of the hollow of heel.

*FL23. Three Yang Vein *San Yan Lo* (Figs. 3–37, 3–39).

Location. In the muscle groove, 2 tsun below the tubercle of the radius for the lateral ligament, lateral to the forearm.

Method. See p. 260.

Indication. See pp. 260–263.

*FL24. Night Eye *Yeh Yan* (Fig. 3–39).

Location. Medial side of the forelimb, equivalent to the site of the "chestnut" (probably a little cranial to the chestnut).

Method. See p. 260.

Indication. See pp. 260–263.

Trunk (T)

T1. Wither Armor *Ch'i Chia* (Figs. 3–28, 3–30, 3–31).

Location. On the midline 1.5 tsun cranial to the highest point of the wither, between the 3rd and the 4th thoracic vertebrae.

Method. Hao chen is inserted 3 tsun.

Indication. Cough, asthma.

T2. Hundred Meetings *Pai Hui* (Figs. 3–28 to 3–31, 3–40, 3–43).

Location. At the depression above the lumbosacral space. This is an important point for the thoracic and hindlimb region.

Method. Hao chen is inserted about 2.5 tsun, or a hot needle 1.5–1.7 tsun.

Indication. Lumbar rheumatism, twisted pelvic joint,

spasm of bowel, intestinal dilatation, diarrhea, paralysis of the hindquarter; common cold, stroke, tetanus.

T3. Kidney God *Shen Shu* (Fig. 3–31).

Location. A straight line is drawn from T2 to the tuber coxae, the most prominent area of the external wing of the ilium. Locate a point on this line ⅔ of the distance from T2. From this point, draw a line parallel to the dorsal spines of the vertebrae. Points T3 to T8 are located on this line. On the lateral side of T2, on the line, is T3. Use the distance between T2 and T3 (about 2 tsun) to measure and locate T4 caudal to and T5 cranial to T3. In the same manner, measure from T5 cranially and locate T6, T7, and T8.

Method. A hot needle is inserted 1–1.5 tsun; hao chen, 2 tsun.

Indication. Lumbar rheumatism, paralysis of loin and hindquarter.

T4. Kidney Horn *Shen Chiao* (Fig. 3–31). See T3 for location, method, and indication.

T5. Kidney Bubble *Shen Chi* (Figs. 3–28, 3–31). See T3 for location, method and indication.

T6. Hind Waist *Yao Hou* (Figs. 3–28, 3–31). See T3 for location, method, and indication.

T7. Middle Waist *Yao Chung* (Figs. 3–28, 3–31). See T3 for location, method, and indication.

T8. Front Waist *Yao Ch'ien* (Figs. 3–28, 3–31). See T3 for location, method, and indication.

T9(A–D). Eight Cellars *Pa Chiao* (Figs. 3–28, 3–31, 3–40).

T9A. Upper Cellar *Shang Chiao* (Figs. 3–28, 3–31, 3–40).

Location. From the lateral side of the tail root, draw a straight line parallel to and 1.5 tsun lateral to the dorsal spines of the sacrum. T9(A) is located on this line at the intersection of a perpendicular line drawn from the area between the 1st and 2nd sacral vertebrae (S_1 and S_2). In this manner, T9 (B–D) are located at the intersection of a perpendicular line drawn from the area between S_2 and S_3; S_3 and S_4; and S_4 and S_5.

Method. A hot needle is inserted 8 fen to 1 tsun; hao chen, 1.5 tsun.

Indication. Rheumatism in the lumbar region.

T9B. Medium Cellar *Tzu Chiao* (Figs. 3–28, 3–31, 3–40). See T9A for location, method, and indication.

T9C. Middle Cellar *Chung Chiao* (Figs. 3–28, 3–31, 3–40). See T9A for location, method, and indication.

T9D. Lower Cellar *Hsia Chiao* (Figs. 3–28, 3–31, 3–40). See T9A for location, method, and indication.

*T10. Spleen God *P'i Shu* (Figs. 3–28, 3–31).

Location. In the cleft between the longissimus costarum muscle and the longissimus dorsi muscle at the level of the third intercostal space, counting cranially from the last rib.

Method. A hot needle is inserted at an angle 8 fen to 1 tsun, or hao chen, 1–1.5 tsun.

Indication. Dilatation of intestine, acid stomach, stomach disturbance, spasm of bowel.

*T11. Gate Origin God *Kuan Yuan Shu* (Figs. 3–28, 3–30, 3–31).

Location. In the depression at the intersection between the ventral margin of the longissimus dorsi muscle and the caudal edge of the last rib.

Method. Hao chen is inserted at an angle 2–2.5 tsun. Electrical stimulation is supposed to be best.

Indication. Constipation, intestinal dilatation, indigestion, stomach dilatation.

T12. Lung God *Fei Shu* (Figs. 3–28, 3–30, 3–31).

Location. In the cleft of longissimus costarum muscle and longissimus dorsi muscle at the level of the 9th intercostal space.

Method. Hao chen is inserted about 1 tsun, or a hot needle at an angle 8 fen to 1 tsun.

Indication. Cough, bronchitis, pleuritis, pneumonia.

T13. Carriage Vein *Tai Mai* (Fig. 3–28).

Location. On the blood vessel, 2 tsun caudal to the elbow.

Method. The medium, wide needle is inserted into the blood vessel to bleed 100–300 cc.

Indication. Enteritis, bowel spasm, sunstroke.

T14. Piercing Jaundice *Ch'uan Huang* (Figs. 3–28, 3–34B).

Location. At the skin fold on the lower margin of the chest on the midline.

Method. See Chapter Two on the use of the piercing jaundice needle.

Indication. Edema of the chest.

T15. Yellow Water *Huang Shui.*

Location. The ventral abdominal area caudal to the sternum and cranial to the prepuce or mammary gland.

Method. Use a large, wide needle, and avoid large blood vessels; random insertion 3 fen deep.

Indication. Edema of the chest.

T16. Cloud Door *Yun Men* (Figs. 3–28, 3–36).

Location. Five fen lateral to the midline of the abdomen and 3 tsun cranial to the umbilicus.

Method. The large, wide needle is inserted to pierce through the skin. A tube is inserted for drainage of ascitic fluid.

Indication. Ascites.

Hind Limb (HL)

HL1. Expectation Mountain *Pa Shan* (Figs. 3–28, 3–29, 3–31, 3–43).

Location. The midpoint of a line joining T2 and the medium trochanter of the femur. Bilateral.

Method. A hot needle is inserted 1–1.5 tsun; hao chen, 2 tsun.

Indication. Rheumatism of the hindlimb, twisted pelvic joint, myositis of biceps femoris muscle, paralysis of sciatic nerve.

HL2. Trail Thigh *Lu Ku* (Figs. 3–28, 3–29, 3–31, 3–43).

Location. Two tsun caudal and ventral to HL2.

Method. Same as HL1.

Indication. Same as HL1.

*HL3. Resident Bone *Chu Liao* (Figs. 3–28 to 3–30).

Location. At the depression of the inferior margin of the gluteal muscles and anterior to the medium trochanter of the femur.

Method. Hao chen is inserted 2–2.5 tsun.

Indication. Same as HL1.

*HL4. Jumping Circle *Huan T'iao* (Figs. 3–28 to 3–30, 3–43).

Location. At the depression of the inferior margin of the gluteal muscles and anterior to the medium trochanter of the femur.

Method. Same as HL3.

Indication. Same as HL1.

*HL5. Middle Circle *Huan Chung* (Figs. 3–28, 3–29, 3–31).

Location. Cranial and dorsal to the medium trochanter of the femur. In the furrow of muscles, at the midpoint of a line joining the tuber coxae of the ilium and the posterior margin of the thigh.

Method. A hot needle or hao chen is inserted 1.6–1.8 tsun.

Indication. Same as HL1.

*HL6. Hind Circle *Huan Hou* (Figs. 3–28 to 3–31).

Location. Cranial and dorsal margin of the greater trochanter of the femur, and caudal and ventral to HL5.

Method. A hot needle or hao chen is inserted 1.5–1.7 tsun.

Indication. Same as HL1.

HL7. Great Mount *Ta K'ua* (Figs. 3–28 to 3–30, 3–43).

Location. In the depression cranial and ventral of the medium trochanter of the femur.

Method. A hot needle or hao chen is inserted 1–1.5 tsun.

Indication. Same as HL1.

HL8. Lesser Mount *Hsiao K'ua* (Figs. 3–28 to 3–30, 3–43).

Location. At the depression caudal and ventral to the 3rd trochanter of the femur.

Method. Same as HL7.

Indication. Rheumatism of the hindlimbs; infection of the biceps femoris muscle; paralysis of the femoral, tibial and fibular nerves; myositis of the biceps femoris.

*HL9. Evil Ch'i *Hsieh Ch'i* (Figs. 3–28, 3–29, 3–31, 3–41, 3–43).

Location. In the muscle cleft between the biceps femoris muscle and the semitendinosus, 2 tsun dorsal to the tuber ischii.

Method. A hot needle is inserted 1.5 tsun, or hao chen 2 tsun.

Indication. Same as HL1.

*HL10. Meeting Yang *Hui Yang* (Figs. 3–28, 3–29, 3–31).

Location. At the upper terminal end of the muscle

furrow between the biceps femoris muscle and the semitendinosus.

Method. Same as HL3.

Indication. Same as HL1.

°HL11. Sweat Furrow *Han Kou* (Figs. 3–28, 3–29, 3–41, 3–43).

Location. About 3 tsun ventral to HL9 in the same furrow. It forms an equilateral triangle with HL9 and the middle trochanter of the femur.

Method. Same as HL9.

Indication. Same as HL1.

°HL12. Imbricated Tiles *Yi Wa* (Figs. 3–28, 3–29, 3–43).

Location. About 3 tsun below HL11 along the same muscle furrow.

Method. Same as HL9.

Indication. Same as HL1.

HL13. Bounded Kidney *Ch'ien Shen* (Figs. 3–28, 3–29, 3–41 to 3–43).

Location. About 2 tsun below HL12 in the muscle furrow. Slightly higher than HL14.

Method. Same as HL9.

Indication. Rheumatism of the hindlegs, arthritis of the hindlegs.

°HL14. Flipping Grass *Lueh T'ao* (Figs. 3–28, 3–30, 3–42).

Location. In the depression between the middle and lateral patellar ligaments at the cranial and ventral margin of the knee cap.

Method. Hao chen is inserted at a caudal and dorsal angle 1.5 tsun.

Indication. Twisted knee, rheumatism of the knee, arthritis of the knee.

°HL15. Kidney Mansion *Shen T'ang* (Figs. 3–35A, 3–35C).

Location. At the saphenus veins about 4 tsun below the fold on the thigh.

Method. A medium, wide needle is quickly inserted 3 fen. Bleed 300–500 cc.

Indication. Twisted pelvic joint, twisted knee.

°HL16. Crooked Bond *Ch'u Ch'ih* (Figs. 3–28, 3–35C, 3–42).

Location. At the saphenous vein, slightly medial and cranial to the tarsal joint.

Method. A medium, wide needle is inserted 3 fen to bleed 100–300 cc.

Indication. Swelling and pain in the tarsal joint.

°HL17. Hind Sea *Hou Hai* (Fig. 3–35A).

Location. In the depression ventral to the tailhead and dorsal to the anus.

Method. A hot needle is inserted in a dorsal and cranial direction for 2–2.5 tsun.

Indication. Diarrhea and gaseous dilation of the intestine.

HL18. Root of Tail *Wei Ken* (Figs. 3–28, 3–30, 3–31, 3–40, 3–43).

Location. In the depression between the 1st and 2nd coccygeal vertebrae.

Method. The tail is swung to locate the area between the movable and nonmovable vertebral joints. A straight insertion is made using a hot needle 4–5 fen, or hao chen 1 tsun.

Indication. Lumbar rheumatism, rheumatism of the hindlimbs, arthritis of the hindlimbs and lumbar region.

HL19. Tail Foundation *Wei Pen* (Figs. 3–28, 3–35A, 3–43).

Location. At the tail vein, two tsun from the tailhead.

Method. A medium, wide needle is inserted upward into the blood vessels 3 fen to bleed.

Indication. Twisted lumbosacral region, twisted gluteal region.

HL20. Tail of Tail *Wei Chien* (Figs. 3–28, 3–29).

Location. At the tip of the tail, unpaired.

Method. A medium, wide needle is inserted 4–5 fen, or the tip of the tail is cut with a cross line.

Indication. Seizure, sunstroke.

HL21. See FL19.

HL22. See FL20.

HL23. See FL21.

HL24. Hind Depression (Celestial Depression) *Hou Chiu (T'ien Chiu)* (Fig. 3–35A).

Location. The pit in the hollow depression at the middle of the caudal surface of the hoof.

Method. A medium, wide needle is inserted 3 fen to slightly bleed.

Indication. Pain of the hollow of heel.

CATTLE

Chinese Veterinary Handbook[3] *(Figs. 3–44 to 3–48)*

Head and Neck (HN)

°HN1. Celestial Gate *T'ien Men* (Figs. 3–44, 3–47).

Location. In the depression slightly caudal to the midpoint of a line joining the roots of the two horns. Single point.

Method. A medium, wide needle is inserted in caudal and ventral direction, 5–8 fen.

Indication. Congestion of cerebral vessels, epilepsy.

°HN2. Tip of Ear (Blood Print) *Erh Chien* (*Hseuh Yin*) (Fig. 3–47).

Location. On the dorsal tip of the three parallel blood vessels on the medial surface of the ear, three points on each ear.

Method. A medium, wide needle is inserted into blood vessels to bleed.

Indication. Sunstroke, abdominal pain, cold.

°HN3. The Great Yang *T'ai Yang* (Figs. 3–44, 3–45).

Location. On the blood vessel, 1 tsun caudal to the lateral canthus.

Method. A medium, wide needle is inserted into blood vessel 3–5 fen, to bleed.

Indication. Conjunctivitis, keratitis, sunstroke, cold.

HN4. Brightened Sight (Swift Sight) *Ching Ming* (*Ching Ling*) (Figs. 3–44, 3–45).

Location. At the lower margin of the upper eyelid, inside the medial canthus.

Method. A small, wide needle is inserted caudal and ventral, 1.5–2 fen.

Indication. Conjunctivitis, keratitis.

°HN5. Root of the Mountain (Middle of Man) *Shan Ken* (*Jen Chung*) (Figs. 3–44, 3–45, 3–48).

Location. There are 3 points, one at the middle of the upper margin of the hairless area of the nose. The other two are on the dorsal surface of each nostril.

Method. A small, wide needle is inserted 2–3 fen.

Indication. Sunstroke, cough, intestinal pain.

HN6. Middle Nose (Three Gates) *Pi Chung* (*San Kuan*) (Figs. 3–44, 3–45, 3–48).

Location. At the middle of a line joining the medial edges of the nostrils.

Method. A small, wide needle is inserted 2–3 fen for bleeding.

Indication. Loss of appetite, epidemic fever.

HN7. Thoroughfare Gate (Knowing Sweat, Tongue Bottom) *T'ung Kuan* (*Chih Kan, She Ti*) (Fig. 3–34A).

Location. On the blood vessels at the lateral sides of the ventral surface of the tongue.

Method. The tongue is pulled out and turned upside down. A small, wide needle or prism needle is inserted about 1.5 fen. Bleed.

Indication. Loss of appetite, laryngitis, sunstroke.

HN8. Receiving Fluid (Fate Tooth) *Ch'eng Chiang* (*Ming Ya*) (Figs. 3–44, 3–48).

Location. On the middle of the lower lip at the border of the hairy and nonhairy areas.

Method. A medium, wide needle is inserted in a caudal and dorsal direction 2–3 fen. Bleed.

Indication. Inflammation of oral mucosa, laryngitis, stomach and intestinal disturbances.

HN9. *Gate Switch* (Tooth Gate) *K'ai Kuan* (*Ya Kuan*) (Figs. 3–44, 3–45).

Location. At the rostral margin of the masseter muscle, slightly caudal and dorsal to the last molar.

Method. A medium, wide needle is inserted 5–8 fen.

Indication. Trismus.

°HN10. Neck Vein (Large Vein) *Ching Mai* (*Tai Mai*) (Figs. 3–44, 3–45).

Location. On the large blood vessel 2 tsun ventral to the larynx.

Method. The vessel is held off and the large, wide needle is inserted 3–5 fen. Bleed.

Indication. Pneumonia, cerebral vessel congestion, sunstroke, acute poisoning.

Forelimb (FL)

°FL1. Shoulder Well (Middle Arm, Collide Arm) *Chien Ching* (*Chung Po, Ch'uang P'ang*) (Figs. 3–44 to 3–46).

Location. In the depression dorsal and lateral to the shoulder joint.

Method. A medium (or small), wide needle or hot needle is inserted ventral and caudal direction 1–1.5 tsun.

Indication. Twisted shoulder joint, front limb rheumatism, front limb arthritis, myositis of the front limb and shoulder.

°FL2. Wind Chase (Medium Wrist) *Ch'ang Feng* (*Chung Wan*) (Figs. 3–44, 3–45).

Location. In the depression caudal and ventral to the shoulder joint, in the deepest part of the depression formed by the long head and lateral head of the triceps and deltoid.

Method. A medium, wide needle or hot needle is inserted 1–2 tsun.

Indication. Same as FL1.

FL3. Elbow God (Lower Wrist) *Chou Shu (Hsia Wan)* (Figs. 3–44, 3–45).

Location. 2.5 tsun caudal and ventral to FL2.

Method. A medium, wide needle or hot needle is inserted 1 tsun.

Indication. Swelling, rheumatism, or arthritis of carpus.

FL4. Pectoral Hall *Hsiung T'ang* (Figs. 3–44, 3–45, 3–48).

Location. On the blood vessel, lateral to the sternum and cranial to the axillary fossa.

Method. A medium, wide needle is inserted into the blood vessel 3–5 fen. Bleed.

Indication. Shoulder pain, twisted shoulder.

***FL5.** Hind Wrist (Chasing Wind) (Crooked Pond) *Wan Hou (Chiu Feng)* (Chu Chih) (Figs. 3–44, 3–45).

Location. On the caudal surface of the carpus slightly medial to the midpoint.

Method. Medium, (or small) wide needle, 5–8 fen.

Indication. Rheumatism or arthritis of front limb, twisted front limb.

FL6. Eye of Knee *Hsi Yen* (Figs. 3–44, 3–48).

Location. Slightly lateral to the cranial and ventral margin of the carpus joint.

Method. A medium, wide needle is inserted in a caudal direction 3 fen.

Indication. Carpitis.

FL7. Knee Vein *Hsi Mai* (Figs. 3–44, 3–45).

Location. On the blood vessel, 2 tsun ventral to the carpus on the medial side.

Method. A medium, wide needle is inserted 3 fen into the blood vessel.

Indication. Rheumatism of the carpus.

FL8. Wrist Entangled (Son of Ankle) *Ch'an Wan (Ch'un Tzu)* (Figs. 3–44, 3–45).

Location. In the depression, about 5 fen dorsal and medial or lateral to the accessory digits. One point at each surface of each limb for a total of 8 points.

Method. A medium, wide needle is inserted into the blood vessel 5–8 fen. To bleed or release synovial fluid.

Indication. Twisted fetlock joint.

FL9. Swelling Well *Yung Ch'uan* (Front Limb) (Figs. 3–44, 3–45, 3–48).

Location. At the middle of the cranial surface of the foot slightly dorsal to the joining of the digits.

Method. A medium, wide needle is inserted in a caudal and ventral direction 3 fen. Bleed.

Indication. Twisted fetlock joint, inflammation of coronary corium.

***FL10.** Hoof head (Eight Point) *T'i T'ou (Pa Tzu)* (Figs. 3–44, 3–45, 3–48).

Location. At the junction of the hairy and the non-hairy area of each digit at the middle of the cranial surface.

Method. A medium, wide needle is inserted in a ventral and caudal direction 3 fen. Bleed.

Indication. Laminitis, cold, abdominal pain.

Trunk (T)

T1. Green Field *Tan T'ien* (Figs. 3–44, 3–46, 3–47).

Location. On the midline of the back in the depression between the 1st and 2nd thoracic vertebral spines.

Method. A medium, wide needle is inserted 5–8 fen.

Indication. Sunstroke, exhaustion.

***T2.** Three Platforms *San T'ai* (Figs. 3–44, 3–46, 3–47).

Location. In the depression between the 3rd and 4th thoracic vertebral spines on the most elevated area of the withers, or in the depression caudal to the depression at the intersection point between the upward extension line of the spine of scapula and the midline of the back.

Method. A medium, wide needle is inserted 5–8 fen.

Indication. Rheumatism of the front limb, cough.

T3. Peaceful Blessing *An Fu* (Figs. 3–44, 3–46, 3–47).

Location. In the depression between the 10th and the 11th thoracic vertebral spines.

Method. A medium, wide needle is inserted 5–8 fen.

Indication. Pneumonia, diarrhea, rheumatism.

T4. Celestial Peace *T'ien P'ing* (Figs. 3–44, 3–46, 3–47).

Location. In the depression between the 13th thoracic vertebral and 1st lumbar vertebral spines.

Method. A medium, wide needle is inserted 5–8 fen.

Indication. Anuria, enteritis, loss of appetite.

T5. Hind Green Field *Hou Tan T'ien* (Figs. 3–44, 3–46, 3–47).

Location. In the depression between the 1st and the 2nd lumbar vertebral spines.

Method. A hot needle is inserted 5–8 fen.

Indication. Loss of appetite, lumbar rheumatism, hindlimb anuria.

*T6. Awakening Ch'i *Su Ch'i* (Figs. 3–44, 3–46, 3–47).

Location. There are 7 points. The unpaired point is located at the depression between the 8th and 9th thoracic vertebral spines. The 3 bilateral points are located in the 10th, 11th, and 12th intercostal spaces (or the 4th, 5th, and 6th spaces counted from caudal to cranial), slightly dorsal to the extension line from the 3 points of T13.

Method. A medium, wide needle is inserted straight 5–8 fen in bilateral points and in a cranial and ventral direction 5–8 fen in unpaired points.

Indication. Acute bronchitis, lung congestion.

*T7. Hundred Meetings (Thousand Gold) *Pai Hui (Chien Ching)* (Figs. 3–44, 3–46, 3–47).

Location. In the depression at the lumbosacral space.

Method. A medium, wide needle or hot needle is inserted 1–1.5 tsun.

Indication. Rheumatism of lumbar and hindlimb region, arthritis hindlimb joints.

*T8. Kidney God *Shen Shu* (Figs. 3–44, 3–46, 3–47).

Location. In the muscle furrow about 2.5 tsun lateral to T7.

Method. A medium, wide needle or hot needle is inserted 5 fen to 1 tsun.

Indication. Rheumatism of lumbar and hindlimb region, arthritis of the lumbar and hindlimb joints.

*T9. Middle Lumbar (Lumbar Belt) *Yiu Chung (Yiu Dai)* (Figs. 3–44, 3–46, 3–47).

Location. In the muscle cleft about 2.5 tsun lateral to the 3rd lumbar intervertebral space.

Method. A medium, wide needle is inserted 1–1.5 tsun, or a hot needle, 5–8 fen.

Indication. Lumbar rheumatism.

*T10. Carriage Vein *Tai Mai* (Figs. 3–44, 3–45).

Location. On the blood vessel about 3 tsun caudal to the elbow.

Method. A medium, wide needle is inserted 3 fen to bleed.

Indication. Enteritis, abdominal pain, cold, sun stroke.

*T11. Spleen God *Pi Shu* (Figs. 3–44, 3–46).

Location. In the muscle cleft between the longissimus dorsi and longissimus costarum muscles at the 11th intercostal space (or 3rd, counted from caudal to cranial).

Method. A medium, wide needle or hot needle is inserted in a ventral direction 1–1.5 tsun.

Indication. Gaseous distension of stomach, abdominal pain, loss of appetite.

T12. Lung God *Fei Shu* (Fig. 3–47).

Location. In the 9th right intercostal area (or 5th, counted from caudal to cranial) at the muscle cleft of the longissimus dorsi and longissimus costarum muscles. Single point, on right side only.

Method. A medium, wide needle is inserted in a ventral direction, 1–1.5 tsun.

Indication. Cough, lung congestion.

*T13. Six Vein *Liu Mai* (Figs. 3–44, 3–46, 3–47).

Location. In the 10th, 11th, and 12th intercostal spaces (or 1st, 2nd, and 3rd caudal to cranial) at the muscle cleft of the longissimus dorsi and longissimus costarum muscles; three points on each side. Another name for the most anterior point on each side is T11, *Pi Shu.*

Method. A medium, wide needle is inserted in a ventral direction 5–8 fen (see also T11).

Indication. Loss of appetite, gaseous distension of stomach (see also T11).

*T14. Knee God (Ch'i Needle) *Ch'ien Shu (Ch'i Chien)* (Figs. 3–44, 3–45).

Location. At the middle of the left para lumbar fossa; single point on left side only.

Method. A syringe with a regular hypodermic needle is inserted in a ventral direction 1–3 tsun to release gas.

Indication. Gaseous distension of rumen.

*T15. Dripping Bright *T'i Ming* (Fig. 3–44).

Location. On the blood vessel at the depression, 5 tsun cranial and 4 tsun lateral to the umbilicus.

Method. A medium, wide needle is inserted 3 fen to bleed.

Indication. Gaseous distension.

T16. Gate of Sea (Cloud Door) *Yuen Men (Hai Men)* (Figs. 3–44, 3–45).

Location. 1 tsun lateral to the umbilicus.

Method. A medium, wide needle is used to cut through the skin.

Indication. Ascites.

T17. Piercing Yellow (Hanging Yellow) *Ch'uan Huang (Teil Huang)* (Figs. 3–44, 3–45, 3–48).
Location. On the skin fold at the middle of the cranial margin of the sternum.
Method. See Chapter Two for the use of the piercing jaundice needle.
Indication. Edema of the chest.

Hind Limb (HL)

*HL1. Middle Circle *Huon Chung* (Figs. 3–44 to 3–46).
Location. In the muscle cleft, anterior and superior to the major trochanter.
Method. A hot needle is inserted 1.6–1.8 tsun.
Indication. Twisted pelvic joint, hindlimb rheumatism, arthritis of hindlimb joints.

*HL2. Hind Circle *Huan Hou* (Figs. 3–44 to 3–46).
Location. At the cranial and dorsal edge of the major trochanter of the femur, and caudal and ventral to HL1.
Method. A hot needle is inserted straight 1.5–1.7 tsun.
Indication. Same as HL1.

HL3. Evil Ch'i (Yellow Gold) *Hsieh Ch'i (Huang Chin)* (Figs. 3–44, 3–45).
Location. In the muscle cleft between the biceps femoris and the semitendenous muscles and dorsal to the ischium.
Method. A hot needle is inserted 1 tsun.
Indication. Same as HL1.

*HL4. Sweat Furrow *Hun Kou* (Figs. 3–44, 3–45).
Location. In the muscle cleft between the biceps femoris and semitendenous muscles and ventral to the ischium.
Method. Same as HL3.
Indication. Same as HL1.

HL5. Imbricated Tile (Pulling Legs) *Yi Wa (Ch'ih Chiao)* (Figs. 3–44, 3–45).
Location. In the muscle cleft 2 tsun below HL4.
Method. Same as HL3.
Indication. Same as HL1.

HL6. Flipping Grass *Lueh Ts'ao* (Figs. 3–44 to 3–46).
Location. In the depression ventral and slightly lateral to the stifle joint.
Method. A hot needle is inserted in a caudal and dorsal direction 8 fen.
Indication. Twisted stifle joint, hindlimb rheumatism, arthritis of hindlimb joints.

*HL7. Pectoral Hall *Shen T'ang* (Figs. 3–35A, 3–35C).
Location. On the blood vessel at the upper portion of the medial surface of the hindlimb.
Method. A medium, wide needle is inserted 3 fen to bleed.
Indication. Twisted pelvic or stifle joint, painful and swollen hindlimb.

HL8. Crooked Pond (Supporting Mountain) *Ch'u Ch'ih (Cheng Shan)* (Fig. 3–44).
Location. On the blood vessel, cranial and slightly medial to the stifle joint.
Method. A medium, wide needle is inserted 3–5 fen to bleed.
Indication. Rheumatism or arthritis of the stifle joint.

HL9. Root of Tail *Wei Ken* (Figs. 3–44, 3–46).
Location. On the midline in the depression cranial to the tailhead, at the sacrococcygeal junction.
Method. A medium, wide needle or hot needle is inserted 3 fen.
Indication. Constipation.

HL10. Tail Foundation *Wei Pen* (Figs. 3–44, 3–45).
Location. On the tail vein at the midline on the ventral surface of the tailhead.
Method. A medium, wide needle is inserted 3 fen to bleed.
Indication. Abdominal pain, constipation.

HL11. Tip of Tail (Pearls Dangling) *Wei Chien (Ch'ui Chu)* (Figs. 3–44, 3–45).
Location. At the tip of the tail.
Method. A medium, wide needle is inserted 3 fen to bleed.
Indication. Sunstroke, overexhaustion.

HL12. Hind Sea (Inner Nest) *Hou Hai (Chiao Ch'ao)* (Figs. 3–44, 3–45).
Location. At the depression on the midline midway between the tailhead and anus.
Method. A hot needle is inserted in a cranial and dorsal direction 1–1.5 tsun.
Indication. Diarrhea, constipation.

HL13. Dripping Water *Ti Shui* (Figs. 3–44, 3–45, 3–48).
Location. At the middle of the cranial surface of the foot, slightly dorsal to the joining of the digits.
Method. A medium, wide needle is inserted in a caudal and ventral direction 3 fen to bleed.
Indication. Twisted fetlock joint, inflammation of coronary corium.

PIG

Chinese Veterinary Handbook[3] *(Figs. 3–49 to 3–64)*

Head and Neck (HN)

°**HN1.** Celestial Gate *T'ien Men* (Figs. 3–50, 3–51).

Location. At the middle of the occipital fossa—that is, the depression at the middle of the line joining the caudal margin of the roots of the two ears.

Method. Hao chen is inserted in a caudal and ventral direction 3–5 fen.

Indication. Epilepsy, encephalitis, wheezing, sunstroke, tetanus, cerebral congestion.

°**HN2.** Tip of the Ear (Bloody Print) *Erh Chien (Hsueh Yin)* (Figs. 3–49 to 3–52).

Location. At the blood vessel 1 tsun away from the pointed edge on the medial surface of the ear. Three points on each ear.

Needle sensation. Feeling of excitement, sense of comfort.

Method. Scratch the skin; bleed about 50 cc.

Indication. Sunstroke, cold, abdominal pain, fever, food poisoning.

HN3. Ear Proper *K'a Erh* (Figs. 3–49 to 3–51, 3–53).

Location. The middle of the proximal part of the ear.

Method. A medium, wide needle is inserted 6–8 fen, either from the lateral or the medial surface of the ear. Blood vessels should be avoided, and drugs may be injected in the subcutaneous site.

Indication. Cold, fever.

HN4. The Great Yang *T'ai Yang* (Figs. 3–50, 3–51, 3–53).

Location. Eight fen to 1 tsun caudal to the lateral canthus.

Method. A small, wide needle is inserted 3 fen to bleed.

Indication. Common cold, influenza, keratitis, epilepsy, fever.

HN5. Brain God (Brain Transparency) *Nao Shu (T'au Nao)* (Figs. 3–51, 3–53).

Location. At the rostral and dorsal margin of the mandibular joint in the suture between the squamous temporal bone and the parietal bone, rostral and dorsal to HN4.

Method. Hao chen is inserted in a caudal and ventral direction 1–2 tsun.

Indication. Encephalitis, epilepsy, cold.

HN6. Brightened Sight (Swift Sight) *Ching Ming (Ching Ling)* (Figs. 3–50, 3–51, 3–53).

Location. In the depression below the medial canthus.

Method. Hao chen is inserted in a ventral direction 3 fen.

Indication. Conjunctivitis, keratitis, influenza, abdominal pain.

°**HN7.** Eye God *Ching Yu* (Figs. 3–50, 3–51, 3–53).

Location. At the middle of the dorsal curved margin of the snout and 5 fen to the right and left. Three points.

Method. A small, wide needle is inserted 2–3 fen.

Indication. Sunstroke, cold, stroke, indigestion, rheumatism, asthma.

HN9. Middle Nose (Nose Mountain) *Pi Chung (Pi Liang)* (Fig. 3–49).

Location. At the midpoint between the nostrils.

Method. A small, wide needle is inserted 2–3 fen to bleed.

Indication. Loss of appetite, fever.

HN10. Jade Mansion *Yu T'ang* (Fig. 3–33A; see also HN15—Horse).

Location. At right and left midlines of the hard palate.

Method. The mouth is opened and a small, wide needle is inserted 3 fen at an angle from the corner of the mouth to bleed.

Indication. Gastritis, lingual ulcer, fever.

HN11. Holding Chin *So K'ou* (Figs. 3–49 to 3–51, 3–53).

Location. 5 fen caudal to the corner of the mouth.

Method. Hao chen is inserted in caudal and dorsal direction 5 fen to 1 tsun.

Indication. Trismus, facial palsy, swollen chin.

HN12. Gate Switch (Gate of Teeth) *K'ai Kuan (Ya Kuan)* (Figs. 3–49 to 3–51, 3–53).

Location. At the anterior margin of the masseter muscle, or the midpoint between the last pair of upper and lower molars—that is, at the intersection between a perpendicular line from the lateral canthus and the extension line from the mouth.

Method. Hao chen is inserted in a caudal direction 5 fen to 1 tsun.

Indication. Same as HN11.

*HN13. Wind Pond *Feng Ch'in* (Fig. 3–49).

Location. In the depression behind the ears at both sides of the ligamentum nuchae.

Method. Hao chen is inserted in a ventral direction 3–5 fen.

Indication. Cold, fever, sunstroke.

HN14. Yellow Neck *Ching Huang* (Fig. 3–49).

Location. At the midpoint between mandible and shoulder joint.

Method. A medium, wide needle is inserted 6–8 fen; drug may be injected in the subcutaneous site.

Indication. Cold, rheumatism, fever.

HN15. Receiving Fluid *Cheng Chiang* (Figs. 3–50, 3–51, 3–53).

Location. At the middle of the lower lip at the junction between the hairy and the non-hairy areas; at the depression, 5 fen below the lip, the needle is inserted on the oricularis oris muscle.

Method. A small, wide needle or prism needle is inserted in a caudal and dorsal direction (at the direction of the root of the tongue) 3–5 fen until blood is seen.

Indication. Indigestion, gastritis, oral mucosal ulcer.

HN16. Door of Ear *Fan Men* (Figs. 3–50, 3–51, 3–53).

Location. At the depression between the parotid gland and the base of the ear.

Method. Hao chen is inserted in a slightly ventral direction 5–10 fen.

Indication. Common cold, influenza, sunstroke, epidemic fever.

HN17. Locked Larynx *So Hou* (Figs. 3–50, 3–51, 3–53).

Location. Slightly caudal to the first tracheal ring, in the muscle.

Method. Hao chen is inserted horizontally at the same level as the shoulder joint 5–10 fen. It should be particularly cautioned that the needle not be inserted into the trachea.

Indication. Laryngitis, laryngeal paralysis.

HN18. Door of Ear *Ehr Men* (Figs. 3–50, 3–51, 3–53).

Location. At the depression below the root of the ear at the upper border of the parotid gland and posterior border of the mandible.

Method. Hao chen is inserted in a ventral direction 5–8 fen.

Indication. Facial palsy.

HN19. Root of Ear *Erh Ken* (Figs. 3–50, 3–51, 3–53).

Location. In the depression slightly caudal to the caudal margin of the ear.

Method. Hao chen is inserted in a ventral direction 5–8 fen.

Indication. Sunstroke, influenza, general malaise, fever.

Forelimb (FL)

*FL1. Wind Chase (Shoulder God) *Ch'ang Feng (Kuang Shu)* (Figs. 3–49 to 3–51, 3–56).

Location. Three tsun caudal to the shoulder joint in the muscle furrow of the caudal margin of the deltoid muscle, between the long and lateral heads of the triceps.

Method. Hao chen is inserted 1 tsun.

Indication. Twisted front limb, rheumatism or arthritis of front limb.

FL2. Celestial Rush *Ch'ung T'ien* (Fig. 3–49).

Location. In the muscle cleft 1.5 tsun dorsal to FL1.

Method. Same as FL1.

Indication. Same as FL1.

FL3. Elbow God *Chou Yu* (Fig. 3–49).

Location. In the depression 5 fen cranial to the elbow.

Method. Same as FL1.

Indication. Same as FL1.

FL4. Seven Stars *Ch'i Hsing* (Fig. 3–58).

Location. There are 5 or 7 black spots caudal to the fetlock joint. The needle is inserted into the middle black spot.

Method. The forelimb is raised and hao chen is inserted 2–3 fen.

Indication. Rheumatism, bronchitis, indigestion, painful and swollen ankle, food poisoning (for ½ month to 2 month old pig, this point is most frequently used).

*FL5. Wrist Entangled (Son of Ankle) *Ch'an Wan (Ch'un Tsu)* (Figs. 3–49 to 3–51, 3–55B, 3–57, 3–58).

Location. In the depression lateral and medial to the dewclaw. Two points on each of the limbs.

Method. A small, wide needle is inserted 3–5 fen into blood vessels to bleed.

Indication. Arthritis and rheumatism of the fetlock joint, twisted fetlock joint.

*FL6. Swelling Well *Yung Chuan* (Figs. 3–49 to 3–51, 3–55A, 3–57B).

Location. On the cranial midline 3 fen dorsal to the hoof bifurcation.

Method. A small, wide needle is inserted into the blood vessel to bleed.

Indication. Rheumatism and arthritis of fetlock joint, twisted fetlock joint, cold, loss of appetite, sunstroke, laminitis, abdominal pain.

FL7. Hoof Head (Letter 8) *T'i T'ou (Pa Tzu)* (Fig. 3–49).

Location. Three fen from the midline at two sides of the hoof bifurcation at the junction between the hairy and the nonhairy keratin of the hoof.

Method. A small, wide needle is inserted 2–3 fen to bleed.

Indication. Twisted hoof, painful swelling of hoof, abdominal pain.

FL8. Body Pillar *Shen Chu* (Figs. 3–49 to 3–51).

Location. At the depression between the 3rd and 4th thoracic vertebrae.

Method. Hao chen is inserted 1–1.5 tsun.

Indication. Encephalitis, epilepsy, influenza, cough, bronchitis.

FL9. Tip of Shoulder (Shoulder Well) *Po Chien (Chien Ch'ung)* (Figs. 3–50, 3–51, 3–54).

Location. At the cranial angle of the scapula in the depression 1.5 tsun from the vertebral column.

Method. The needle is inserted 8–10 fen in a ventral and caudal direction at 15 degrees.

Indication. Front limb paralysis, pain in the thorax and shoulder, paralysis of the scapular region.

FL10. Shoulder Fence (Middle Shoulder) *Po Lan (Chien Chung)* (Figs. 3–50, 3–51, 3–54).

Location. At the caudal angle of the scapula in the depression 2.5 tsun from the vertebral column.

Method. Hao chen is inserted 2.5 tsun in a cranial and ventral direction at 15 degrees.

Indication. Same as FL9.

FL11. Gate of Wind *Fei Men* (Figs. 3–50, 3–51, 3–54).

Location. At the cranial border of the scapular bone.

Method. Hao chen is inserted 8–10 fen in a caudal direction at 15 degrees.

Indication. Rheumatism of the shoulder, pneumonia, emphysema.

FL12. Lung Approach *Fei P'an* (Figs. 3–50, 3–51, 3–54).

Location. Cranial and ventral to FL10. The needle is inserted at the upper third of the caudal border of the trapezius muscle into the long head of the triceps muscle.

Method. Hao chen is inserted 8–10 fen in a cranial and ventral direction at a 15-degree angle.

Indication. Same as FL11.

FL13. Front Leg Hoof Fork *Chien T'i Ch'a* (Figs. 3–50, 3–57).

Location. At the middle of the upper end of the hoof bifurcation. There are four points.

Method. Hao chen is inserted in a caudal and ventral direction 2–3 fen.

Indication. Pain in the hoof, paralysis, rheumatism and arthritis in the four limbs.

FL14. Lamp Stand *Deng Chan* (Fig. 3–57).

Location. In the depression at the middle of the two dewclaws.

Method. Hao chen is inserted in a dorsal direction 2–3 fen.

Indication. Laminitis, paralysis.

FL15. Gate of Hoof *T'i Men* (Fig. 3–57).

Location. In the depression, slightly dorsal to the corium on the two sides of the hoof cleft.

Method. A small, wide needle is inserted in a cranial direction 2–3 fen to bleed.

Indication. Inflammation of the hooves, indigestion, abdominal pain, constipation, sunstroke, bladder retention.

Trunk (T)

*T1. Great Vertebrae *Ta Chui* (Figs. 3–49 to 3–51).

Location. On the midline between the vertebral spines of the 6th and 7th cervical vertebrae and at the level of the cranial margin of the scapula.

Method. Hao chen is inserted 1.5 tsun in a slightly cranial and ventral direction.

Indication. Asthma, cold, hematuria, vomiting, epilepsy.

T2. Three Platforms *San T'ai* (Figs. 3–49 to 3–51).

Location. On the dorsal midline at the depression between the 2nd and 3rd thoracic vertebral spines at the level of the caudal border of scapula.

Method. Same as T1.

Indication. Rheumatism and arthritis of front limbs, a twisted front limb.

°T3. Awakening Chi *Su Ch'i* (Figs. 3–49 to 3–51).

Location. There are 7 points, 3 bilateral and 1 unpaired, on the dorsal midline in the depression between the spines of the 4th and the 5th thoracic vertebrae. Three are at the 7th, 8th, and 9th intercostal spaces counted from caudal to cranial in the cleft of the longissimus costarum muscle.

Method. Hao chen is inserted in a slightly cranial and ventral direction 1.5 tsun for the unpaired one. Hao chen is inserted 5–8 fen for the other bilateral points.

Indication. Cold, pneumonia, asthma, cough.

°T4. Hundred Meetings (Thousand Gold) *Pai Hui* (*Chien Ching*) (Figs. 3–49 to 3–51).

Location. In the depression immediately behind the lumbosacral junction.

Method. Hao chen is inserted 8 fen to 1 tsun.

Indication. Rheumatism of lumbar and hindlimb regions, motor dysfunction of the hindlimbs, anurea and constipation, paralysis, wheezing, rectal prolapse.

T5. Upper Cellar (T6A) *Shang Tzu* (Fig. 3–49).

T6. Middle Cellar (T6B) *Chung T'zu* (Fig. 3–49).

T7. Lower Cellar (T6C) *Hsia T'zu* (Fig. 3–49).

Location. In the pelvic region at the intersection of a line extending from the area in between the 1st and 4th sacral vertebral spines laterally and the horizontal line of the sacroiliac joint. The 1st point (T5) is lateral to the 1st and 2nd sacral vertebral spaces, the middle point (T6) lateral to the 2nd and 3rd, and the last point (T7) lateral to the 3rd and 4th.

Method. Hao chen is inserted 1 tsun.

Indication. Rheumatism and arthritis of hindlimb, rheumatism of the lumbar and hindlimb region, paralysis of hindlimb, lack of sexual drive, urine retention, urogenital diseases.

T8. Wind Release *Kai Feng* (Figs. 3–49 to 3–51).

Location. A depression between the 3rd and the 4th sacral vertebral spines or the 3rd depression caudal to T5.

Method. Hao chen is inserted 5 fen to 1 tsun.

Indication. Rheumatism and arthritis of the hindlimb; gastritis, constipation, urogenital and gastrointestinal diseases.

°T9. Lung God *Fei Shu* (Figs. 3–49 to 3–51).

Location. At the intersection of a line extended from the sacroiliac (parallel to the spine) and the 6th intercostal space (counted from caudal to cranial).

Method. Hao chen is inserted in a ventral direction 5–8 fen.

Indication. Asthma, cough, cold, rhinitis, bronchitis, pulmonary congestion.

°T10. Six Veins *Liu Mai* (Figs. 3–49 to 3–51).

Location. At the 1st, 2nd, and 3rd intercostal spaces counted from caudal to cranial in the muscle cleft between the longissimus dorsi and longissimus costarum muscles.

Method. Hao chen is inserted 5–8 fen.

Indication. Gastritis.

°T11. Platform Middle *T'an Chung* (Figs. 3–49, 3–59, 3–60).

Location. On the ventral midline between the two front limbs.

Method. Hao chen is inserted in a cranial and dorsal direction 2–3 fen.

Indication. Asthma, cough, pneumonia, abdominal pain, spasm.

°T12. Middle Channel *Chung Wan* (Figs. 3–49 to 3–51, 3–60).

Location. On the ventral midline at the midpoint between the caudal border of the sternum and the umbilicus.

Method. Hao chen is inserted 2–3 fen or moxibustion for 3–5 min.

Indication. Gastritis, acid stomach, cough.

T13. Upper Channel *Shang Wan* (Figs. 3–49 to 3–51, 3–60).

Location. On the ventral midline at the midpoint between the caudal corner of sternum and T11.

Method. Same as T11.

Indication. Same as T11.

T14. Lower Channel *Hsia Wan* (Figs. 3–49 to 3–51).

Method. Same as T11.

Indication. Same as T11.

T15. Celestial Control (Gate of Sea) *T'ien Shu (Hai Men)* (Figs. 3–49 to 3–51).

Location. 1 tsun lateral to the umbilicus.

Method. Hao chen is inserted 5 fen to 1 tsun.

Indication. Diarrhea in baby pig, anuria.

T16. Supernatural Tower *Ling Tai* (Figs. 3–50, 3–51).

Location. On the dorsal midline in the depression between the 5th and the 6th thoracic vertebral processes.

Method. Hao chen is inserted 5 fen to 1.5 tsun.

Indication. Rheumatism of scapular muscles, paralysis of the shoulder.

T17. Liver God *Kan Shu* (Figs. 3–50, 3–51).

Location. In the 4th intercostal space counted from caudal to cranial, in the muscle cleft between the longissimus dorsi and longissimus costarum muscles.

Method. Hao chen is inserted 6–10 fen at a 45-degree angle in a caudal and posteroventral direction.

Indication. Hepatitis, eye diseases, indigestion.

T18. Spleen God *Pi Shu* (Fig. 3–59).

Location. At the intercostal space, counting from caudal to cranial and in the muscle cleft between the longissimus dorsi and longissimus costarum muscles two tsun from the midline, unpaired on the left side.

Method. Hao chen is inserted at a 45-degree angle in a ventral direction.

Indication. Indigestion, diaphragmatic spasm, distention of stomach and intestine.

T19. Interrupted Blood *Tuan Hsueh* (Figs. 3–50, 3–51).

Location. On the midline in the last thoracic and 1st two lumbar intervertebral spaces.

Method. Hao chen is inserted 5–8 fen.

Indication. Hemorrhage after castration, hematuria, blood in stool.

T20. Door of Kidney *Shen Men* (Figs. 3–50, 3–51).

Location. On the midline cranial to T4 in the depression between the 3rd and 4th lumbar vertebrae.

Method. Hao chen is inserted 5–10 fen.

Indication. Rheumatism of the lumbar region, anuresis, inflammation of the bladder, indigestion.

T21. Hind Knot *Hou Ger Dai* (Fig. 3–61).

Location. At the subcutaneous tendon cranial to the stifle joint.

Method. A small, wide needle is inserted at the subcutaneous location of the tendon.

Indication. Constipation, gaseous distension.

T22. Yang Light *Yang Ming* (Figs. 3–50, 3–51, 3–61).

Location. Five fen lateral to the most caudal two pairs of nipples. There are four points.

Method. Hao chen is inserted 5–6 fen in a cranial direction.

Indication. Bladder retention, mastitis.

Hind Limb (HL)

HL1. Middle Circle *Huan Chung* (Figs. 3–49, 3–51).

Location. Cranial and dorsal to the greater trochanter of the femur in the muscle cleft at the midpoint of a line joining the most elevated area of the tuber coxae and the caudal extremity of the thigh.

Method. Hao chen is inserted 1 tsun.

Indication. Rheumatism of the hindlimb, arthritis of the hindlimb.

HL2. Hind Circle *Huan Hou* (Fig. 3–49).

Location. At the caudal and dorsal margin of the greater trochanter of the femur, caudal and slightly ventral to HL1.

Method. Same as HL1.

Indication. Same as HL1.

HL3. Sweat Furrow *Hon Kou* (Fig. 3–49).

Location. In the muscle cleft between the bicep femoris and semitendinosus muscles slightly ventral to the sciatic notch.

Method. Same as HL1.

Indication. Same as HL1.

HL4. Crooked Pond *Chu Ch'ih* (Fig. 3–49).

Location. At the blood vessel, cranial and slightly medial to the tarsal joint.

Method. A small, wide needle is inserted 3 fen into the blood vessel to bleed.

Indication. Swollen pain of the tarsal joint.

HL5. Four Great Wind Gate *Tzu Ta Feng Men* (Fig. 3–60).

Location. On the front limb at the tip of the posterior margin in the scapular bone; on the hindlimb at the tip of the angle of the ilium.

Method. The small, wide needle is inserted 3 tsun. On the forelimb the needle is inserted subcutaneously vertically along the posterior margin of the scapula bone. On the hindlimb, the needle is inserted subcutaneously vertically toward the knee along the angle of the ilium.

Indication. Paralysis of front limb and hindlimb.

HL6. Final Three Miles *Hou San Li* (Figs. 3–50, 3–51, 3–62, 3–64).

Location. Lateral to the tibia in the depression formed by the muscle cleft, 2 tsun below the patella.

Method. Hao chen is inserted 5–8 fen caudal to the depression in the area between the tibia and fibula.

Indication. Indigestion, loss of appetite, diarrhea, abdominal pain, hindlimb paralysis.

HL7. Greater Hind *Ta K'ua* (Figs. 3–50, 3–51).

Location. At the muscle cleft on the cranial margin of the biceps femoris muscle, caudal and ventral to the greater trochanter.

Method. Hao chen is inserted 5–10 fen.

Indication. Pain, paralysis and rheumatism of the hindlimbs.

HL8. Lesser Hind *Shiao K'ua* (Figs. 3–50, 3–51).

Location. In the muscle cleft on the cranial margin of the biceps femoris muscle 1 tsun cranial and ventral to HL7.

Method. Hao chen is inserted 5–10 fen.

Indication. Rheumatism and paralysis of hindlimbs.

HL9. Flipping Glass *Lieh Ts'ao* (Figs. 3–50, 3–51).

Location. In the depression underneath the patella.

Method. Hao chen is inserted 5–6 fen in a caudal direction; moxibustion is used on the needles.

Indication. Rheumatism of the knee, contusion, crippling.

HL10. Gate of Hoof *T'i Men* (Fig. 3–57A).

Location. In the depression slightly dorsal to the corium on the two sides of the hoof cleft (same as FL15).

Method. A small, wide needle is inserted in a cranial direction 2–3 fen to bleed.

Indication. Inflammation of the hooves, indigestion, abdominal pain, constipation, sunstroke, bladder retention.

HL11. Root of Tail *Wei Ken* (Figs. 3–49 to 3–51).

Location. On the dorsal midline in the depression between the 4th sacral and the 1st coccygeal vertebrae.

Method. Hao chen is inserted 2–3 fen.

Indication. Rheumatism and arthritis of the lumbar region and hindlimbs, indigestion, constipation, influenza.

HL12. Tail Foundation *Wei Pen* (Figs. 3–49 to 3–51, 3–63).

Location. At the blood vessel about 5 fen from the tailhead at the middle of the ventral surface of the tail.

Method. A small, wide needle is inserted 2–3 fen to bleed.

Indication. Rheumatism and arthritis of the lumbar region and hindlimbs, sunstroke, urine retention, abdominal pain.

°HL13. Tip of Tail *Wei Chien* (Figs. 3–49 to 3–51, 3–63).

Location. On the ventral midline 5 fen from the tip of the tail.

Method. The tip of the tail is raised and a small, wide needle is inserted through the tip to bleed.

Indication. Sunstroke, fever, abdominal pain, loss of appetite.

HL14. Tail Notch *Wei Chieh* (Figs. 3–50, 3–51).

Location. On the dorsal midline in the depression between the 1st and the 2nd coccygeal vertebrae, a vertebral segment caudal to Wei Ken (HL11). When the tail is raised, the unpaired point is located at the middle of the second skin fold.

Method. Hao chen is inserted 3–5 fen.

Indication. Constipation, anuresis, rheumatism and arthritis of the hindlimb, common cold.

HL15. Tail Trunk *Wei Kan* (Figs. 3–50, 3–51).

Location. In the depression between the 2nd and 3rd coccygeal vertebrae, a vertebral segment caudal to Wei Chien (HL13). When the tail is raised, the unpaired point is located at the middle of the 3rd skin fold.

Method. Same as HL13. In clinical application, HL12, HL13, and HL14 are prescribed as a group.

Indication. Same as HL13.

HL16. Yin God *Yin Shu* (Figs. 3–62, 3–63).

Location. On the midline located between the vagina and the anus (female), or in the middle of the anal opening (male).

Method. Hao chen is inserted 3–5 fen.

Indication. Cystitis, urine retention.

HL17. Inner Nest (Hind Sea) *Chiao Ch'ao (Hou Hai)* (Figs. 3–49 to 3–51, 3–63).

Location. On the midline at the depression, cranial and medial to the tarsal joint.

Method. Hao chen is inserted to 5 fen in a caudal direction.

Indication. Rheumatism and arthritis of the tarsal joint, indigestion, gastroenteritis.

HL19. Hind Leg Hoof Fork *Hou T'i Ch'a* (Figs. 3–50, 3–57B).

Location. At the middle of the upper end of the hoof bifurcation. There are four points (same as FL13).

Method. Hao chen is inserted 2–3 fen in a caudal and ventral direction.

Indication. Hoof pain, paralysis, rheumatism and arthritis in the four limbs.

HL20. Lamp Stand *Deng Chan* (Fig. 3–57A).

Location. In the depression at the middle of the two dewclaws (same as FL14).

Method. Hao chen is inserted 2–3 fen in a dorsal direction.

Indication. Laminitis, paralysis.

HL21. Letter Eight *Pa Tzu* (Figs. 3–50, 3–51, 3–57B, 3–64).

Location. At the midpoint of the border of the

hairy and nonhairy areas of the hoof (same as FL7).

Method. A small, wide needle is inserted 2–3 fen in a ventral direction to bleed.

Indication. Rheumatism and arthritis of four limbs, paresis, contusion, abdominal pain, influenza, sunstroke.

HL22. Dripping Water *T'i Shui* (Figs. 3–49 to 3–51, 3–55A, 3–57B).

Location. On the cranial midline 3 fen dorsal to the bifurcation of the hoof (same as FL6).

Method. A small, wide needle is inserted into the blood vessel to bleed.

Indication. Rheumatism and arthritis of fetlock joint, twisted fetlock joint, cold, loss of appetite, sunstroke, laminitis, abdominal pain.

HL23. Wrist Entangled (Son of Ankle) *Ch'an Wan (Ch'un Tsu)* (Figs. 3–49 to 3–51, 3–55A, 3–57A and B, 3–58).

Location. In the depression lateral and medial to the dewclaw; two points on each of the limbs (same as FL5).

Method. A small, wide needle is inserted 3–5 fen into blood vessels to bleed.

Indication. Arthritis and rheumatism of fetlock joint, twisted fetlock joint.

GOAT

Chinese Veterinary Handbook[3] *(Figs. 3–65 to 3–70)*

Head and Neck Region (HN)

HN1. Celestial Gate *T'ien Men* (Fig. 3–68).

Location. At the occipital fossa where the hair is spirally arranged; unpaired.

Method. A hot needle or hao chen is inserted 2–3 fen in a caudal and ventral direction, or moxibustion is used 10–15 min.

Indication. Epilepsy.

HN2. Thorough Heaven *Tung T'ien* (Figs. 3–67, 3–68).

Location. The midpoint of a line joining the proximal ends of ears.

Method. A hot needle or hao chen is inserted 5 fen in a caudal and ventral direction, or moxibustion is used for 3 min.

Indication. Paralysis of the facial muscles, epilepsy.

*HN3. Tip of Ear (Bloody Print) *Erh Chien (Hsueh Yin)* (Figs. 3–65, 3–68).

Location. On the blood vessel of the medial surface of the ear, 1 tsun from the distal end of the ear.

Method. The prism needle or small, wide needle is inserted until blood is seen.

Indication. Sunstroke, cold, abdominal pain, gaseous distension.

HN4. The Greater Yang *T'ai Yang* (Figs. 3–65, 3–66).

Location. On the blood vessel 5 fen caudal to the lateral canthus.

Method. The vein is held off. A small, wide needle or prism needle is inserted 1–2 fen until blood is seen.

Indication. Conjunctivitis, keratitis.

HN5. Brightened Sight (Swift Sight) *Ching Ming (Ching Ling)* (Figs. 3–65, 3–66).

Location. In the depression rostral and ventral to the medial canthus; bilateral.

Method. Hao chen is inserted 3 fen in a ventral direction.

Indication. Conjunctivitis.

HN6. Three Rivers *San Chiang* (Figs. 3–65, 3–66, 3–70).

Location. On the blood vessel about 5 fen below the medial canthus.

Method. A small, wide needle is inserted 3 fen until blood is seen.

Indication. Abdominal pain.

°HN7. God of Nose (Over the Mountain) *Pi Yu (Kuo Liang)* (Figs. 3–65, 3–66, 3–70).

Location. Slightly dorsal to the nostril.

Method. Hao chen or a prism needle is inserted horizontally, piercing through the nostril until blood is seen.

Indication. Cold, cough.

°HN8. Root of Mountain (Watery River) *San Ken (Shui K'ou)* (Fig. 3–70).

Location. At the middle of the hairy and the non-hairy junction of the mouth and nostril area.

Method. A small, wide needle or hao chen is inserted 2–3 fen.

Indication. Cold, sunstroke, abdominal pain, loss of appetite.

HN9. Outer Lip Ying *Wai Ch'un Ying* (Fig. 3–70).

Location. In the middle of the philtrum, below HN8.

Method. A small, wide needle is inserted 2 fen.

Indication. Loss of appetite.

°HN10. Inner Lip Ying *Nei Ch'un Ying* (Fig. 3–68).

Location. On the blood vessel at the ventral surface of the upper lip.

Method. A prism needle is inserted 2 fen until blood is seen.

Indication. Loss of appetite, abdominal pain.

HN11. Jade Mansion *Yu T'ang* (Fig. 3–33A).

Location. Three fen, lateral to the midline of the 3rd ridge of the hard palate inside the mouth.

Method. A prism needle is inserted at an angle 1 fen to bleed.

Indication. Loss of appetite, vomiting.

HN12. Thoroughfare Gate *T'ung Kuan (Chih Kan, She Ti)* (Fig. 3–34A).

Location. On the blood vessel lateral to the midline on the ventral surface of the tongue.

Method. The tongue is pulled out and turned up-side down, and a prism needle is inserted 2 fen until blood is seen.

Indication. Loss of appetite, ulcer of the tongue.

Forelimb Region (FL)

FL1. Shoulder Well (Middle Arm, Collide Arm) *Chien Ching (Chung Po, Ch'uang P'ang)* (Figs. 3–65 to 3–67, 3–70).

Location. In the depression dorsal to the shoulder joint.

Method. Hao chen or a hot needle is inserted 8 fen in a ventral direction.

Indication. Twisted shoulder joint; rheumatism, arthritis, or myositis of front limb.

°FL2. Wind Chase (Medium Wrist) *Ch'ang Feng (Chung Wan)* (Figs. 3–65, 3–66).

Location. Caudal to the shoulder joint in the muscle cleft formed by the caudal margin of the deltoid muscle, of the long head, and of the lateral head of the triceps muscle.

Method. Hao chen or a hot needle is inserted 5 fen to 1 tsun.

Indication. Same as FL1.

FL3. Elbow God (Lower Wrist) *Chou Yu (Hsia Wan)* (Figs. 3–65 to 3–67).

Location. In the depression dorsal to the elbow.

Method. A hot needle is inserted 3 fen.

Indication. Pain in the elbow.

FL4. Eye of Knee *Hsi Yen* (Figs. 3–65, 3–66, 3–70).

Location. In the depression slightly lateral to the cranial margin of the carpus.

Method. A small, wide needle is inserted in a dorsal direction 2–3 fen.

Indication. Swollen carpus.

°FL5. Wrist Entangled (Son of Ankle) *Ch'an Wan (Ch'un Azu)* (Figs. 3–65 to 3–67, 3–70).

Location. In the depression lateral and dorsal to the dewclaw, one point on the medial and lateral side.

Method. A small, wide needle is inserted 2–3 fen to bleed.

Indication. Rheumatism of the fetlock joint, twisted fetlock joint.

FL6. Swelling Well *Yung Chuan* (Figs. 3–65, 3–66, 3–70).

Location. On the cranial surface slightly dorsal to the joining of the claws.

Method. A small, wide needle is inserted 2 fen in

a caudal and ventral direction until blood is seen.

Indication. Loss of appetite, abdominal pain, gaseous distension.

°FL7. Hoof Head *T'i T'ou* (Figs. 3–65, 3–70).

Location. On the blood vessels at the lateral and medial side of the foot slightly above the hairline of the hooves.

Method. A small, wide needle is inserted 2 fen in a caudal and ventral direction until blood is seen.

Indication. Loss of appetite, abdominal pain, gaseous distension, infection of the hooves.

Trunk Region (T)

°T1. Hundred Meetings (Thousand Gold) *Pai Hui (Chien Ching)* (Figs. 3–65 to 3–68).

Location. At the lumbosacral space.

Method. Hao chen or a hot needle is inserted 4–5 fen.

Indication. Rheumatism of lumbar region or hindlimb; arthritis of hindlimb, diarrhea.

°T2. Lung God *Fei Shu* (Figs. 3–65 to 3–68).

Location. In the 6th intercostal area (counted from caudal to cranial) in the muscle cleft of the longissimus dorsi and longissimus costarum muscles.

Method. Hao chen or a hot needle is inserted 3–5 fen in a ventral direction.

Indication. Asthma, cough.

T3. Awakening Chi *Su Ch'i* (Figs. 3–65, 3–68).

Location. In the 4th and 5th intercostal area (counted from caudal to cranial) in the muscle cleft of the longissimus dorsi and longissimus costarum muscles.

Method. Hao chen or a hot needle is inserted 4 fen in a ventral direction, or moxibustion is used.

Indication. Same as T2.

°T4. Spleen God *P'i Shu* (Figs. 3–65, 3–68).

Location. In the 3rd intercostal area, counted from caudal to cranial, in the muscle cleft of the longissimus dorsi and longissimus costarum muscles.

Method. Hao chen or a hot needle is inserted 5 fen in a ventral direction.

Indication. Diarrhea, gaseous distension, loss of appetite.

T5. Abdominal God (Abdominal Corner) *Ch'ien Shu (Tu Chiao)* (Fig. 3–65).

Location. At the middle of the left paralumbar fossa.

Method. A regular hypodermic needle is inserted 1–2 tsun for the drainage of gas.

Indication. Gaseous distension of the rumen.

T6. Kidney God *Shen Shu* (Figs. 3–66, 3–68).

T7. Kidney Horn *Shen Chiao* (Figs. 3–66, 3–68).

T8. Kidney Bubble *Shen Cha* (Figs. 3–66, 3–68).

Location. On a line from T1 and the tuber coxae of the ilium ⅔ of the distance from T1, draw a line parallel to the spine. T6, T7, and T8 are located on this line. Lateral to T1 is T6. The distance between T1 and T6 is taken as the distance caudad to locate T7 and craniad to locate T8.

Method. Hao chen or a hot needle is inserted 4–5 fen.

Indication. Rheumatism, arthritis, or pain of the lumbar region, myositis of the lumbar muscles.

T9. Front Umbilicus *Ch'i Ch'ien* (Fig. 3–69).

Location. On the ventral midline 1 tsun cranial to the umbilicus.

Method. Hao chen is inserted 3 fen, or moxibustion is used.

Indication. Diarrhea, loss of appetite, constipation.

T10. Middle Umbilicus (Door of Abdomen) *Ch'i Chung (Tu K'ou)* (Fig. 3–69).

Location. In the middle of the umbilicus.

Method. No needle insertion; moxibustion is used for 10–15 min.

Indication. Diarrhea, stomach pain, loss of appetite.

°T11. Celestial Control (Gate of Sea) *T'ien Shu (Hai Men)* (Fig. 3–69).

Location. One tsun lateral to the umbilicus.

Method. Hao chen is inserted 2–3 fen.

Indication. Diarrhea, gaseous distension.

T12. Behind Umbilicus *Ch'i Hou* (Fig. 3–69).

Location. On the ventral midline 1 tsun caudal to the umbilicus.

Method. Hao chen is inserted 2–3 fen, or moxibustion is used for 10–15 min.

Indication. Diarrhea, intestinal pain.

Hind Limb Region (HL)

°HL1. Middle Circle *Huan Chung* (Figs. 3–65, 3–66).

Location. At the midpoint of a line joining the tuber coxae and the tuber ischii.

Method. A hot needle or hao chen is inserted 5–6 fen.

Indication. Rheumatism, arthritis, or myositis of the hindlimb; twisted hindlimb.

*HL2. Hind Circle *Huan Hou* (Figs. 3–65, 3–66).

Location. Caudal and ventral to HL1, or cranial and dorsal to the greater trochanter of the femur.

Method. A hot needle or hao chen is inserted 3–4 fen.

Indication. Same as HL1.

HL3. Evil Chi *Hsieh Ch'i* (Figs. 3–65, 3–66).

Location. One tsun lateral to the sacral vertebrae in the muscle cleft of the biceps femoris and semitendinosus muscles.

Method. A hot needle or hao chen is inserted 5 fen in a ventral and cranial inferior direction.

Indication. Rheumatism, arthritis, or myositis of hindlimb; twisted hindlimb.

HL4. Sweat Furrow *Hon Kou* (Figs. 3–65, 3–66).

Location. 1.5 tsun ventral to HL3, in the muscle cleft of the biceps femoris and semitendinous muscle.

Method. Same as HL3.

Indication. Same as HL3.

HL5. Imbricated Tiles *Yi Wa* (Figs. 3–65, 3–66).

Location. At 1.5 tsun ventral to HL4 in the muscle cleft of the biceps femoris and semitendinous muscles.

Method. Same as HL3.

Indication. Same as HL3.

HL6. Kidney Mansion *Shen T'ang* (Figs. 3–35A, 3–35C).

Location. On the blood vessel at the medial and proximal surface of the hindlimb.

Method. A small, wide needle is inserted 2–3 fen until blood is drawn.

Indication. Erythema, swelling due to twisted sacropelvic region.

*HL7. Flipping Grass *Lueh Ts'ao* (Figs. 3–65, 3–67).

Location. At the depression slightly lateral to the cranial-ventral margin of the patella.

Method. A hot needle is inserted 4–5 fen in a caudal and dorsal direction.

Indication. Pain from a swollen stifle; rheumatism, arthritis, or myositis of the hindlimb.

HL8. Crooked Pond *Ch'u Ch'ih* (Figs. 3–65).

Location. On the blood vessel cranial and slightly medial to the tarsal joint.

Method. A small, wide needle is inserted 3 fen to bleed.

Indication. Pain from a swollen tarsal joint.

HL9. Hind Sea (Inner Nest) *Hou Hai (Chiao Ch'ao)* (Fig. 3–65).

Location. On the midline in the depression below the tailhead and above the anus.

Method. Hao chen or a hot needle is inserted 1 tsun in a cranial and dorsal direction.

Indication. Constipation, gaseous distension, diarrhea.

HL10. Root of Tail *Wei Ken* (Figs. 3–65, 3–67).

Location. On the midline in the depression between the 1st and 2nd coccygeal vertebrae.

Method. Hao chen is inserted 2–3 fen in a cranial direction, or moxibustion is used for 15 min.

Indication. Diarrhea, gaseous distension, abdominal pain.

HL11. Tail Foundation *Wei Pen* (Fig. 3–65).

Location. On the blood vessel at the middle of the ventral surface of the tail, 1 tsun from the tailhead.

Method. A small, wide needle is inserted 2 fen until blood is seen.

Indication. Abdominal pain.

*HL12. Tip of Tail *Wei Chien* (Figs. 3–65, 3–67).

Location. At the tip of the tail.

Method. A small, wide needle is inserted 3 fen to draw blood.

Indication. Abdominal pain, gaseous distension, sunstroke.

HL13. Dripping Water *Ti Shui* (Figs. 3–65, 3–66, 3–70).

Location. On the cranial surface slightly dorsal to the joining of the claws.

Method. A small, wide needle is inserted 2 fen in a caudal and ventral direction until blood is seen.

Indication. Loss of appetite, abdominal pain, gaseous distension.

HL14. Hoof Head *T'i T'ou* (Figs. 3–65, 3–70).

Location. On the blood vessels at the lateral and medial side of the foot slightly above the hairline of the hooves.

Method. A small, wide needle is inserted 2 fen in a caudal and ventral direction until blood is seen.

Indication. Loss of appetite, abdominal pain, gaseous distension, infection of the hooves.

CAMEL

Chinese Veterinary Handbook[3] *(Figs. 3–71 to 3–72)*

Head and Neck (HN)

*HN1. Bright Sight *Ching Ming* (Figs. 3–71, 3–72).

Location. On the blood vessel 5 fen rostral to the medial canthus, bilateral.

Method. A small, wide needle is inserted 3 fen in a dorsal direction to bleed.

Indication. Conjunctivitis.

HN2. Three River *San Chiang* (Figs. 3–71, 3–72).

Location. On the blood vessel 1.5 tsun rostral to the medial canthus.

Method. A small, wide needle is inserted 3 fen to bleed.

Indication. Abdominal pain, conjunctivitis, keratitis.

*HN3. Hall of Mansion *Hsueh T'ang* (Fig. 3–71).

Location. On the blood vessel inside the dorsal surface of the nostril.

Method. A small, wide needle is inserted 2 fen to bleed.

Indication. Abdominal pain, running nose.

HN4. God of Nose (Sea of Ch'i) *Pi Shu (Ch'i Hai)* (Figs. 3–71, 3–72).

Location. One tsun dorsal to the nostril.

Method. A small, wide needle is inserted 5 fen to bleed.

Indication. Fever, indigestion.

HN5. Inner Bright Sight *Nei Ching Ying* (Fig. 3–33B).

Location. On the blood vessel at the inner surface of the lip, slightly off the midline; bilateral.

Method. A small, wide needle is inserted 2 fen to bleed.

Indication. Respiratory infection.

*HN6. Thoroughfare Gate *T'ung Kuan* (Fig. 3–34A; see also HN16 Horse).

Location. On the blood vessels lateral to the ventral midline of the tongue.

Method. The tongue is pulled out and a small, wide needle is inserted into the blood vessels on the ventral surface of the tongue to bleed.

Indication. Oral mucosal inflammation, abdominal pain.

*HN7. Eye Vein *Yen Mai* (Figs. 3–71, 3–72).

Location. Two tsun caudal and ventral to the lateral canthus.

Method. A small, wide needle is inserted 3 fen to bleed.

Indication. Conjunctivitis, keratitis.

*HN8. Tip of the Ear *Erh Chien* (Figs. 3–71, 3–72).

Location. On the blood vessel at the distal end of the ear.

Method. A small, wide needle is inserted 3 fen to bleed.

Indication. Cold.

*HN9. Nine Divisions *Chiu Wei* (A-I) (Fig. 3–72).

Location. HN9A is located 3 tsun behind the ear; the HN9I is located 1.5 tsun cranial to the cranial angle of the scapula. The distance between the two points is divided into 8 equal parts for the location of the 7 points along the lower margin of the rhomboideus muscle.

Method. A hot needle is inserted 1 tsun.

Indication. Rheumatism of the neck.

*HN10. Ku Mai *Ching Mai* (Figs. 3–71, 3–72).

Location. On the blood vessel, 3.5 tsun below the mandible.

Method. A large, wide needle is inserted 3 fen to bleed.

Indication. Pneumonia, fever.

Forelimb (FL)

FL1. Tip of Shoulder *Po Chien* (Figs. 3–71, 3–72).

Location. At the cranial angle of the scapula.

Method. A hot needle is inserted 1.5 tsun.

Indication. Rheumatism of the front limb, arthritis of joints of front limbs.

FL2. Shoulder Fence *Po Lan* (Figs. 3–71, 3–72).

Location. Three tsun below FL1.

Method. A hot needle is inserted 1.5 tsun.

Indication. Rheumatism of neck muscles and shoulder, arthritis of neck.

*FL3. Wind Chase *Ch'ang Feng* (Figs. 3–71, 3–72).

Location. In the depression 4 tsun below the shoulder joint.

Method. A hot needle is inserted 2 tsun.

Indication. Twisted shoulder joint, strained muscles of shoulder and carpus, rheumatism or arthritis of the front limb.

*FL4. Celestial Rush *Chung T'ien* (Figs. 3–71, 3–72).

Location. In the depression 3.5 tsun caudal and dorsal to FL3.

Method. A hot needle is inserted 1.5 tsun.

Indication. Twisted shoulder joint, rheumatism or arthritis of the shoulder, thoracic and shoulder pain.

FL5. Gas Releasing *Chia Ch'i* (Fig. 3–34B).

Location. At two lateral sides of the cranial end of the sternum in the axillary fossa.

Method. The sick limb is lifted and dragged forward and outward; the skin along the point is cut and the chia ch'i needle is inserted backward and upward 7–8 tsun. The needle is then withdrawn and the limb is swayed several times.

Indication. Chronic shoulder lameness, paralysis of the scapular nerve.

°FL6. Pectoral Hall *Hsiung T'ang* (Fig. 3–34B; see also FL16 Horse).

Location. On the blood vessel cranial and lateral to the sternum.

Method. A medium, wide needle is inserted 3 fen to bleed.

Indication. Twisted shoulder joint, pain in the thorax and shoulder region.

°FL7. Wrist Entangled *Ch'an Wan* (Figs. 3–71, 3–72).

Location. On the blood vessel between the tendon and cone, slightly dorsal to the fetlock joint on the lateral side.

Method. A medium, wide needle is inserted 3 fen to bleed.

Indication. Twisted fetlock joint.

FL8. Swelling Well *Yung Ch'uan* (Fig. 3–71).

Location. At the dorsal surface of the foot between the toes.

Method. A medium, wide needle is inserted 3 fen in a ventral direction to bleed.

Indication. Painful, swollen foot.

Trunk (T)

°T1. Front Mountain *Ch'ien Fen* (Figs. 3–71, 3–72).

Location. Cranial and ventral to the front hump, and 3 tsun caudal and dorsal from FL1.

Method. A hot needle is inserted 1.5 tsun.

Indication. Rheumatism or arthritis of front limb and neck regions.

T2. Green Field *T'an T'ien* (Figs. 3–71, 3–72).

Location. On the midline between the two humps, at the 2nd depression cranial to the posterior hump.

Method. A hot needle is inserted 1.5 tsun.

Indication. Rheumatism of the lumbar region, arthritis of vertebral joints, seizures.

°T3. Hundred Meetings *Pai Hui* (Figs. 3–71, 3–72).

Location. On the midline in the depression between the lumbar and sacral vertebrae.

Method. A hot needle is inserted 2 tsun.

Indication. Rheumatism of lumbar region and hindlimb, arthritis of vertebral and hip joints, diarrhea, abdominal pain, constipation.

°T4. Lung God *Fei Shu* (Figs. 3–71, 3–72).

Location. At the 5th intercostal area (counting from caudal to cranial) in the muscle cleft of the longissimus dorsi and longissimus costarum muscles.

Method. A hot needle is inserted 1 tsun.

Indication. Asthmatic bronchitis.

°T5. Spleen God *Pi Shu* (Figs. 3–71, 3–72).

Location. At the 3rd intercostal area (counting from caudal to cranial) in the muscle cleft of the longissimus dorsi and longissimus costarum muscles.

Method. A hot needle is inserted 1 tsun.

Indication. Indigestion, abdominal pain, gaseous distension.

°T6. Kidney God *Shen Shu* (Figs. 3–71, 3–72).

Location. Two tsun lateral and slightly cranial and ventral to T3.

Method. A hot needle is inserted 1 tsun.

Indication. Rheumatism of lumbar region and limbs, arthritis of lumbar vertebral joints.

°T7. Kidney Bubble *Shen Cha* (Figs. 3–71, 3–72).

Location. Two tsun cranial to T6.

Method. A hot needle is inserted 1 tsun.

Indication. Same as T6.

T8. Hind Waist *Yao Hou* (Figs. 3–71, 3–72).

Location. Two tsun cranial to T7.

Method. A hot needle is inserted 1 tsun.

Indication. Same as T6.

°T9. Carriage Vein *Tai Mai* (Fig. 3–71).

Location. Two tsun behind the elbow on the blood vessel at the lateral side of the rib cage.

Method. A medium, wide needle is inserted 3 fen to bleed.

Indication. Indigestion, enteritis.

T10. Cloud Door *Yun Men* (Figs. 3–71, 3–72).

Location. One tsun cranial and slightly lateral to the umbilicus.

Method. A large, wide needle is used to cut through the skin, and a drainage tube inserted.

Indication. Ascites.

Hind Limb (HL)

HL1. Hind Circle *Huan Hou* (Figs. 3–71, 3–72).

Location. In the depression behind the greater trochanter of the femur.

Method. A hot needle is inserted 1.5–2 tsun.

Indication. Rheumatism of hindlimb.

HL2. Lesser Mount *Hsia K'ua* (Figs. 3–71, 3–72).

Location. About 4 tsun below HL1, caudal and ventral to the greater trochanter of the femur.

Method. A hot needle is inserted 1–1.5 tsun.

Indication. Same as HL1.

HL3. Imbricated Tiles *Yi Wa* (Figs. 3–71, 3–72).

Location. In the muscle cleft about 3 tsun caudal and ventral to HL2.

Method. A hot needle is inserted 1–1.5 tsun.

Indication. Same as HL1.

°HL4. Sweat Furrow *Hon Kou* (Figs. 3–71, 3–72).

Location. In the muscle cleft 2 tsun dorsal to HL3.

Method. A hot needle is inserted 1–1.5 tsun.

Indication. Same as HL1.

°HL5. Kidney Mansion *Shen T'ang* (Figs. 3–35A, 3–35C; see also Horse, HL15, p. 95).

Location. The medial side of the thigh on the blood vessel, 2 tsun ventral to the abdomen.

Method. A medium, wide needle is inserted 3 fen to bleed.

Indication. Twisted lumbopelvic region.

°HL6. Flipping Grass *Lueh Ts'ao* (Figs. 3–71, 3–72).

Location. Cranial and lateral to the stifle.

Method. A hot needle is inserted 1 tsun in a caudal direction.

Indication. Twisted stifle, rheumatism of the hindlimb.

°°HL7. Hind Sea *Hou Hai* (Fig. 3–35A).

Location. On the midline in the depression between the tailhead and the anus.

Method. A hot needle is inserted 1 tsun in a cranial and slightly dorsal direction.

Indication. Twisted lumbopelvic region.

HL8. Tail Side *Wei P'ang* (Figs. 3–71, 3–72).

Location. One tsun from the anus, lateral to the tailhead.

Method. A hot needle is inserted 1 tsun in a cranial and ventral direction.

Indication. Twisted lumbopelvic region.

°HL9. Tail Foundation *Wei Pen* (Figs. 3–71, 3–72).

Location. The middle of the ventral surface of the tail, on the vein.

Method. A small, wide needle is inserted 3 fen; bleed.

Indication. Abdominal pain, twisted lumbopelvic region.

HL10. Tip of Tail *Wei Chien* (Figs. 3–71, 3–72).

Location. At tip of tail.

Method. A small, wide needle is inserted 1 tsun.

Indication. Abdominal pain.

HL11. Dripping Water (Hindlimb) *T'i Shui* (Fig. 3–71).

Location. At the dorsal surface of the foot between the toes.

Method. A medium, wide needle is inserted 3 fen in a ventral direction, to bleed.

Indication. Painful, swollen foot.

Acupuncture Points in Small Animals

DOG

Five sets of charts are presently available in the United States.[5, 15, 17, 18, 19] They are among the charts following this chapter.

The only published description of acupuncture points in the dog that contains anatomical locations, methods of needle insertion and indications for the various points was produced by Chen in 1976.[5] His work is reproduced on pages 113–118.

POINT NO.	NAME	LOCATION	ANATOMY	MANIPULATION	MAIN INDICATIONS
1	Jen chung	At upper third of philtrum	M. Levator naso-labialis, orbicularis oris A. & V. Labialis superior N. Labialis superior	Straight, about 0.5 cm depth	Shock; sunstroke
2	Pi liang	At middle of dorsal surface of nose, just at junction of skin and dorsum nasi	M. Dorsum nasi A. & V. Dorsalis nasi N. External nasi	Bleed; about 0.2–0.5 cm depth	Shock; sunstroke; sinusitis; cold; initial stage of distemper
3	Ta feng men	At middle of posterior border of occipital bone	M. Brachiocephali-cus, rectus capitis dorsalis A. & V. Occipital N. Spinal, cervical	Straight, about 1–3 cm depth	Epileptic attack; distemper; encepha-litis; tetany; convulsion
4	Shang kuan	Above mandibular articulation	M. Temporal A. & V. Temporal N. Zygomatic branch of facial n.	Straight, about 3 cm depth	Facial paralysis; deafness
5	Hsia kuan	Under mandibular articulation	M. Temporal A. & V. Temporal N. Zygomatic branch of facial n.	Straight, about 3 cm depth	Facial paralysis; deafness
6	Ching ming	At medial canthus	M. Orbicularis oculi A. & V. Angularis oculi N. Infratrochlear	Straight, push eye-ball externally about 0.2–0.5 cm depth	Conjunctivitis; keratitis; enlarge-ment of nictitating membranes
7	Cheng chi	At middle of infraorbital process	M. Orbicularis oculi A. & V. Angularis oculi N. Frontalis, infratrochlear	Straight. Push eye-ball upwards, insert about 2–5 cm along the orbit	Acute and chronic conjunctivitis; atrophy of optic nerve; retinitis; cataract
8	Erh chien	At apex of convex surface of auricula	V. Posterior auricular	Blood-shed	Shock; sunstroke; colic and spasm; cold
9	Yi feng	About 3 cm below the ear base	M. Inf. buccal A. & V. Superficial temporal N. Facial	Straight, about 1–3 cm depth	Facial paralysis; deafness
10	Ta chui	Between spinous processes of C_7–T_1	N. Spinales thoracical	Straight, about 0.5–1 cm depth	Fever; neuralgia and rheumatism; bronchitis; epilepsy
11	Tao dao	Between spinous processes of T_1–T_2	N. Spinales thoracical	Angular, slightly anterior and down-ward, about 0.5–1 cm depth	Neuralgia and sprain of shoulder and forelimb; epilepsy
12	Shen chu	Between spinous processes of T_3–T_4	N. Spinales thoracical	Angular, anterior and downward about 1–1.5 cm depth	Pneumonia; bronchitis; distem-per; sprain and neuralgia of shoulder

POINT NO.	NAME	LOCATION	ANATOMY	MANIPULATION	MAIN INDICATIONS
13	Ling tai	Between spinous processes of T_6–T_7	N.Spinales thoracical	Angular, anterior and downward, about 1–1.5 cm depth	Hepatitis
14	Chung su	Between spinous processes of T_{10}–T_{11}	N.Spinales thoracical	Straight, about 0.5–1 cm depth	Gastritis; lack of appetite
15	Chi chung	Between spinous processes of T_{11}–T_{12}	N.Spinales thoracical	Straight, about 0.5–1 cm depth	Indigestion; diarrhea; enteritis; lack of appetite
16	Hsuan shu	Between spinous processes of T_{13}–L_1	N. Spinales lumbar	Straight, about 0.5–1 cm depth	Rheumatism and sprain of loin; indigestion; enteritis; diarrhea
17	Ming men	Between spinous processes of L_2–L_3	N. Spinales lumbar	Straight, about 0.5–1 cm depth	Rheumatism and sprain of loin; chronic enteritis; hormonal imbalance; impotence; nephritis and other urinary disorders; lack of appetite
18	Yang kuan	Between spinous processes of L_4–L_5	N. Spinales lumbar	Straight, about 0.5–1 cm	Hypogonadism; endometritis; metritis; ovaritis; cystic ovary; atrophy of ovary and uterus; prolonged estrus; rheumatism and sprain of loin
19	Kuan hou	Between spinous processes of L_5–L_6	N. Spinales lumbar	Straight, about 0.5–1 cm	Endometritis; cystic ovary; cystitis; paralysis of large intestine; constipation
20	Pai hui	Between spinous processes of L_7–K_1	N. Spinal n.	Straight, about 0.5–1 cm depth	All kinds of nervous disorders: sciatica; posterior paralysis; prolapse of rectum
21	Erh yen	At dorsal sacral foramina 1, 2	N. Sacral, great sciatic	Straight, about 1–1.5 cm depth	Posterior paralysis; neuralgia
22	Wei ken	At spinous process of S_1–S_2	N. Spinales coccygeus	Straight, about 0.3–0.5 cm depth	Posterior paralysis; paralysis of tail; prolapse of anus; constipation or diarrhea
23	Wei chieh	Between the spinous processes of S_2–S_3	N. Spinales coccygeus	Straight, about 0.3–0.5 cm depth	Posterior paralysis; paralysis of tail; prolapse of anus; constipation or diarrhea
24	Woei kan	Between the spinous processes of S_3–S_4	N. Spinales coccygeus	Straight, about 0.3–0.5 cm depth	Posterior paralysis; paralysis of tail; prolapse of anus; constipation or diarrhea

POINT NO.	NAME	LOCATION	ANATOMY	MANIPULATION	MAIN INDICATIONS
25	Woei chien	At tip of tail	N. Spinales coccygeus	Straight, needle inserts from the end, about 0.5–1 cm depth	Shock; sunstroke; gastroenteritis
26	Chiao cho	Mid point between anus and tail	M. Rectococcygeus, sphincter int. & ext.	Straight, about 1–1.5 cm depth	Diarrhea; prolapse of rectum; paralysis of sphincter muscles
27	Fei yu	At 2nd intercostal space, about 10 cm down	M. Latissimus dorsi, intercostales ext. & int. A. & V. Intercostalis N. Thoracalis intercostalis	Angular, about 1–2 cm depth, along the intercostal space	Pneumonia; bronchitis; cough
28	Shin yu	At 4th intercostal space and about 25 cm downward from back	M. Intercostal A. & V. Intercostal N. Intercostal	Angular, about 1–2 cm depth; along the intercostal space	Mental stress; heart diseases
29	Kan yu	At 8th intercostal space and about 30 cm down the back	M. Obliquus admoninis externus, intercostales ext. & int. A. & V. Intercostal N. Intercostal	Angular, along the intercostal space about 1–2 cm depth	Hepatitis; jaundice; eye diseases
30	Wei yu	At 10th or last 3rd intercostal space and about 15 cm down the back	M. Obliquus abdominis externus, intercostal ext. & int. A. & V. Intercostal N. Intercostal	Angular, along intercostal space about 1–2 cm depth	Gastritis; stomach distension; indigestion; lack of appetite; enteritis
31	Shiao chang yu	At last intercostal space and about 20 cm down the back	M. Obliquus abdominis externus, intercostal ext. & int. A. & V. Intercostal N. Intercostal	Angular, along intercostal space about 1–2 cm depth	Enteritis; intestinal spasm; diarrhea
32	Pi yu	At posterior border of last rib (13th), and about 10 cm down the back	M. Obliquus abdominis ext. & int. A. & V. Lumbar, intercostal N. Lumbar, intercostal	Straight or angular, along posterior border of rib about 1–2 cm depth	Indigestion; chronic diarrhea; lack of appetite
33	Shen yu	About 5 cm lateral to point 17 (ming men)	M. Obliquus abdominis ext. and int. A. & V. Lumbar N. Lumbar	Straight, about 0.5–1 cm depth	Nephritis and other urinary disorders; polyurea; hypogonadism and other sex hormone imbalance; sterility; impotence; rheumatism and sprain of lumbar region
34	Yi yu	About 5 cm ventral to point 33	M. Obliquus abdominis ext. and int. A. & V. Lumbar N. Lumbar	Straight, about 0.5–1 cm depth	Pancreatitis; indigestion; chronic diarrhea; diabetes

POINT NO.	NAME	LOCATION	ANATOMY	MANIPULATION	MAIN INDICATIONS
35	Nuan cho	About 5 cm lateral to the 4th lumbar space (4th and 5th transverse process of lumbar vertebrae)	M. Obliquus abdominis ext. and int. A. & V. ovarian, utero-ovarian N. Ovarian	Straight, about 1.5–3 cm depth	Hypogonadism and ovary hormonal insufficiency; hypotrophy of ovary; ovaritis; cystic ovary
36	Tzu kuan	About 5 cm lateral to the 5th lumbar space	M. Obliquus abdominis ext. and int. A. & V. Utero-ovarian, uterus N. Uterus	Straight, about 1.5–3 cm depth	Cystic uterus; endometritis; metritis; hypotrophy of uterus; rheuma-tism of lumbar region
37	Pung kung yu	About 10 cm lateral to the 6th lumbar space	M. Obliquus abdominis ext. and int. A. & V. Lumbar N. Lumbar	Straight, about 0.5–1 cm depth	Cystitis; hematuria; spasm of bladder; urine retention
38	Tien shu	About 1.5–2 cm lateral to the navel	M. Obliquus abdominis ext. and int. A., V. & N. ventral lumbar	Straight, about 0.5 cm depth	Enteritis; diarrhea; abdominal pain; intestinal spasm
39.	Chung wan	Between the xyphoid process and navel	M. Linea alba A. & V. Ventralis thoracis N. Ventral thoracic	Angular, about 0.5–1 cm depth	Acute gastritis; gastrospasm; gastrorrhagia; gastralgia; dilatation of stomach; vomit-ing; dyspepsia; anorexia
40	Kung tzu	At ventral border of tuber spine of scapula, about 6 cm below the middle of cartilage	M. Deltoid, infraspinatus A. & V. Infrascapular N. Infrascapular	Angular, along tuber spine about 3–5 cm depth	Neuralgia, paralysis, and sprain of shoulder; paralysis of scapular nerve; rheumatism of shoulder
41	Chien ching	Ventral and caudal to the tuber scapulae	M. Brachiocephali-cus, supraspinatus A. & V. Scapular, brachial N. Brachial	Straight, about 2–4 cm depth	Neuralgia and paralysis of shoulder and forelimb; sprain of shoulder; paraly-sis of supraspinatus and brachial nerve
42	Chien juan	Between articular end of scapula and head of humerus	M. Deltoid, caput laterales tricipitis, brachialis A. & V. Posterior circumflex, profound brachii N. Brachii, radialis	Straight, about 2–4 cm depth	Neuralgia and paralysis of shoulder and forelimb; sprain of shoulder; paraly-sis of supraspinatus and brachial nerve
43	Chou yu	Between epicondyle of humerus and olecranon	M. Tensor fascia antibrachii, caput lateralis tricipitis A. & V. Posterior circumflex, profound brachii N. Ulna	Straight, about 2–4 cm depth	Arthritis; neuralgia; paralysis and sprain of elbow and forelimb

POINT NO.	NAME	LOCATION	ANATOMY	MANIPULATION	MAIN INDICATIONS
44	Chih shang	About 1 cm lateral to the condyloid crest	M. Brachialis, extensor carpi radialis A. & V. Brachialis N. Brachialis	Straight, about 2–3 cm depth	Sprain, neuralgia, and paralysis of forelimb; paralysis of brachial and radial nerve
45	Chih chu	Between epicondyle of humerus and fovea capituli of radius	M. Extensor carpi radialis A. & V. Radialis N. Radialis	Straight, about 2–3 cm depth	Sprain, neuralgia, and paralysis of forelimb; paralysis of brachial and radial nerve
46	Ch'ing feng	At the point between points 42 and 43, and about 1.5–2 cm caudal to the humerus	M. Tensor fasciae antibrachii, caput lateralis tricipitis A. & V. Brachialis N. Brachialis	Straight, about 2–3 cm depth	General anesthesia; nervous disorders of forelimb
47	Chien san li	At interosseous space of radius and ulna and about 4–6 cm ventral to the humeroradial joint	M. Extensor carpi radialis A. & V. Radialis N. Radialis. Interosseous	Straight, about 2–3 cm depth	Paralysis of radial and ulna nerves; neuralgia and rheumatism of forelimb
48	Wai kuan	At distal end of interosseous space of radius and ulna; about 4.5 cm dorsal to the ulna carpal bone	M. Extensor carpi radialis A. & V. Radialis N. Radialis. interrosseous	Straight, about 2–3 cm depth	Paralysis of radial and ulna nerves; neuralgia and rheumatism of forelimb
49	Yang chi	About ⅓ the distance to the junction of distal radius and radial carpal bone	M. Extensor carpi radialis A. & V. Radialis N. Radial	Straight, about 0.5–1 cm depth	Sprain of digits; neuralgia and paralysis of forelimb
50	Yang chu	At middle of distal forearm, about 2 cm dorsal to the lateral border of radial carpal bone	M. Extensor carpi radialis A. & V. Proximal collateral, dorsal radial N. Radial	Straight, about 0.5–1 cm depth	Neurologic disorders of thoracic limb; sprain of carpal tendons; paralysis of radial nerve
51	Wan ku	Lateral to the junction of ulna and ulna carpal bone	M. Extensor carpi radialis A. & V. Ulnar N. Ulnar	Straight, needle inserts from lateral side of forearm, about 0.5–1 cm depth	Neurologic disorders of thoracic limb; sprain of carpal tendons; paralysis of radial nerve
52	Pa feng	About 2 cm caudal to the cranial border of interdigital skinfold; 4 points on each leg, total 8 points	N. Dorsal common digitalis, branch of radial (foreleg); branch of superficial peroneal (hindleg)	Angular, about 1–2 cm depth	Sprain and paralysis of digits
53	Nei kuan	About 0.5 cm ventral to the carpal pad	M. Flexors A. & V. Ulnar N. Median	Straight, about 1–2 cm depth	Neurologic disorders of thoracic limb; stomach and intestinal spasm; colic

117 *Animal Acupuncture Points*

POINT NO.	NAME	LOCATION	ANATOMY	MANIPULATION	MAIN INDICATIONS
54	Huan tiao	At trochanter fossa, between trochanter major and head of femur	M. Gluteus superficialis and medius, biceps femoris A. & V. & N. Iliofemoris	Straight, about 3–5 cm depth	Posterior paralysis; neuralgia and paralysis of pelvic limb; sciatica; paralysis of femoral nerve
55	Chi shang	About 0.5 cm above the patella and 0.5 cm lateral	M. Fascia lata, biceps femoralis A. & V. Femoral N. Peroneal, femoral	Straight, about 0.5–1 cm depth	Neurologic disorders of pelvic limb
56	Chi hou	Between medial and lateral condyles	M. Fascia lata, biceps femoralis A. & V. Femoral N. Peroneal, femoral	Straight, about 0.5–1 cm depth	Neurologic disorders of pelvic limb
57	Chi shia	Between patella and tuberosity of tibia, about 0.5 cm laterally	N. Peroneal	Straight, about 0.5–1 cm depth	Sprain, neuralgia, and arthritis of knee
58	Hou san li	At interosseous space of tibia and fibula, about 5 cm ventral to the head of fibula	M. Tibialis anterior, flexor hallucis longus A. & V. Median common interosseous N. Median, Ulnar	Straight, about 1–1.5 cm depth	Posterior paralysis; neuralgia and paralysis of pelvic limb; gastroenteritis; intestinal spasm and colic
59	Chih shi	At the middle of tibia-tibial tarsal joint	N. Superficial peroneal	Straight, about 0.5 cm depth	Sprain, neuralgia, and paralysis of hindfoot
60	Chung fong	About 0.5 cm medial to point 59	N. Deep peroneal	Straight, about 0.5 cm depth	Sprain, neuralgia, and paralysis of hindfoot
61	Hou kon	Plantar surface of hindlimb, about 1 cm medial to the fibular tarsal bone	N. Plantar	Straight, about 0.5 cm depth	Sprain, neuralgia, and paralysis of hindfoot

CAT

The only published description of acupuncture points in the cat is by John Ottaviano,[16] a veterinary acupuncturist currently practicing in California. The numbers for each point are keyed to his chart (Fig. 117).

1. Located between front paw webbing. Used for front leg paralysis.
2. Same as No. 1. Used for front leg paralysis and deafness.
3. Local joint pain.
4. One inch below No. 5 in the crease formed by the muscle. Used for local joint pain, constipation.
5. Located in the crease formed by the elbow. Local pain, paralysis of front limb, constipation, dermatitis, itching, cough.
6. For local pain.
7. Located in the shoulder joint. Used for shoulder pain.
8. Located in the middle of upper lip. Used for emergency and shock. Apply acupuncture by pinching with thumb and index finger [or with needle].
9. Used for difficulty in mastication and local pain.
10. Used for eye problems.
11. Tip of ear. Used for eye problems.
12. One inch behind the ear. Used for cervical problems, and deafness.

13. Located on center line one inch upward and below No. 12. Uses are the same as for No. 12.

14. Located in front of scapula one inch from midline. Used for cervical pain, arthritis in any joint, bone problems in general.

15. Behind scapula one inch from mid-line. Thoracic pain, infections, cleansing of the blood.

16. Located opposite the navel on the spinal area and one inch out from that midline. Used for thoracolumbar pain, urinary problems, kidney and sexual disorders.

17. In front of the ilium one inch from midline. Used for lumbo-sacral pain, pain at the hips, and constipation.

18. Located at the crease formed by the head of the femur and hip joint. Used for hip pain.

19. Located one inch up and 45 degrees out from crease of tail. Used for hip, sacral pain and constipation.

20. Located below the head of the femur. Used for lumbar pain, sacral pain and stifle pain.

21. Located behind the crease formed by flexing the stifle. Used for hind leg paralysis, local pain, and any other weakness of lower limbs.

22. Located one inch below the patella. Used to increase appetite, for paralysis of hind limbs, tonic to entire systems.

23. Used for urinary problems, and as an aid in the delivery of kittens.

24. Used for local pain and lumbar pain.

25. Located at the tip of the tail. Used for all back problems, constipation and hind leg paralysis.

26. Located in hind paw webbing. Used for hind leg paralysis, urinary problems, and as a tonic to give strength to lower limbs.

REFERENCES

1. Anon. 1972. Canton autumn fair marks breakthrough in Sino-U.S. trade. *Business Asia* 3:369–70.
2. Anon. 1972. The man to see about selling chemicals at next fall's Canton Trade Fair. *Chem. Week*, July, 26:54.
3. Anon. 1972. *Chinese Veterinary Handbook.* (in Chinese). pp. 587–670. Compiled by the Lan Chou Veterinary Research Institute. Gan shu, China: The People's Publishing Co.
4. Anon. 1972. The meridians. In *Chung San I Chiang Dun Tsueh (Diagnosis in Chinese Veterinary)* (in Chinese). The Chinese Academy of Agriculture, Research Institute of Chinese Veterinary Medicine. Peking: Agriculture Press.
5. Chen, S. H. 1976. *Veterinary Acupuncture: Anatomical Points of Horse, Cow, Pig and Dog.* Denver, Colorado: University of Oriental Culture.
6. Chen, S. H. 1976. *Veterinary Acupuncture.* Denver, Colorado: University of Chinese Culture.
7. Kothbauer, O. 1974. The bladder meridian of the cow. *Amer. J. Acupuncture* 2:300–305.
8. Kothbauer, O. 1966. Die Provokation einer hyperalgetischen Zone der Haut und eines "Schmerzpunktes" durch Reizung eines Uterushornes beim Rind. *Wien. Tieraerztl. Mschr.* 53:802.
9. Kothbauer, O. 1969. Die Provokation einer hyperalgetischen Zone der Haut und von "Schmerzpunkten" durch Reizung eines Ovars beim Rind. *Wien. Tieraerztl. Mschr.* 56:3–11.
10. Kothbauer, O. 1975. Seventeen years of acupuncture experience—diagnosis and therapy on the cow. *Acupuncture Res.* 2:16–19.
11. Kvirchishvili, V. I. 1974. Projections of different parts of the body on the surface of the concha auriculae in humans and animals. *Amer. J. Acupuncture* 2:208.
12. Milin, J.: L'Acupuncture veterinaire. In *Traité D'Acupuncture*, Tome I, ed. R. De La Fuye, pp. 473–89. Paris: Librairie E. Le Francois.
13. Miyazawa, T. 1974. Personal communication.
14. Morgan, G. 1975. Trading behind the Great Wall. *The New Englander.* March.
15. Ottaviano, J. 1975. Veterinary—anatomy and application. In *Compendium of Veterinary and Human Acupuncture*, ed. by H. E. Warner and R. S. Glassberg, pp. III, 3–III, 9, E. Anaheim, California: National Association for Veterinary Acupuncture.
16. Ottaviano, J. 1976. Acupuncture for cats. In *Cat Catalog*, ed. by J. Fireman, pp. 238–40. New York: Workman Publishing Co.
17. Shin, S. H. 1975. Veterinary—anatomy and application. In *Compendium of Veterinary and Human Acupuncture*, ed. by H. E. Warner and R. S. Glassberg, pp. III, 1–III, 2. Anaheim, California: National Association for Veterinary Acupuncture.
18. Shores, A. 1975. *Canine Acupuncture Chart.* Auburn, Alabama: Box 925.
19. Young, H. G. 1975. *Atlas of Veterinary Acupuncture Charts.* Thomasville, Georgia: Oriental Veterinary Acupuncture Specialties.

Figures to Chapter 3

3–1. Modern Chinese veterinary acupuncture chart for swine.

3–2. Modern Chinese veterinary acupuncture chart for swine.

3–3. Modern Chinese veterinary acupuncture chart for horse.

3–4. Modern Chinese veterinary acupuncture chart for horse.

3–5. Modern Chinese veterinary acupuncture chart for cattle.

3–6. Modern Chinese veterinary acupuncture chart for cattle.

3–7. Modern Chinese veterinary acupuncture chart for chicken.

3–8. Right side of cow.

3–9. Left side of cow.

3–10. Dorsal view of cow.

3–11. Dorsal view of cow.

3–12. Ancient Chinese chart of twelve points (meridians) in the horse.

3–13. Chart of meridian lines and acupuncture points in the horse, as published by Dr. Meiyu Okada.

3–14. Enlarged section of Okada chart: head and neck.

3–15. Enlarged section of Okada chart: caudal section.

3–16. Enlarged section of Okada chart: forelegs.

3–17. Enlarged section of Okada chart: hind legs.

3–18. Enlarged section of Okada chart: feet.

3–19. The Young horse chart: large intestine meridian.

3–20. The Young horse chart: stomach meridian.

3–21. The Young horse chart: small intestine meridian.

3–22. The Young horse chart: bladder meridian.

3–23. The Young horse chart: triple-burner meridian.

3–24. The Young horse chart: gallbladder and liver meridians.

3–25. The Young horse chart: conception vessel.

3–26. The Young horse chart: governing vessel.

3–27. Model of a horse showing acupuncture points.

3–28. Acupuncture chart of the horse (lateral view).

3–29. Acupuncture chart of the horse (lateral view).

3–30. Acupuncture chart of the horse (lateral view).

3–31. Acupuncture chart of the horse (dorsal view).

3–32. Acupuncture chart of the horse (lateral view of the head).

3–33. Acupuncture chart of the horse: a) hard palate; b) dental surface.

3–34. Acupuncture chart of the horse: a) ventral surface of the tongue; b) cranial view.

3–35. Acupuncture chart of the horse: a) caudal view; b) foreleg, medial view; c) hind leg, medial view.

3–36. Acupuncture chart of the horse (ventral view).

3–37. Acupuncture chart of the horse: forelimb (lateral view).

3–38. Acupuncture chart of the horse: forelimb (lateral view).

3–39. Acupuncture chart of the horse: forelimb (lateral view).

3–40. Acupuncture chart of the horse: sacral area (lateral view).

3–41. Acupuncture chart of the horse: hind limb (lateral view).

3–42. Acupuncture chart of the horse: hind limb (lateral view).

3–43. Acupuncture chart of the horse: hind limb (lateral view).

3–44. Acupuncture chart of the cow (lateral view).

3–45. Acupuncture chart of the cow (lateral view).

3–46. Acupuncture chart of the cow (lateral view).

3–47. Acupuncture chart of the cow (dorsal view).

3–48. Acupuncture chart of the cow (cranial view).

3–49. Acupuncture chart of the pig (lateral view).

3–50. Acupuncture chart of the pig (lateral view).

3–51. Acupuncture chart of the pig (lateral view).

3–52. Acupuncture chart of the pig: ear (medial surface).

3–53. Acupuncture chart of the pig: head (lateral view).

3–54. Acupuncture chart of the pig: forelimb (lateral view).

3–55. Acupuncture chart of the pig: a) hind limb (cranial view) b) front limb (cranial view).

3–56. Acupuncture chart of the pig: forelimb (lateral view).

3–57. Acupuncture chart of the pig: a) forefoot (caudal view) b) front foot (cranial view).

3–58. Acupuncture chart of the pig: forelimb (caudal view).

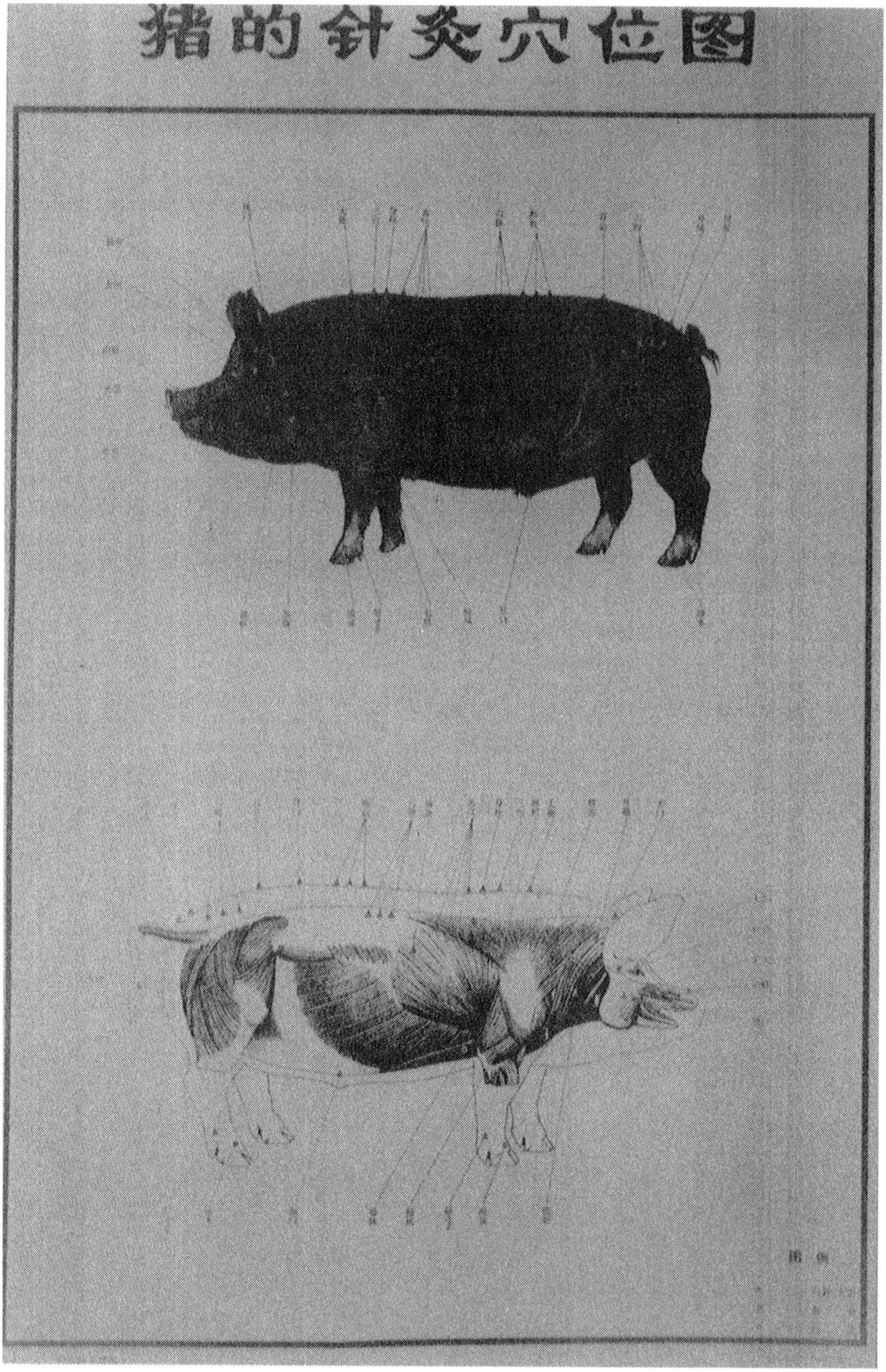

FIGURE 3–1. Modern Chinese veterinary acupuncture chart for pig.

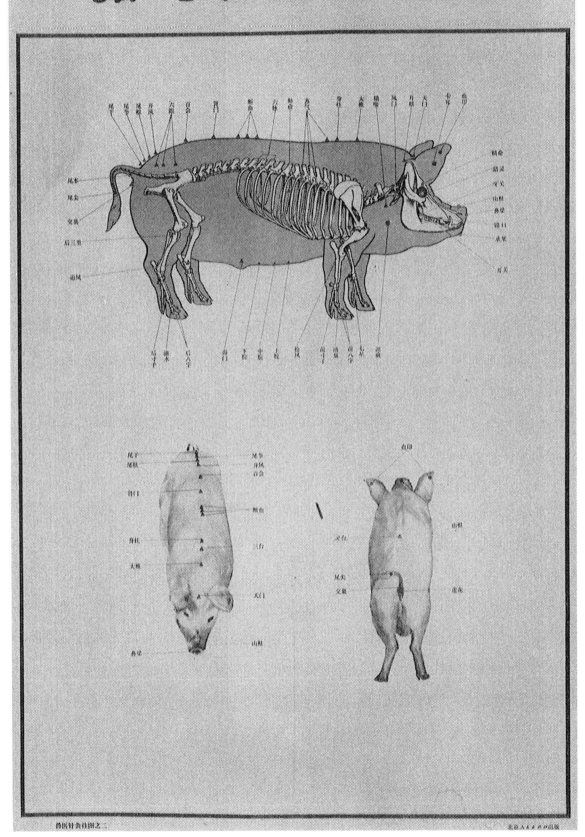

FIGURE 3–2. Modern Chinese veterinary acupuncture chart for pig.

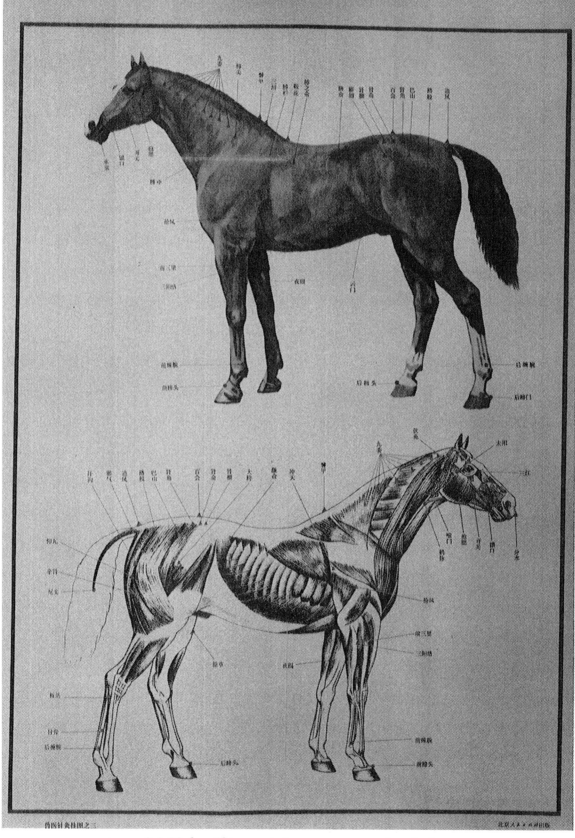

FIGURE 3–3. Modern Chinese veterinary acupuncture chart for horse.

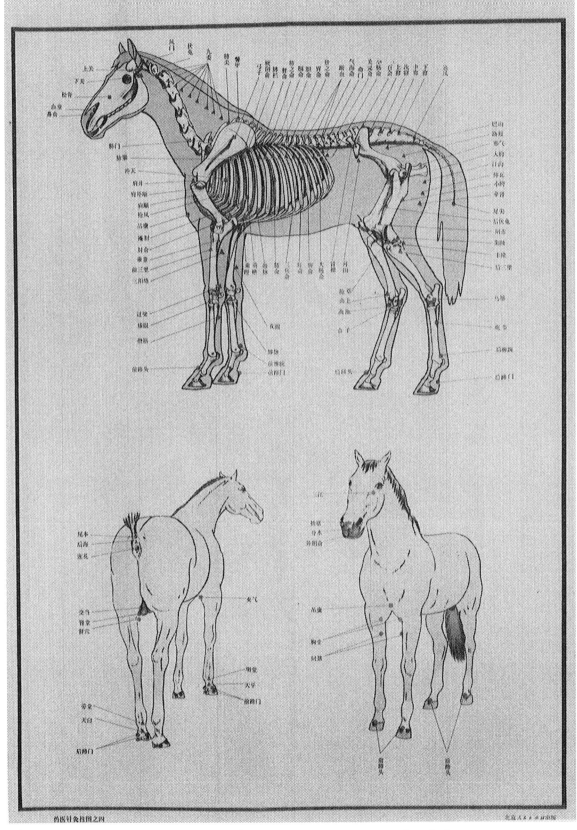

FIGURE 3–4. Modern Chinese veterinary acupuncture chart for horse.

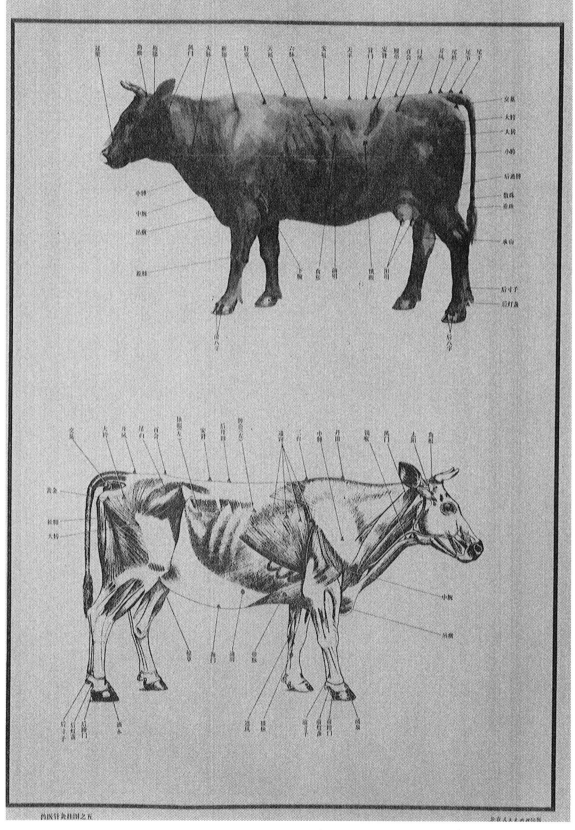

FIGURE 3–5. Modern Chinese veterinary acupuncture chart for cattle.

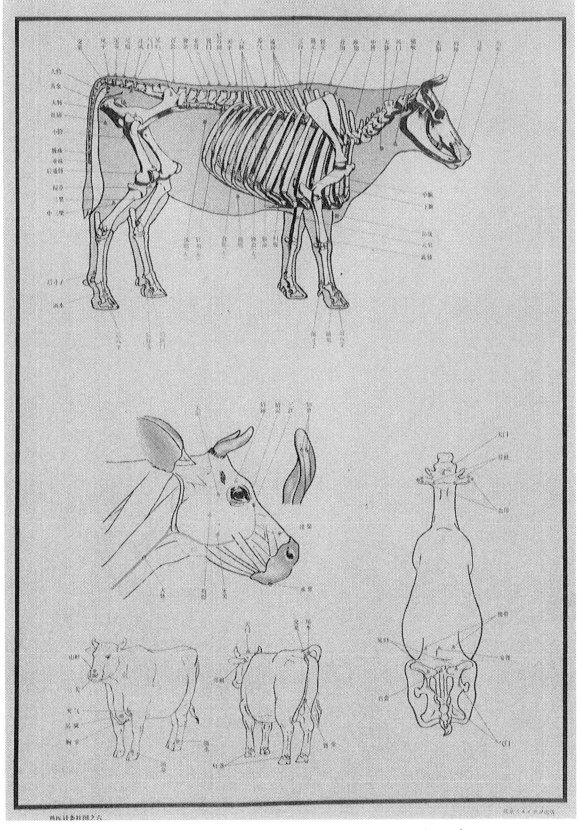

FIGURE 3–6. Modern Chinese veterinary acupuncture chart for cattle.

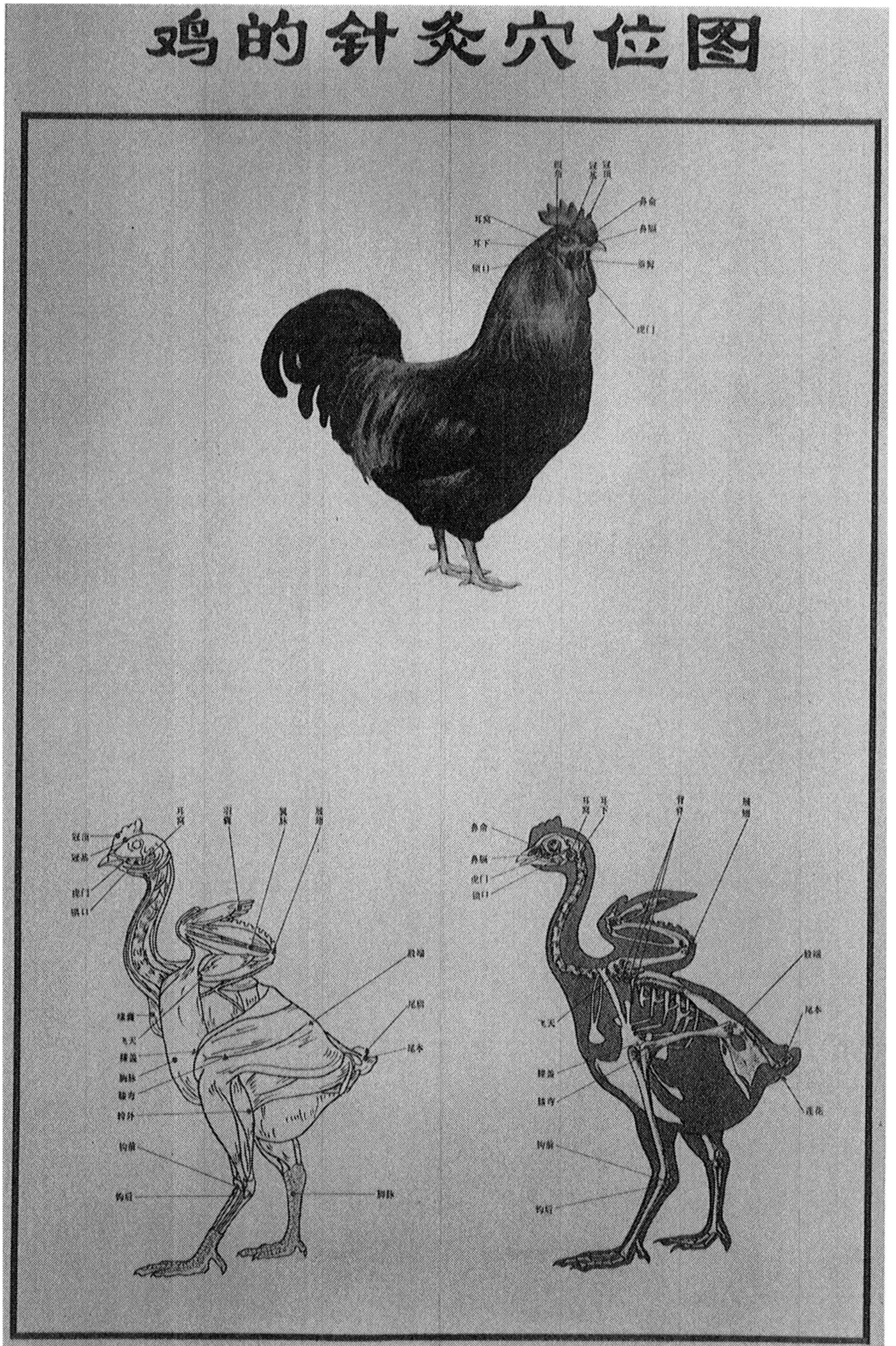

FIGURE 3–7. Modern Chinese veterinary acupuncture chart for chicken.

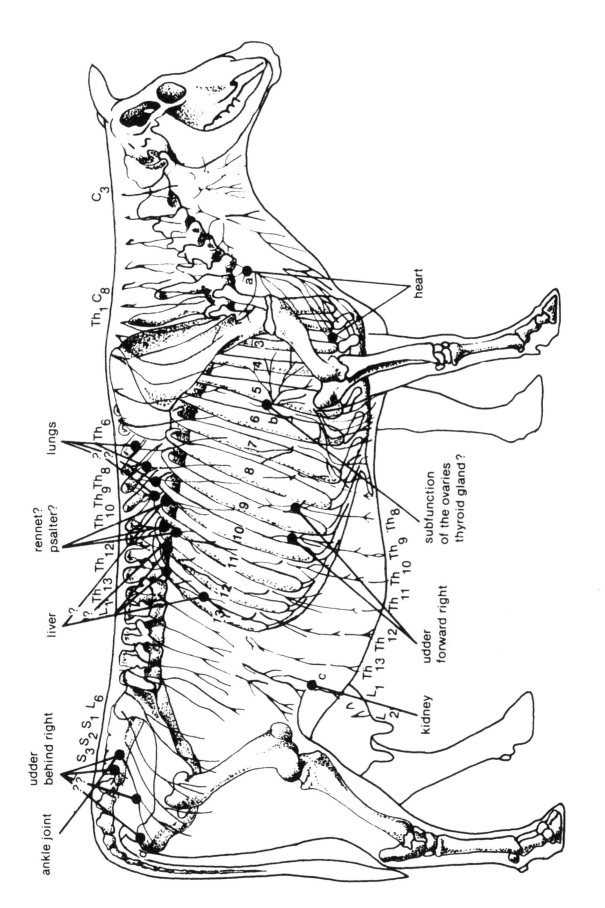

FIGURE 3–8. Right side of cow; chart of acupuncture points reported by Dr. O. Kothbauer and the journal *Acupuncture Research*. (Courtesy of Dr. O. Kothbauer.)

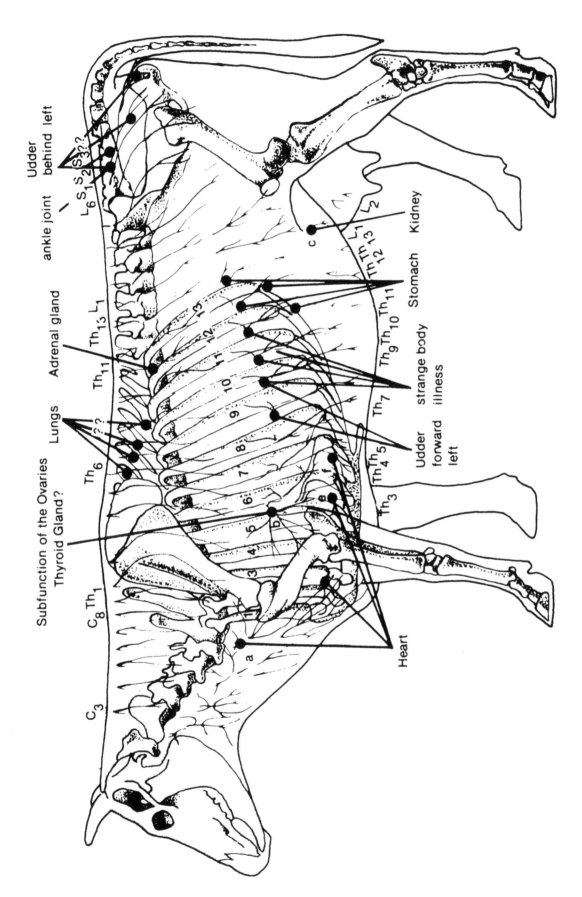

FIGURE 3–9. Left side of cow; chart of acupuncture points reported by Dr. O. Kothbauer. (Courtesy of Dr. O. Kothbauer and the journal *Acupuncture Research.*)

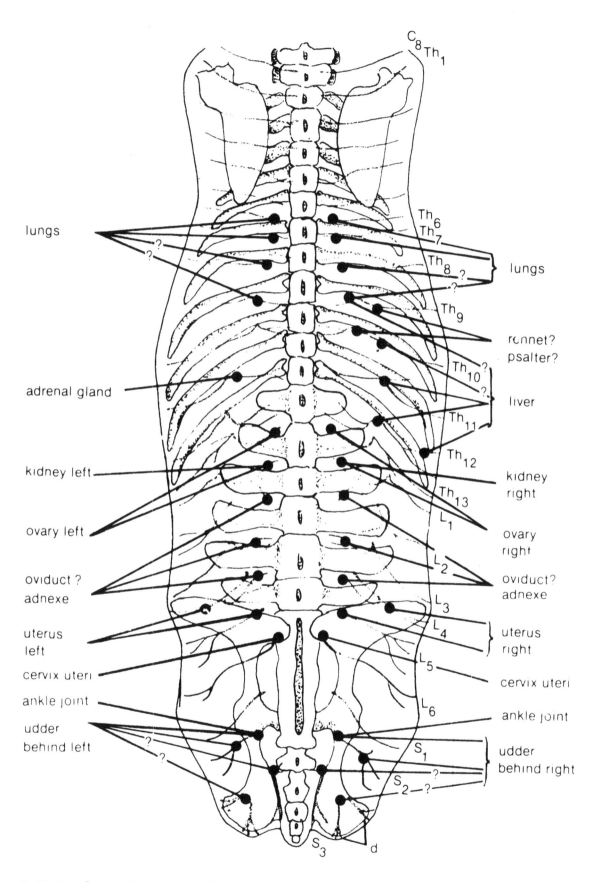

C₈Th₁

lungs

Th₆
Th₇
Th₈ ?
lungs

?
?

Th₉

rennet?
psalter?

adrenal gland

Th₁₀ ?
?

liver

Th₁₁

kidney left

Th₁₂

kidney
right

Th₁₃

L₁

ovary left

ovary
right

L₂

oviduct ?
adnexe

L₃

oviduct?
adnexe

L₄

uterus
left

uterus
right

L₅

cervix uteri

cervix uteri

ankle joint

L₆

ankle joint

udder
behind left

?
?

S₁

udder
behind right

S₂ ?

S₃

d

FIGURE 3–10. Dorsal view of cow; chart of acupuncture points reported by Dr. O. Kothbauer. (Courtesy of Dr. O. Kothbauer and the journal *Acupuncture Research*.)

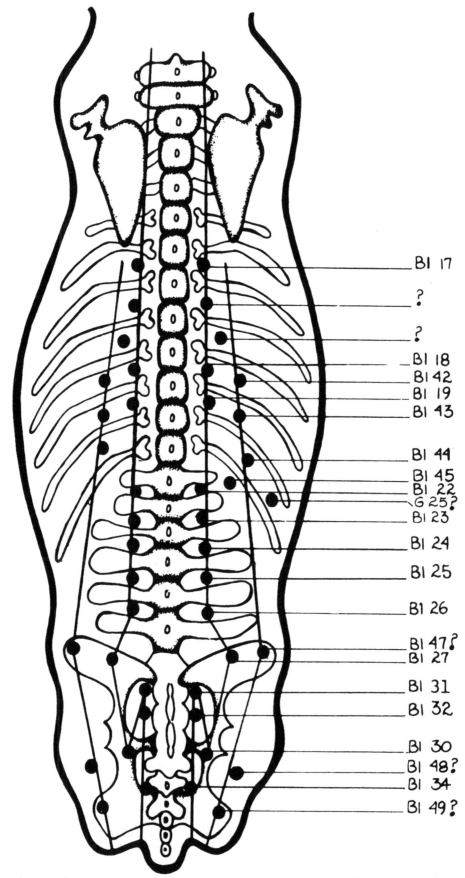

Bl 17
?
?
Bl 18
Bl 42
Bl 19
Bl 43

Bl 44
Bl 45
Bl 22
G 25?
Bl 23

Bl 24

Bl 25

Bl 26

Bl 47?
Bl 27

Bl 31

Bl 32

Bl 30
Bl 48?
Bl 34

Bl 49?

FIGURE 3–11. Dorsal view of cow; chart of acupuncture points reported by Dr. O. Kothbauer. An attempt to label and fit the points found in cattle onto the bladder meridian described in humans. (Courtesy of Dr. O. Kothbauer and the *American J. of Acupuncture* 2:303, 1974.)

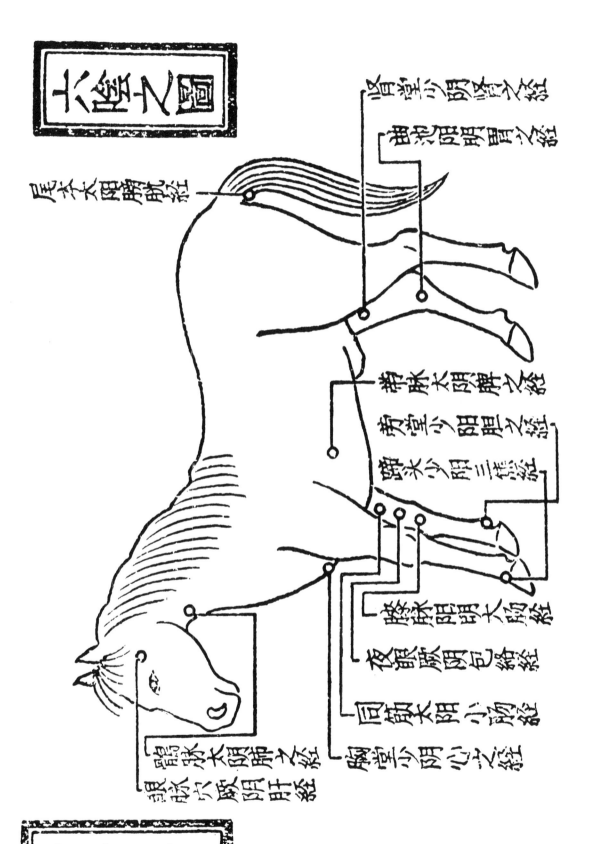

FIGURE 3–12. Ancient Chinese chart of twelve points (meridians) in the horse; each meridian is a single point instead of a line made up of many points.

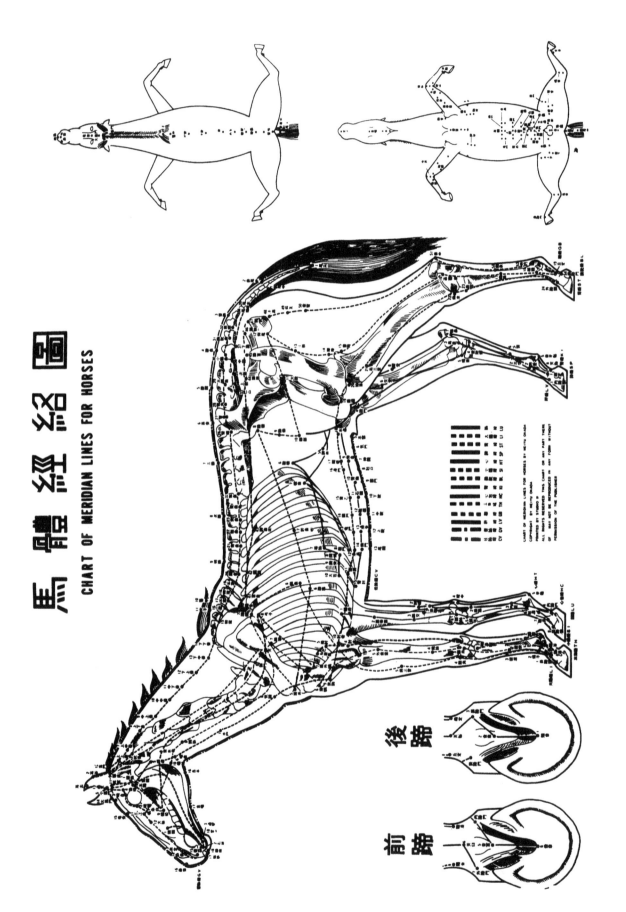

FIGURE 3–13. Chart of meridian lines and acupuncture points in the horse, as published by Dr. Meiyu Okada. (Courtesy of Dr. Meiyu Okada, T. Miyazawa, and the Brethren Corp.)

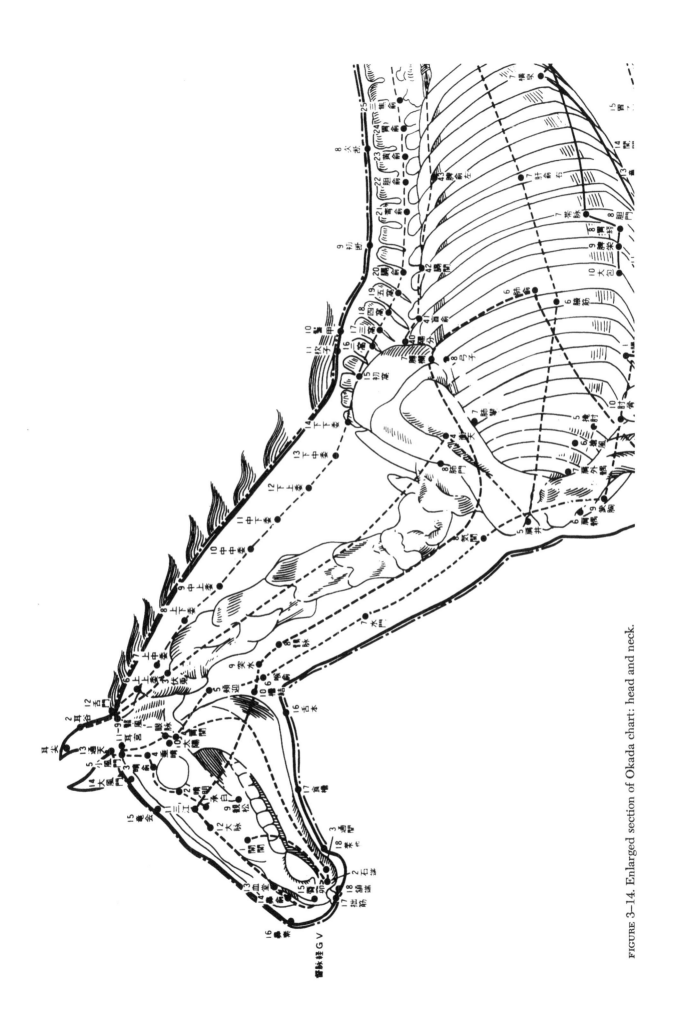

FIGURE 3–14. Enlarged section of Okada chart: head and neck.

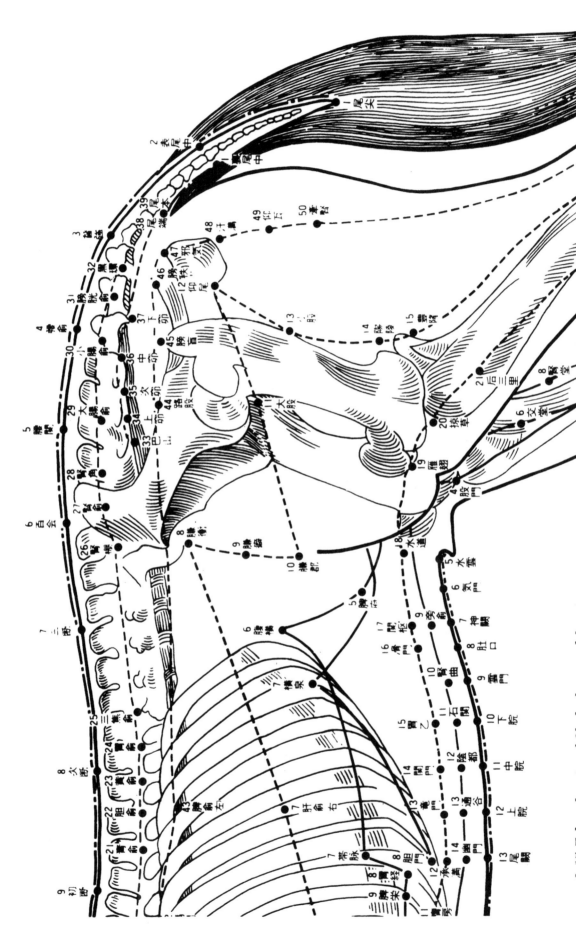

FIGURE 3–15. Enlarged section of Okada chart: caudal section.

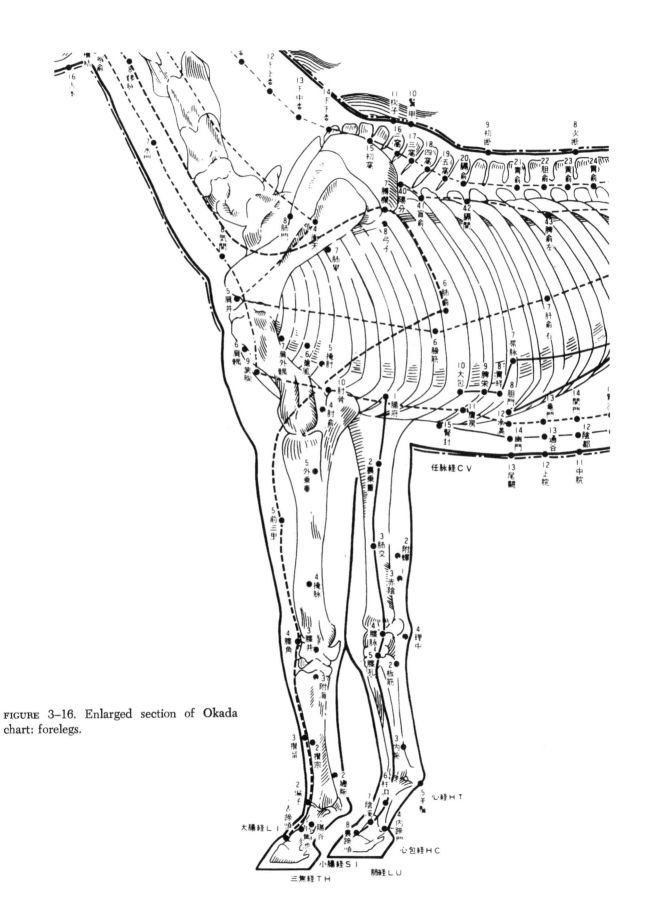

FIGURE 3–16. Enlarged section of Okada chart: forelegs.

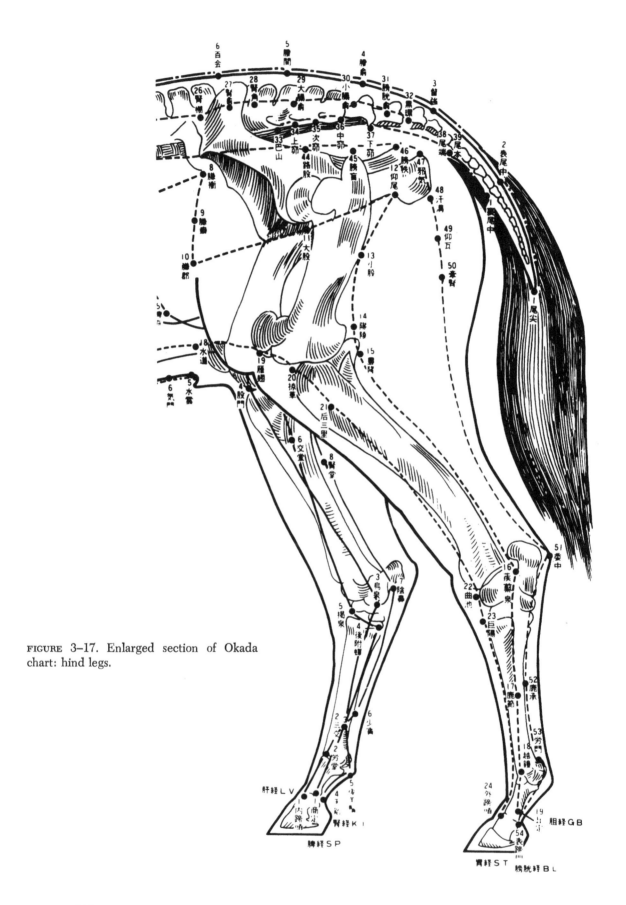

FIGURE 3–17. Enlarged section of Okada chart: hind legs.

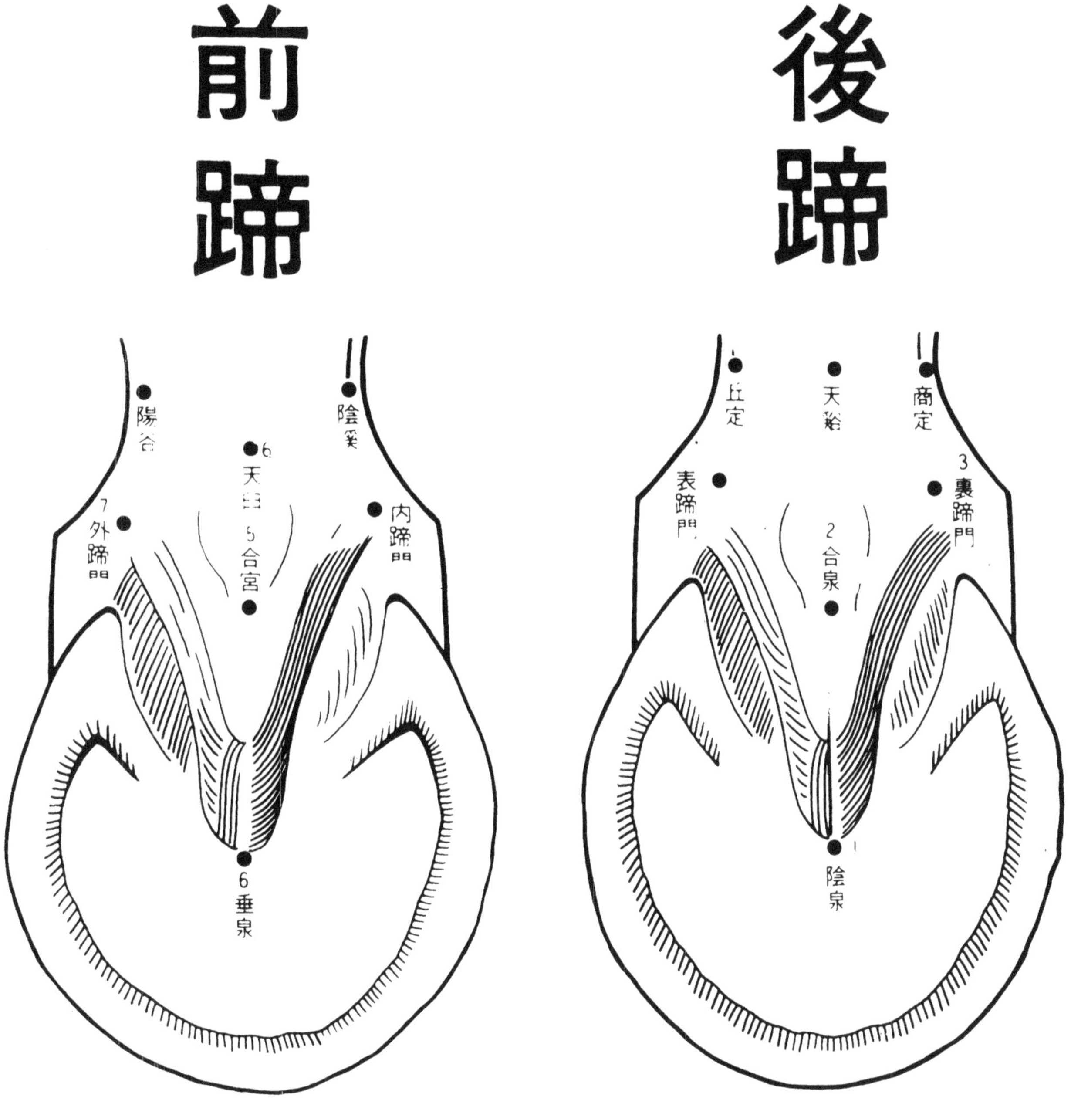

前蹄　　　　　後蹄

FIGURE 3–18. Enlarged section of Okada chart: feet (left side, front foot; right side, hind foot).

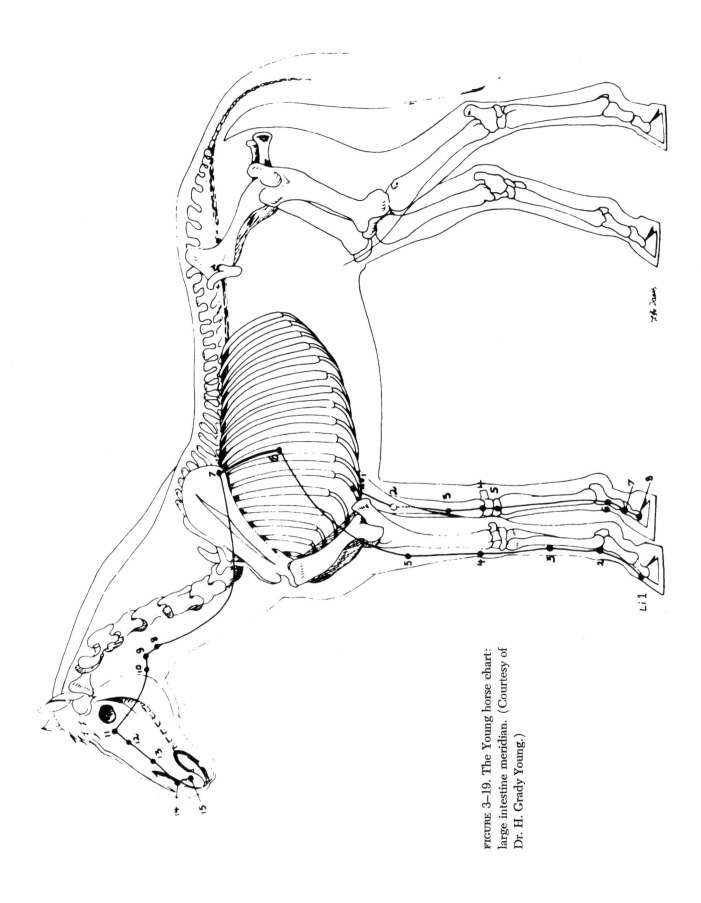

FIGURE 3–19. The Young horse chart: large intestine meridian. (Courtesy of Dr. H. Grady Young.)

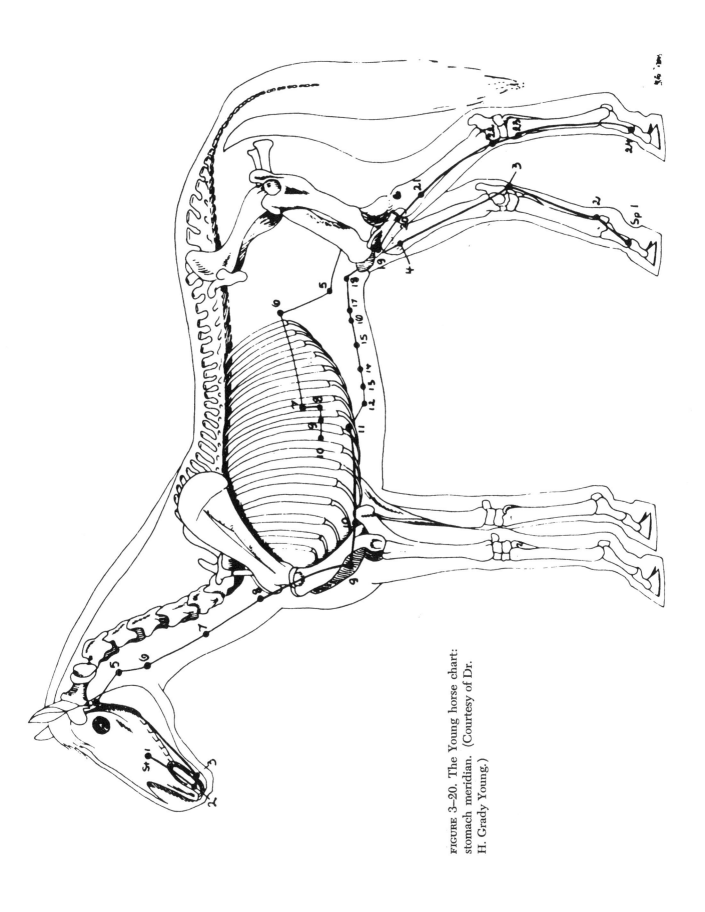

FIGURE 3–20. The Young horse chart: stomach meridian. (Courtesy of Dr. H. Grady Young.)

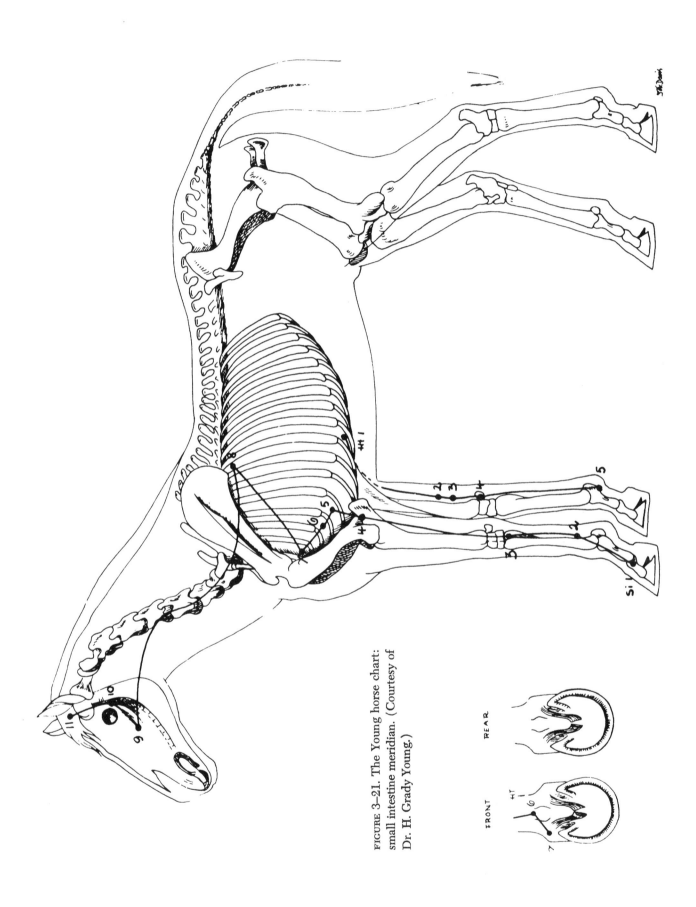

FIGURE 3–21. The Young horse chart: small intestine meridian. (Courtesy of Dr. H. Grady Young.)

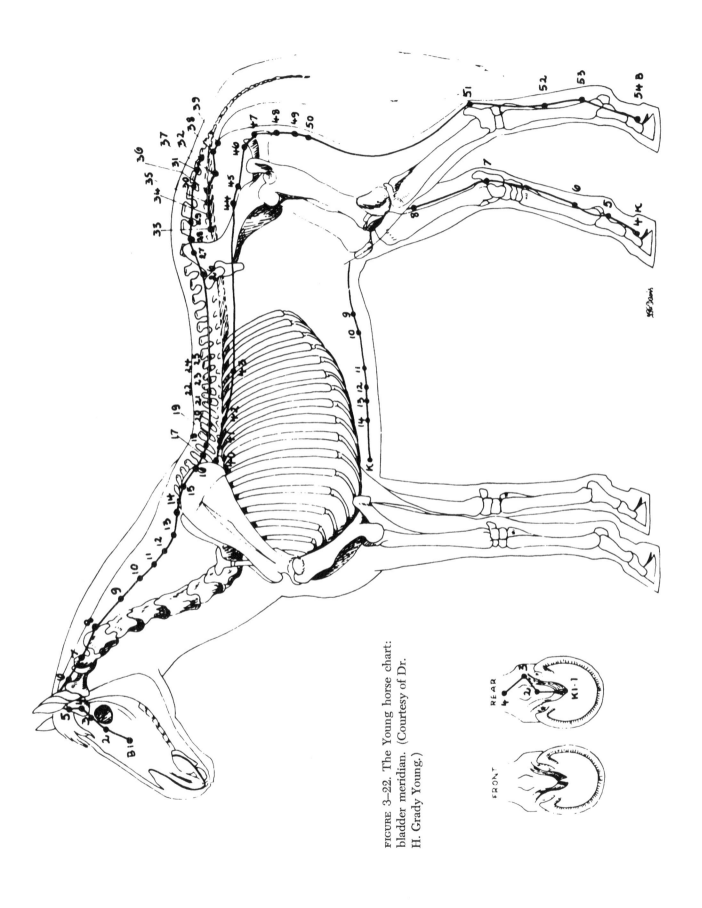

FIGURE 3–22. The Young horse chart: bladder meridian. (Courtesy of Dr. H. Grady Young.)

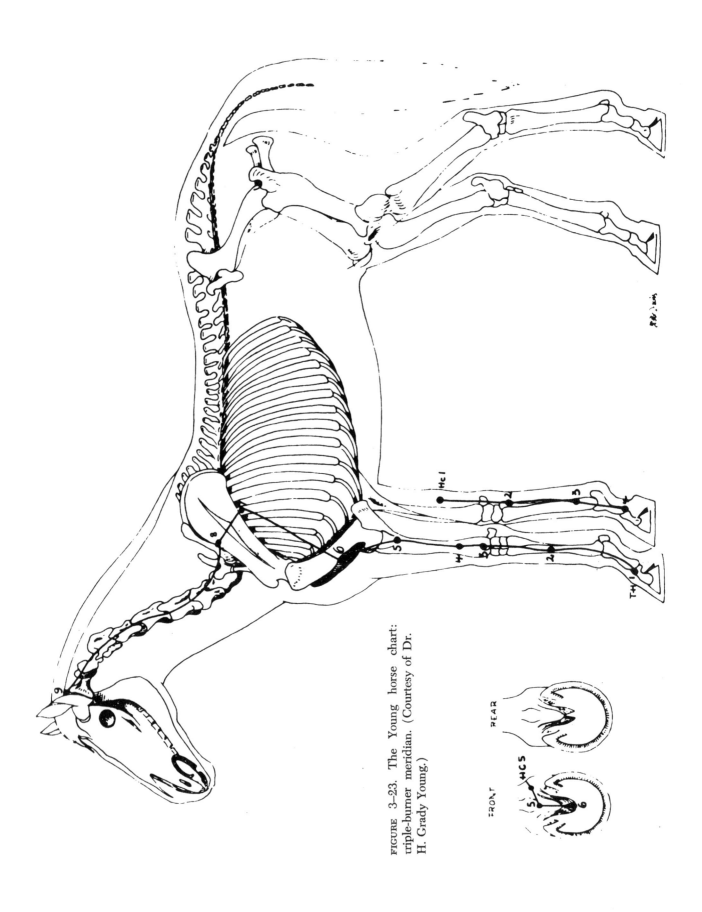

FIGURE 3-23. The Young horse chart: triple-burner meridian. (Courtesy of Dr. H. Grady Young.)

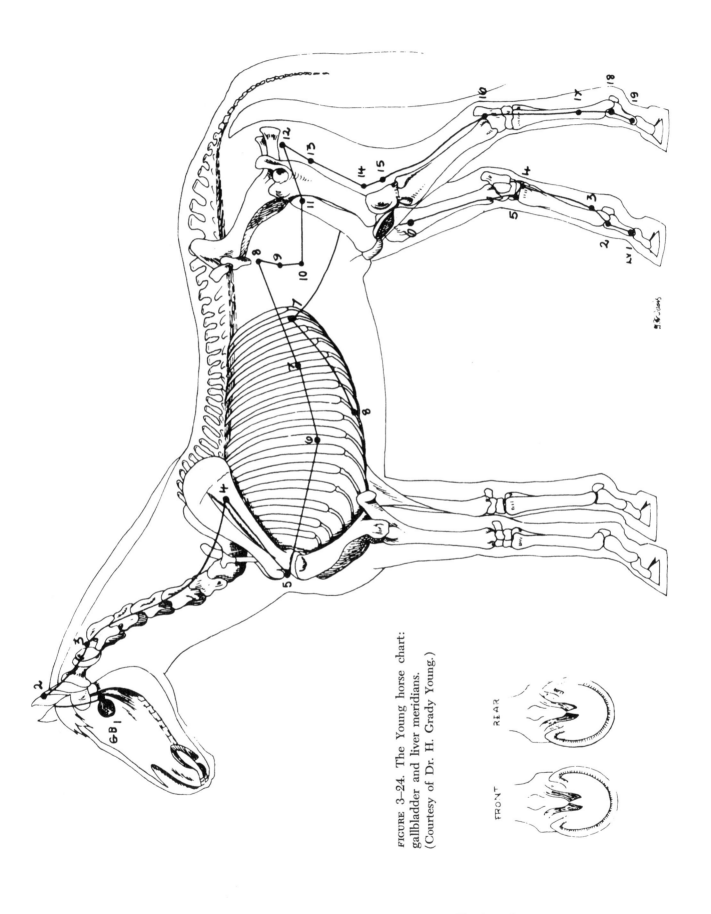

FIGURE 3-24. The Young horse chart: gallbladder and liver meridians. (Courtesy of Dr. H. Grady Young.)

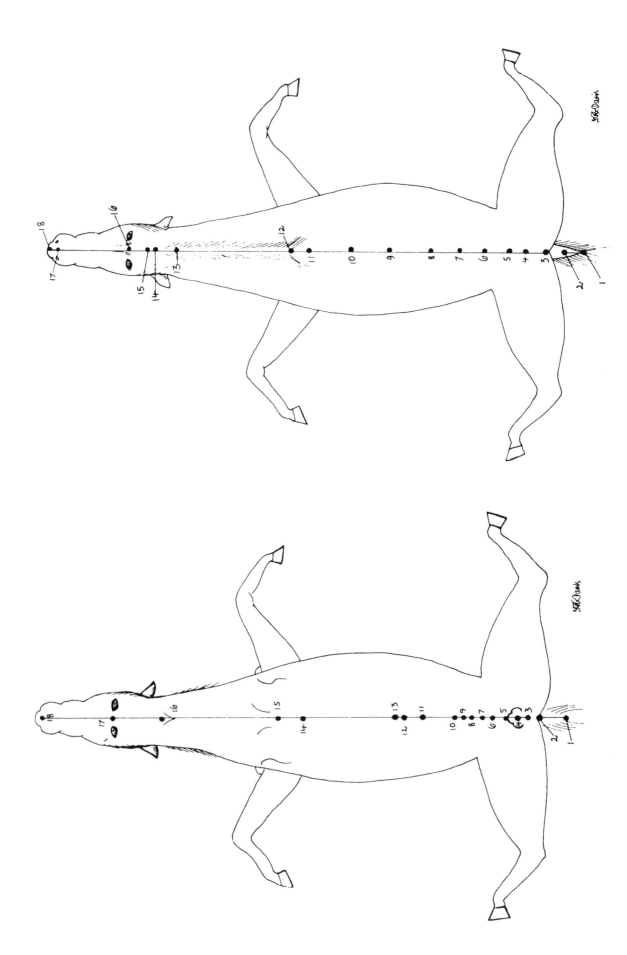

FIGURE 3–26. The Young horse chart: governing vessel. (Courtesy of Dr. H. Grady Young.)

FIGURE 3–25. The Young horse chart: conception vessel. (Courtesy of Dr. H. Grady Young.)

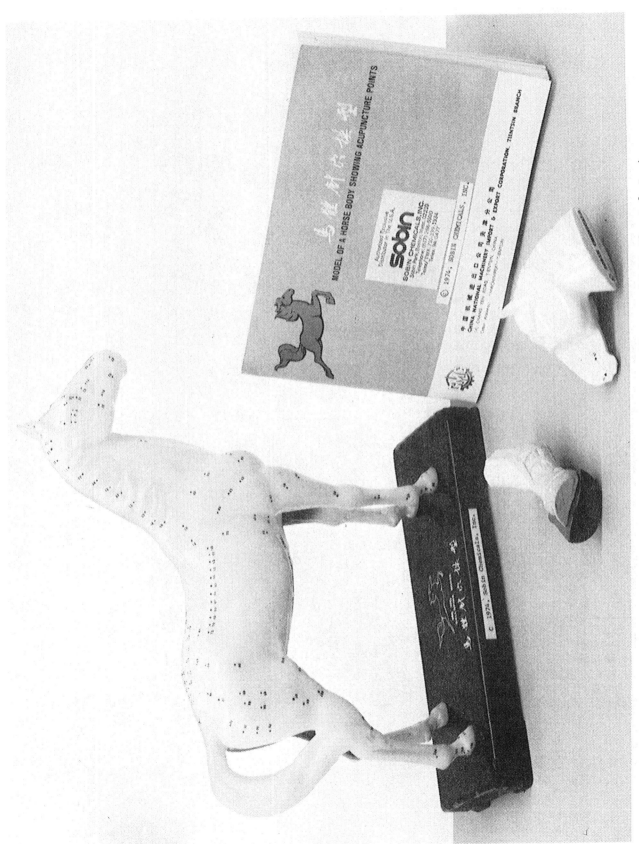

FIGURE 3–27. Model of a horse showing acupuncture points. (Courtesy of Sobin Chemicals, Inc.)

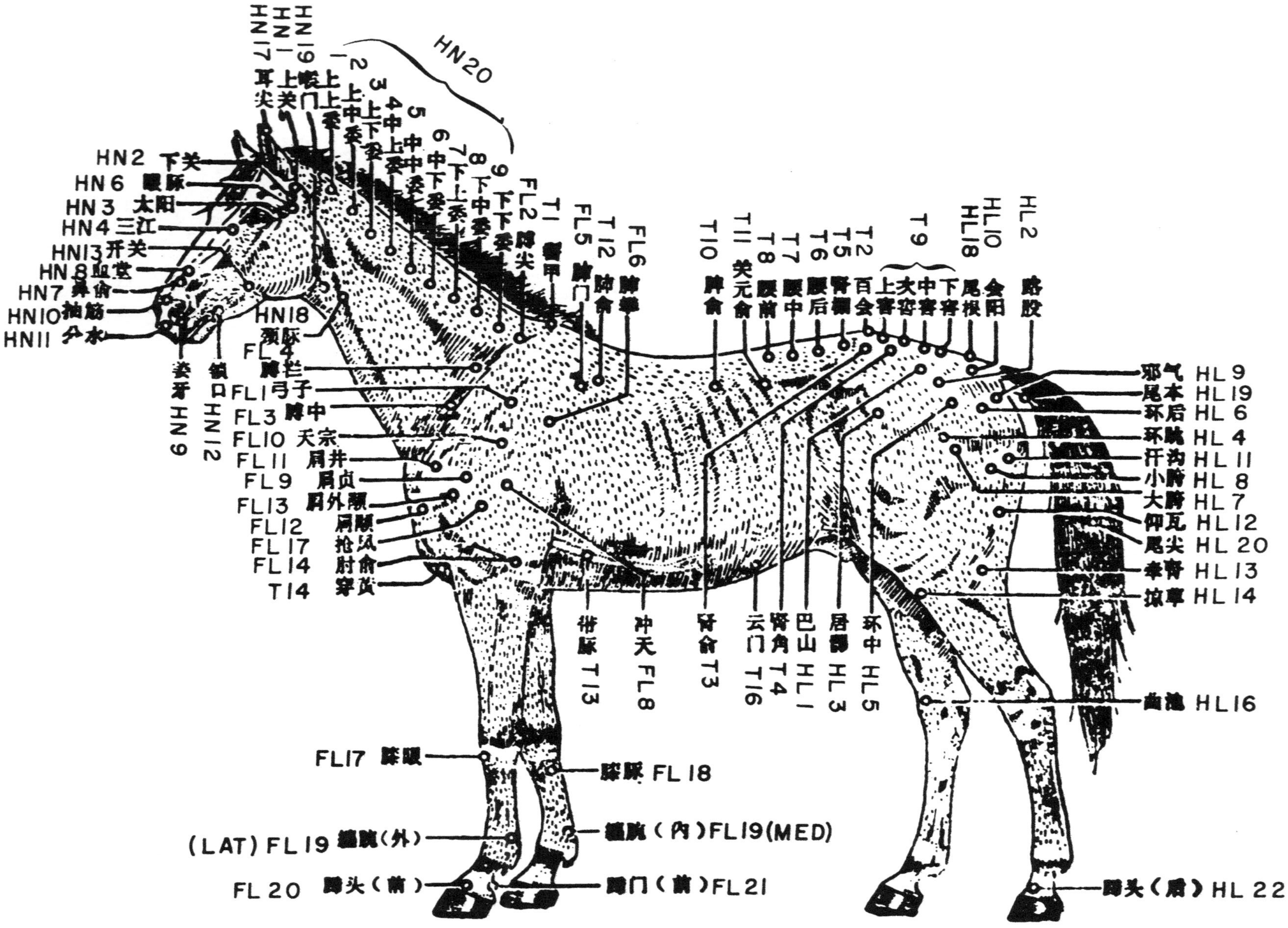

FIGURE 3-28. Acupuncture chart of the horse (lateral view).

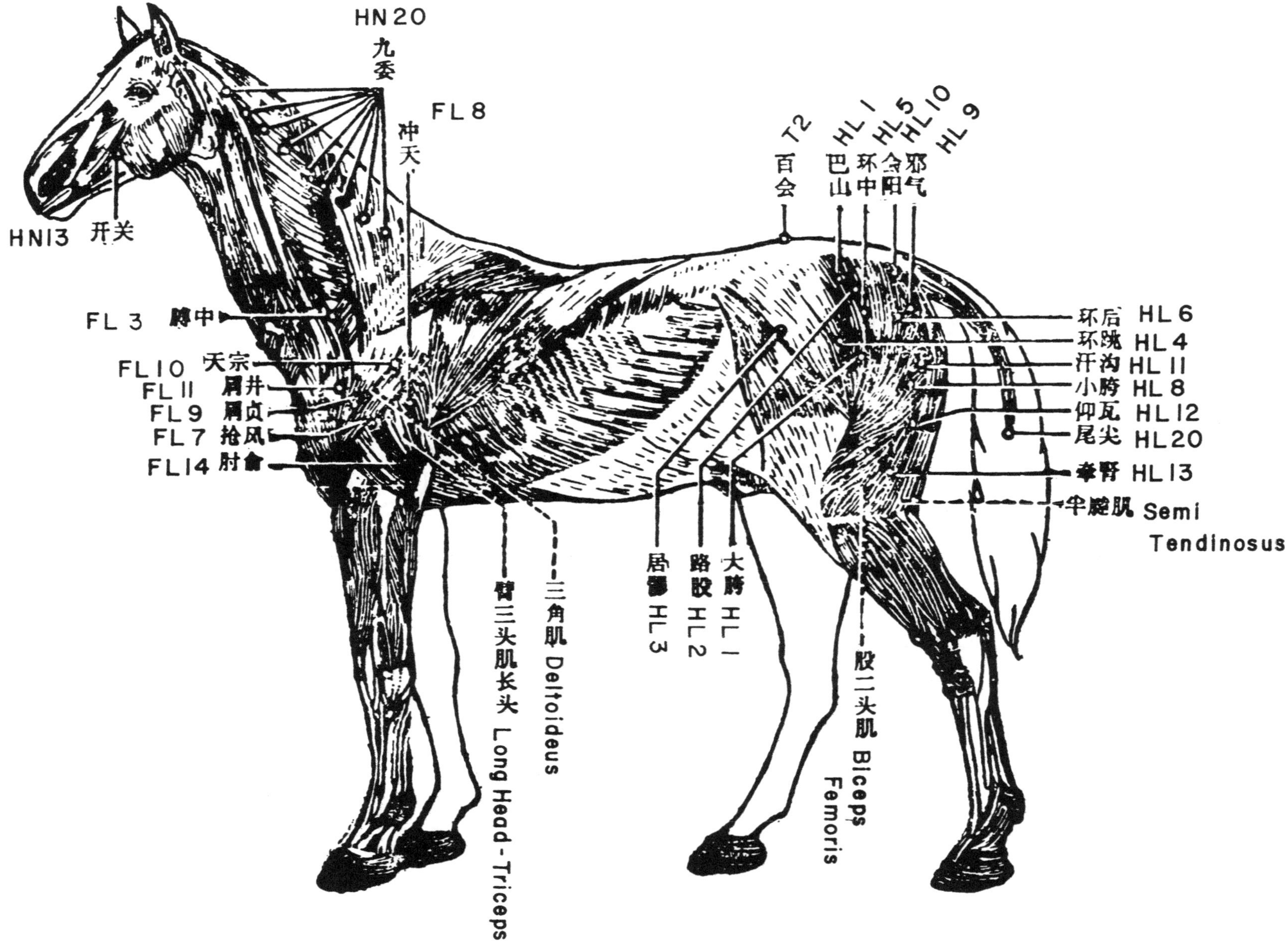

FIGURE 3–29. Acupuncture chart of the horse (lateral view).

环后 HL 6
环跳 HL 4
汗沟 HL 11
小胯 HL 8
仰瓦 HL 12
尾尖 HL 20
掌肾 HL 13
中缝肌 Semi Tendinosus

HL 9
HL 10
HL 5
HL 1
巴 环 合 邪
山 中 阳 气

T 2
百会

股二头肌 Biceps Femoris

大胯 HL 1
路股 HL 2
居髎 HL 3

三角肌 Deltoideus

臂三头肌长头 Long Head - Triceps

HN 20
九委
冲天
FL 8

胸中
天宗
肩井
肩贞
抬风
肘俞
FL 3
FL 10
FL 11
FL 9
FL 7
FL 14

开关
HN 13

149 *Animal Acupuncture Points*

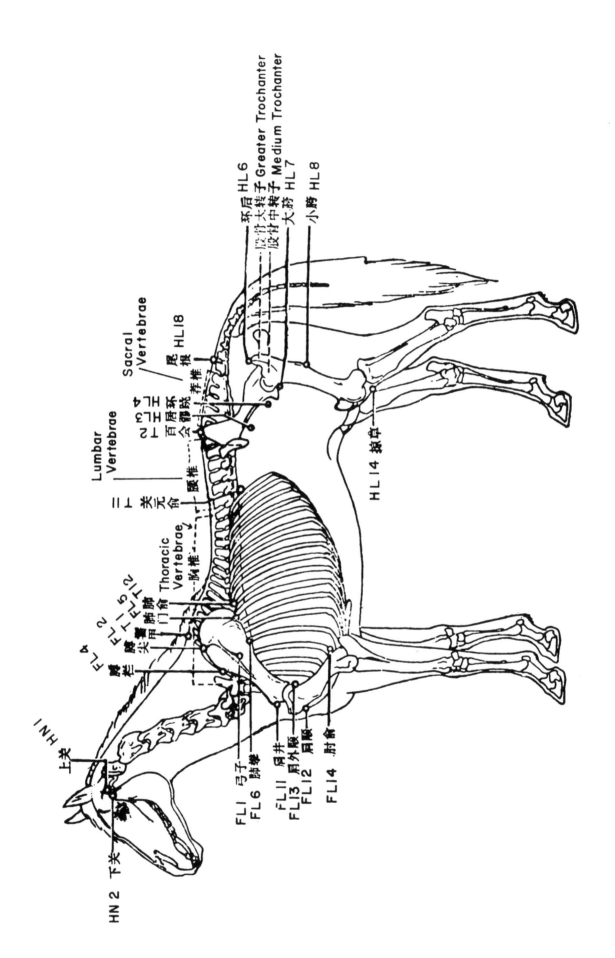

環跳大转子 Greater Trochanter HL6
股后中转子 Medium Trochanter
大胯 HL7
小胯 HL8

尾根 HL18

Sacral Vertebrae 荐椎

Lumbar Vertebrae

合穀腕
百會环
七上王
二五王
三五王

腰椎

命俞
关元俞
玄元俞

HL14 撩草

Thoracic Vertebrae 胸椎

肺 FL1 2
肺门 FL1 1 5 2
脾俞 FL1 2
脾关
膊尖

HN1
上关
HN2 下关

FL1 弓子
FL6 肺攀
FL11 肩井
FL13 肩外顶
FL12 肩顒
FL14 肘俞

FIGURE 3–30. Acupuncture chart of the horse (lateral view).

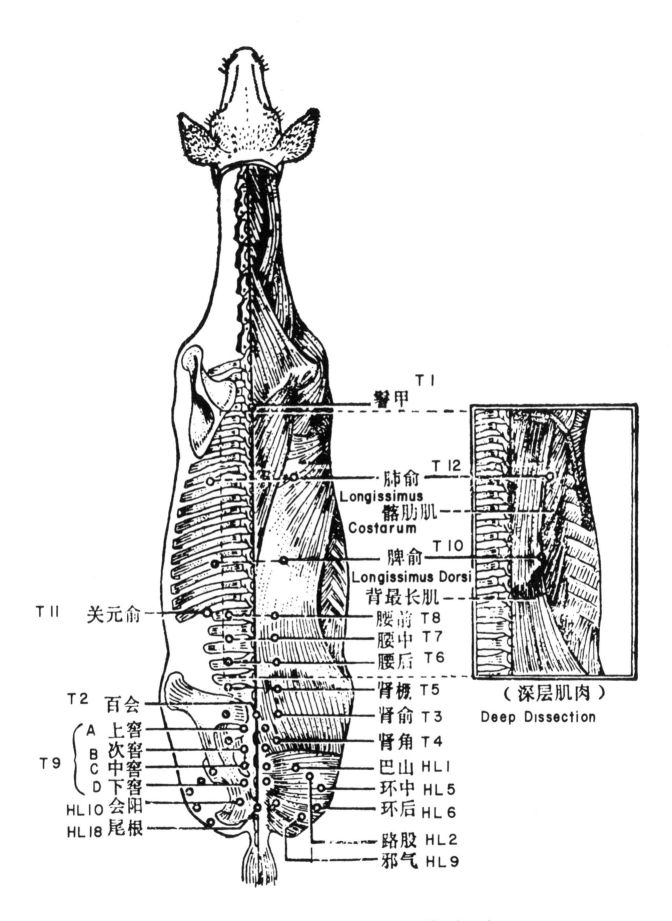

T1

鬐甲

T12
肺俞
Longissimus
髂肋肌
Costarum
T10
脾俞
Longissimus Dorsi
背最长肌

（深层肌肉）
Deep Dissection

T11 关元俞

腰前 T8
腰中 T7
腰后 T6

肾棚 T5

T2 百会
肾俞 T3

A 上窎
肾角 T4
B 次窎
T9
C 中窎
巴山 HL1
D 下窎
环中 HL5
HL10 会阳
环后 HL6
HL18 尾根

跍股 HL2
邪气 HL9

FIGURE 3–31. Acupuncture chart of the horse (dorsal view).

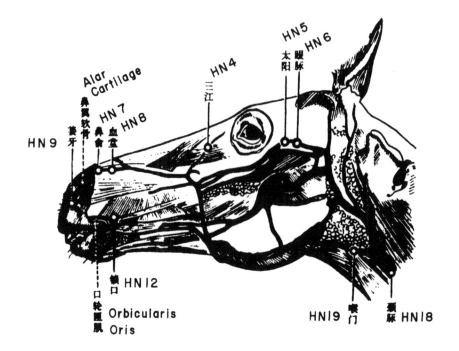

FIGURE 3–32. Acupuncture chart of the horse (lateral view of the head).

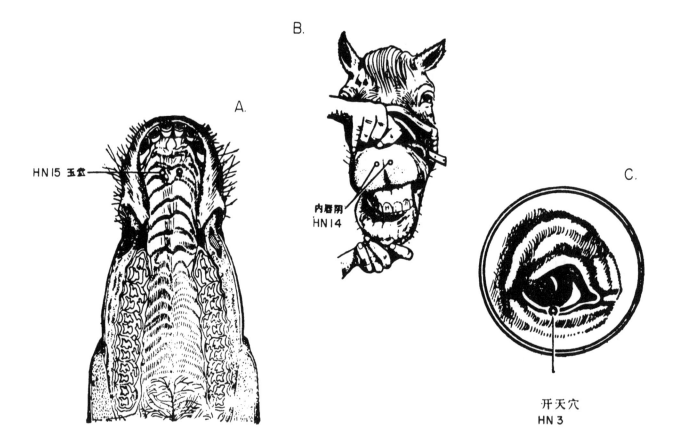

FIGURE 3–33. Acupuncture chart of the horse: a) hard palate; b) dental surface; c) eye.

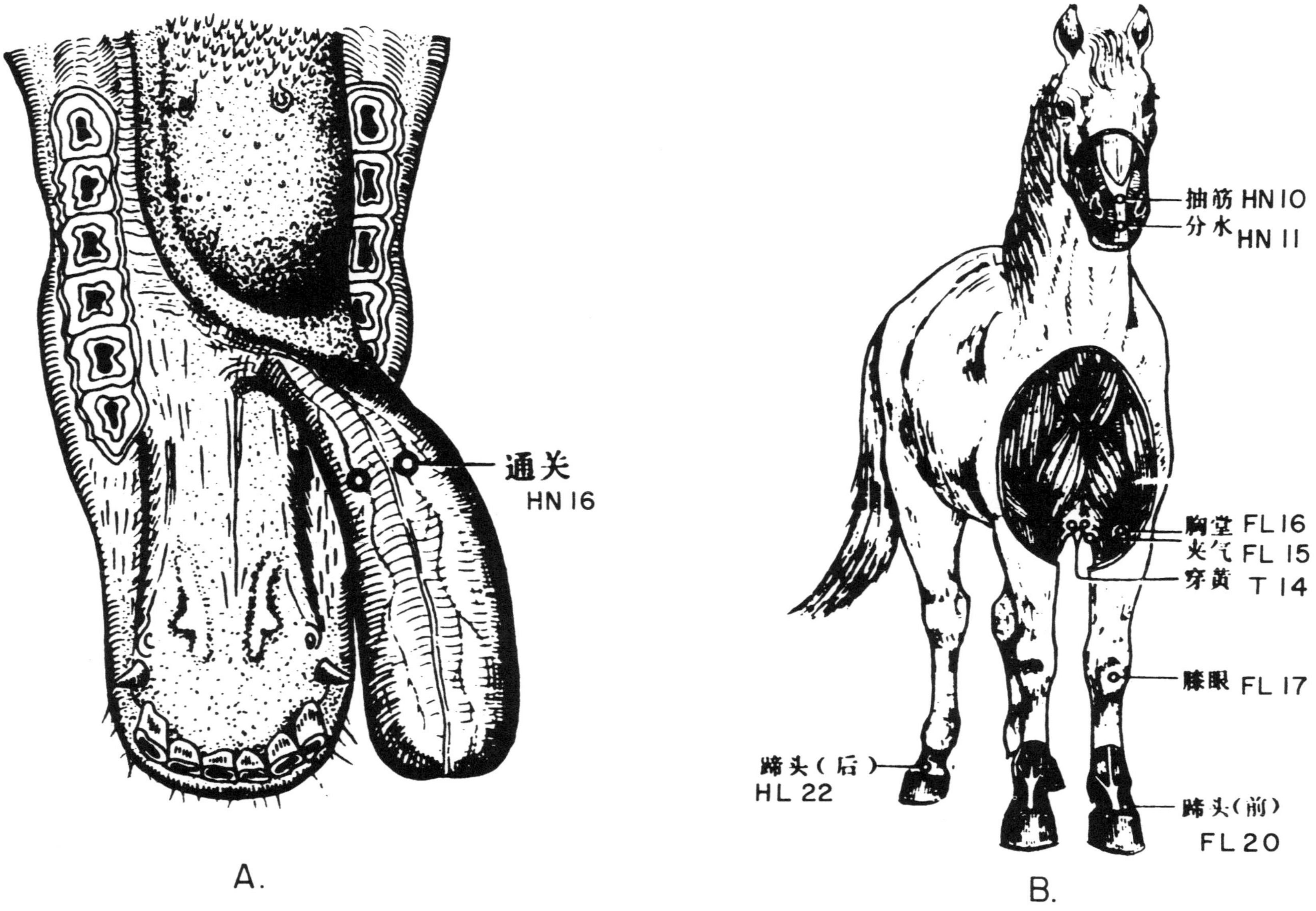

通关
HN 16

抽筋 HN 10
分水 HN 11

胸堂 FL 16
处气 FL 15
牙黄 T 14

膝眼 FL 17

蹄头（前）
FL 20

蹄头（后）
HL 22

B.

A.

FIGURE 3–34. Acupuncture chart of the horse: a) ventral surface of the tongue; b) cranial view.

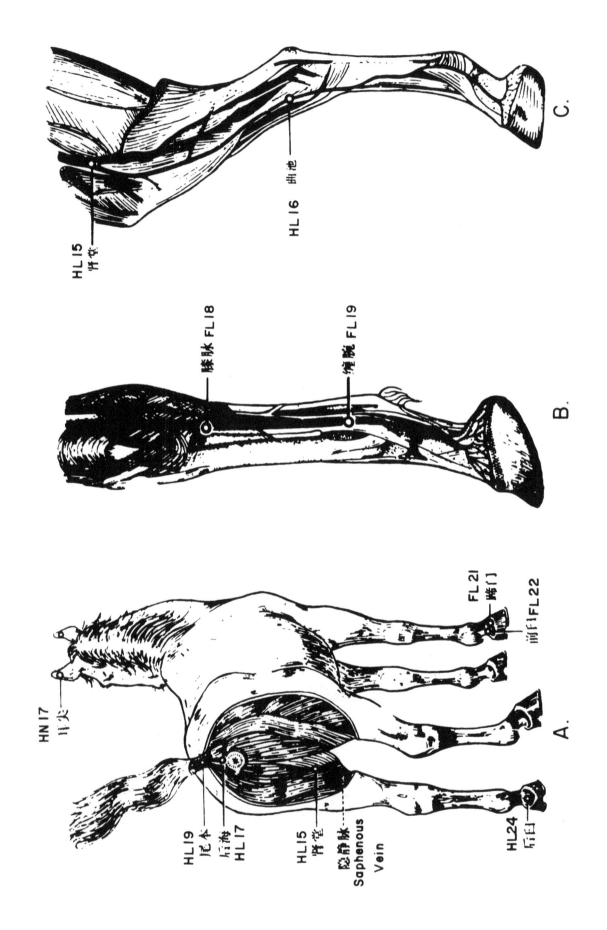

FIGURE 3-35. Acupuncture chart of the horse: a) caudal view; b) foreleg, medial view; c) hind leg, medial view.

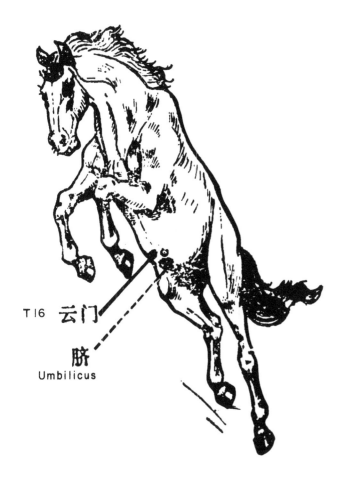

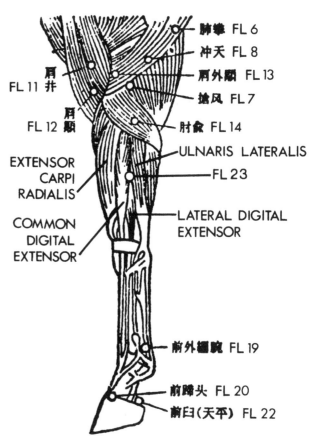

FIGURE 3–36. Acupuncture chart of the horse (ventral view).

FIGURE 3–37. Acupuncture chart of the horse: forelimb (lateral view).

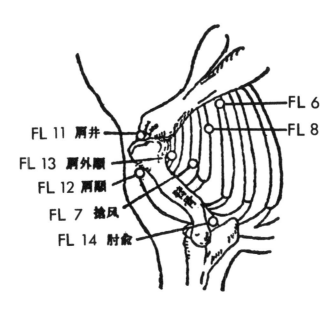

FIGURE 3–38. Acupuncture chart of the horse: forelimb (lateral view).

FIGURE 3–39. Acupuncture chart of the horse: forelimb (lateral view).

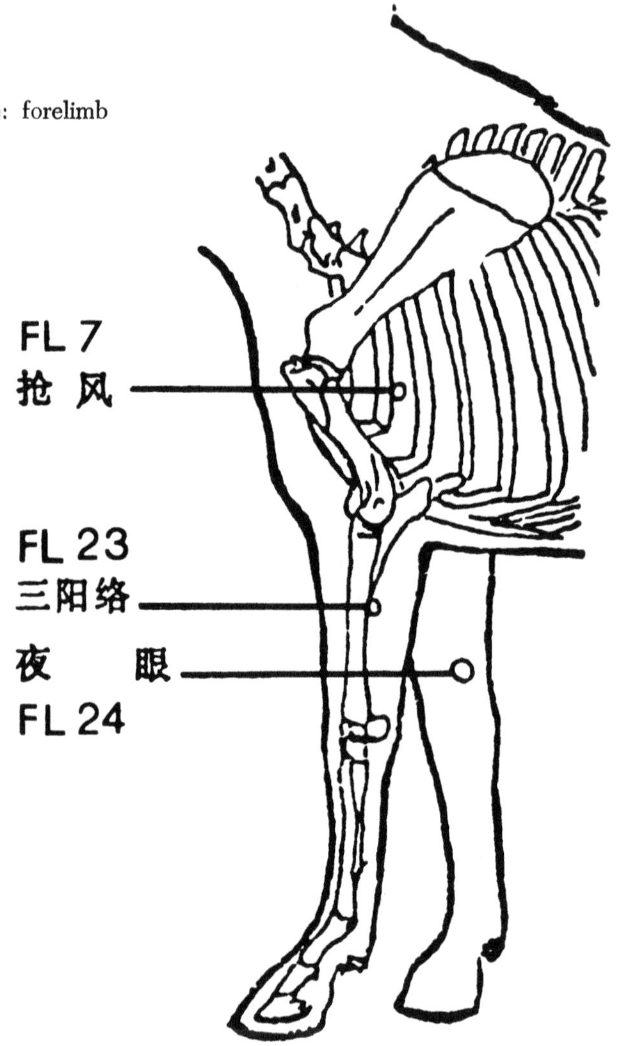

FL 7
抢风

FL 23
三阳络

夜　眼
FL 24

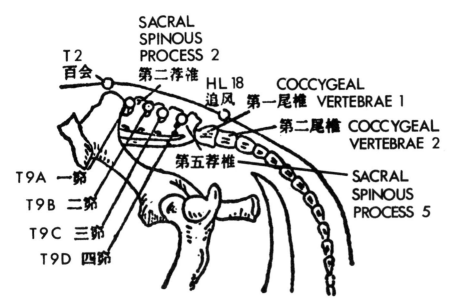

SACRAL
SPINOUS
PROCESS 2

T 2
百会　　第二荐推

HL 18
追风　第一尾椎　COCCYGEAL
VERTEBRAE 1

第二尾椎　COCCYGEAL
VERTEBRAE 2

第五荐椎

SACRAL
SPINOUS
PROCESS 5

T9A 一节

T9B 二节

T9C 三节

T9D 四节

FIGURE 3–40. Acupuncture chart of the horse: sacral area (lateral view).

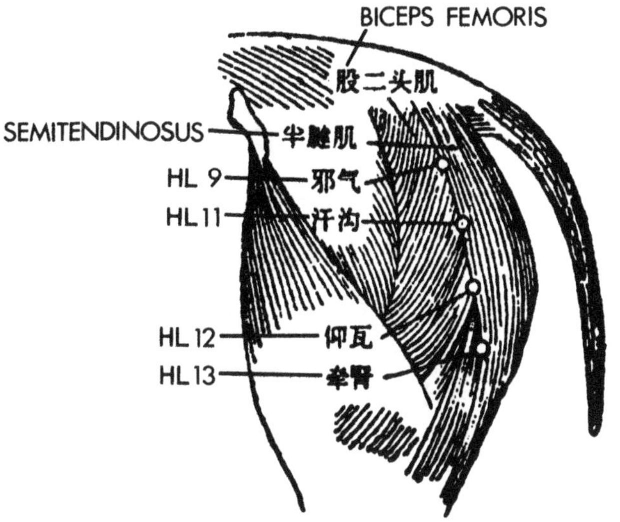

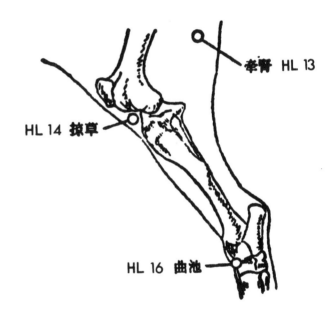

FIGURE 3–41. Acupuncture chart of the horse: hind limb (lateral view).

FIGURE 3–42. Acupuncture chart of the horse: hind limb (lateral view).

FIGURE 3–43. Acupuncture chart of the horse: hind limb (lateral view).

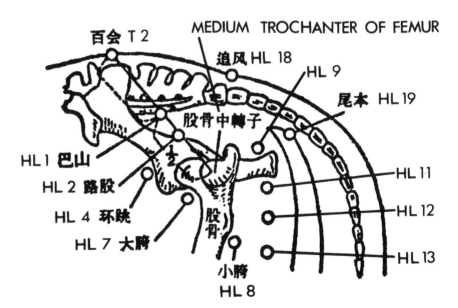

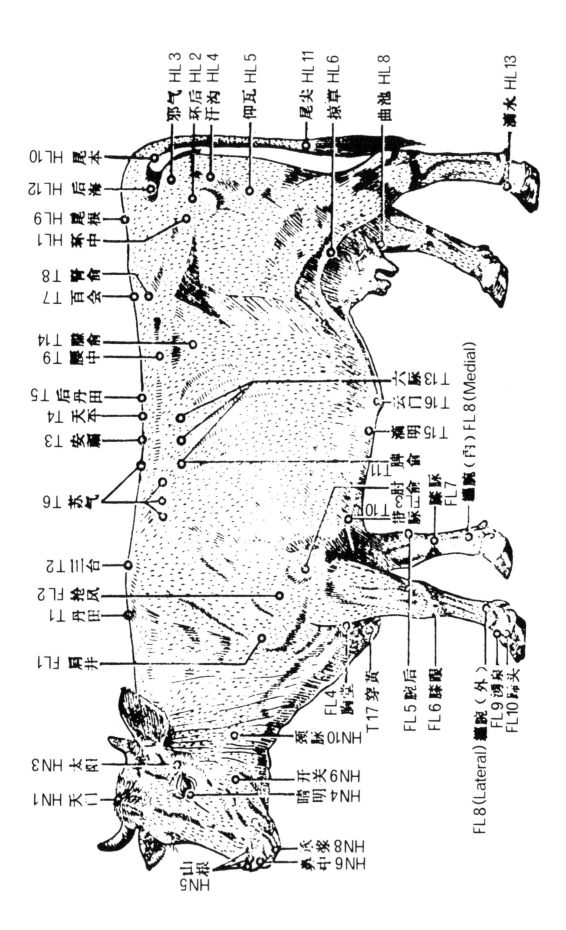

FIGURE 3–44. Acupuncture chart of the cow (lateral view).

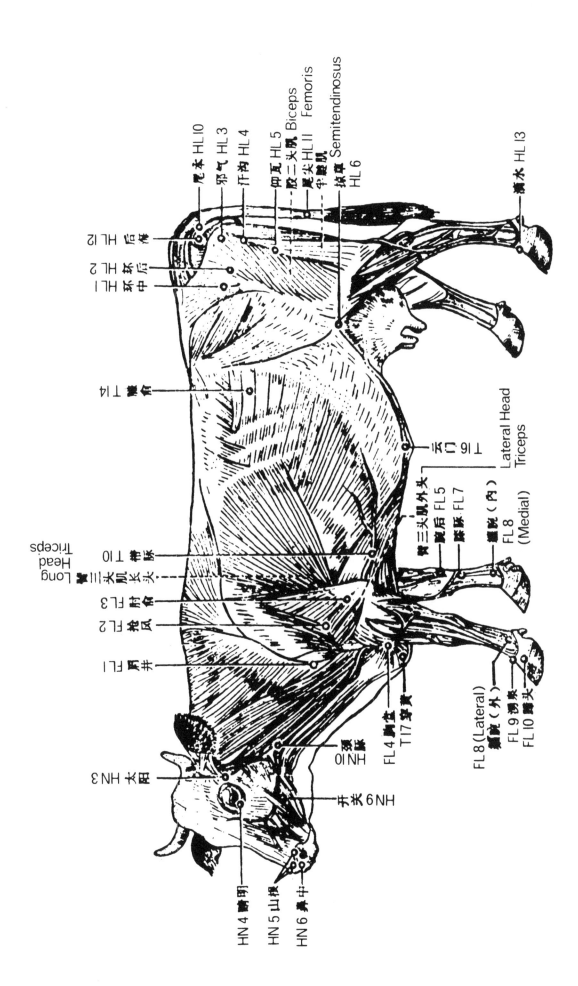

FIGURE 3–45. Acupuncture chart of the cow (lateral view).

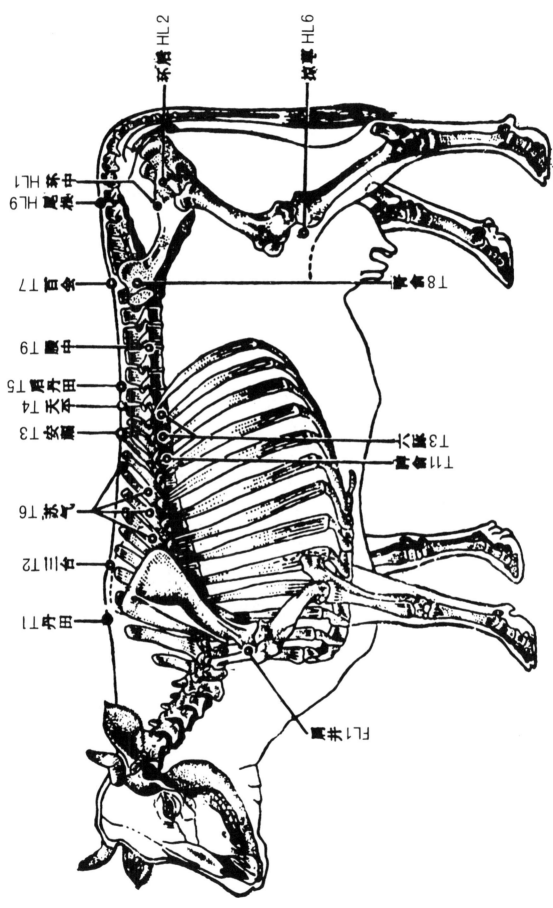

FIGURE 3–46. Acupuncture chart of the cow (lateral view).

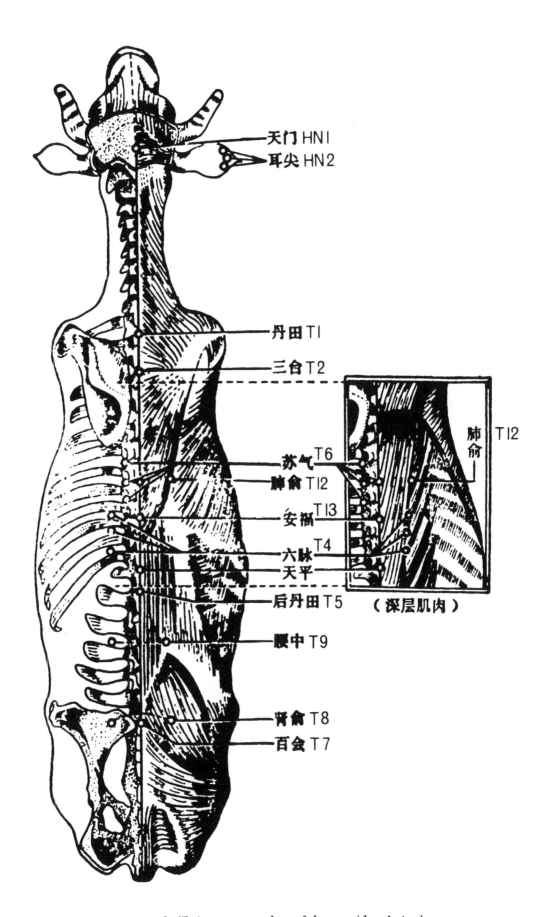

天门 HN1
耳尖 HN2

丹田 T1

三合 T2

肺俞 T12

苏气 T6
肺俞 T12
安福 T13
六脉 T4
天平

后丹田 T5

腰中 T9

肾俞 T8
百会 T7

（深层肌肉）

FIGURE 3–47. Acupuncture chart of the cow (dorsal view).

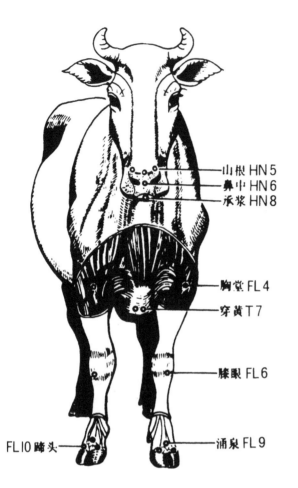

山根 HN 5
鼻中 HN 6
承浆 HN 8

胸堂 FL 4

穿黄 T 7

膝眼 FL 6

FL 10 蹄头

涌泉 FL 9

FIGURE 3–48. Acupuncture chart of the cow (cranial view).

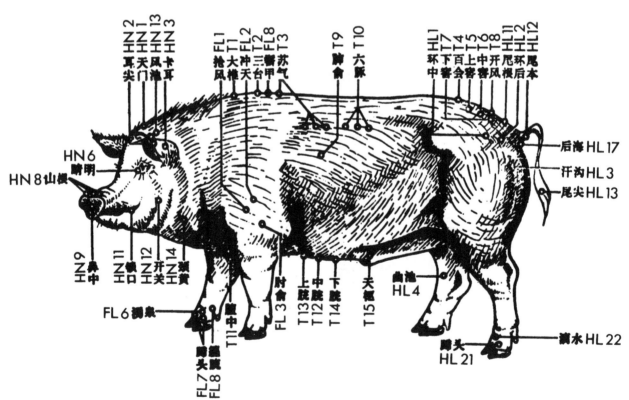

HN 2 耳尖
HN 1 天门
HN 13 风池
HN 3 卡耳

FL 1 抬风
T 1 大椎
FL 2 冲天
T 2 三台
FL 8 警甲
T 3 苏气

T 9 蹄俞
T 10 六脉

HL 1 环中
T 7 下窜
T 4 百会
T 5 上窜
T 6 中窜
T 8 开风
HL 11 尼根
HL 2 环后
HL 12 尾本

后海 HL 17
汗沟 HL 3
尾尖 HL 13

HN 6
HN 8 山根
睛明

HN 9 鼻中
HN 11 锁口
HN 12 银宫
HN 14 开关
HN 14 颈窗

曲池 HL 4

FL 6 涌泉

肘俞 FL 3
T 13 上脘
T 12 中脘
T 14 下脘
T 15 天枢

蹄头 HL 21

滴水 HL 22

蹄头 FL 7
鼠蹊 FL 8
T 11 蹄中

FIGURE 3–49. Acupuncture chart of the pig (lateral view).

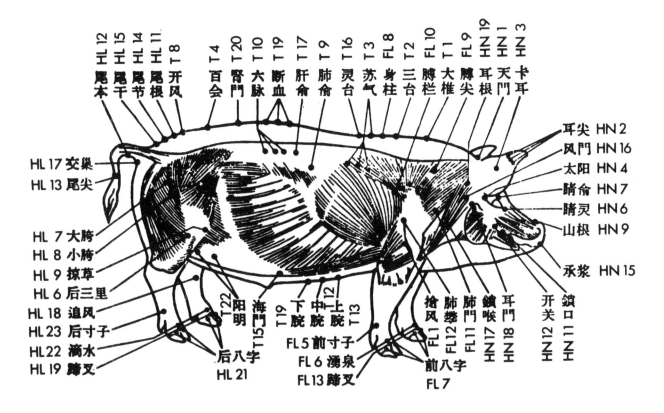

FIGURE 3–50. Acupuncture chart of the pig (lateral view).

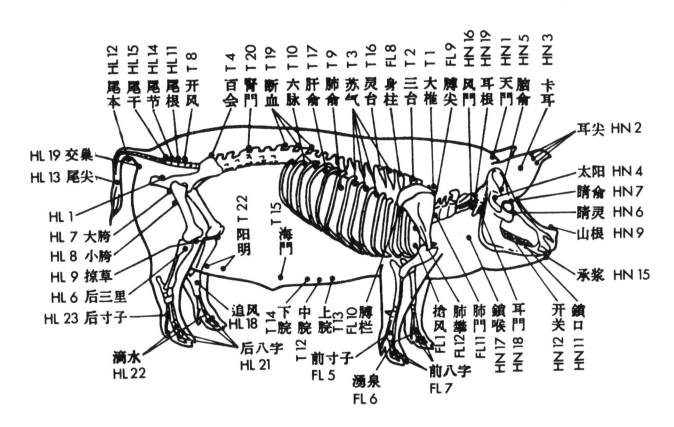

FIGURE 3–51. Acupuncture chart of the pig (lateral view).

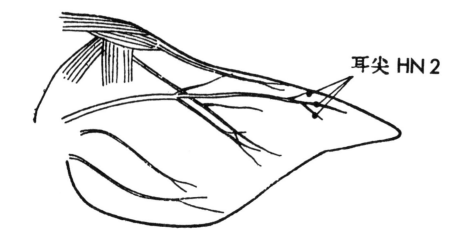

耳尖 HN 2

FIGURE 3–52. Acupuncture chart of the pig: ear, medial surface.

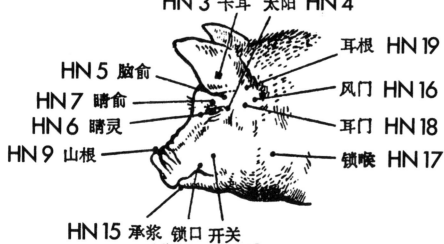
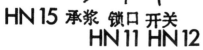

HN 3 卡耳　太阳 HN 4

耳根 HN 19

HN 5 脑俞

风门 HN 16

HN 7 睛俞

HN 6 睛灵

耳门 HN 18

HN 9 山根

锁喉 HN 17

HN 15 承浆　锁口 开关

HN 11 HN 12

FIGURE 3–53. Acupuncture chart of the pig: head (lateral view).

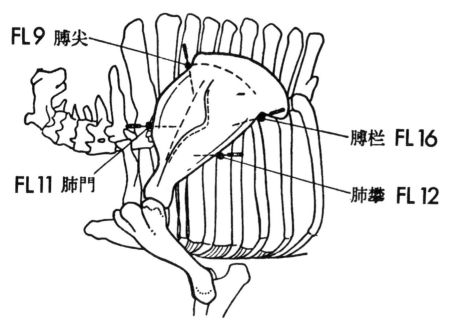

FL 9 膊尖

膊栏 FL 16

FL 11 肺門

肺攀 FL 12

FIGURE 3–54. Acupuncture chart of the pig: forelimb (lateral view).

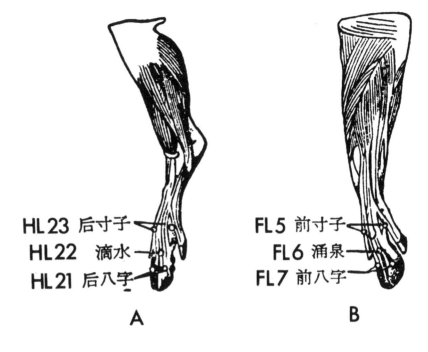

FIGURE 3–55. Acupuncture chart of the pig: a) hind limb (cranial view) b) forelimb (cranial view).

HL 23 后寸子
HL 22 滴水
HL 21 后八字

FL 5 前寸子
FL 6 涌泉
FL 7 前八字

A   B

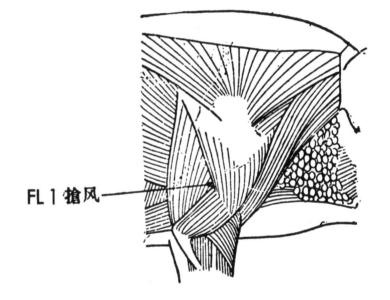

FIGURE 3–56. Acupuncture chart of the pig: forelimb (lateral view).

FL 1 抢风

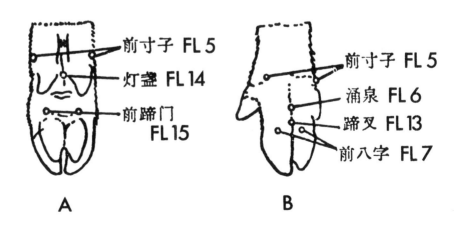

FIGURE 3–57. Acupuncture chart of the pig: a) forefoot (caudal view) b) forefoot (cranial view).

前寸子 FL 5
灯盏 FL 14
前蹄门 FL 15

前寸子 FL 5
涌泉 FL 6
蹄叉 FL 13
前八字 FL 7

A   B

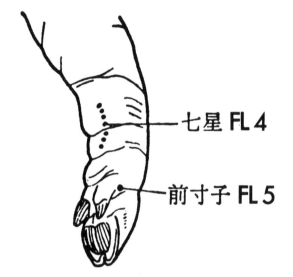

七星 **FL 4**

前寸子 **FL 5**

FIGURE 3–58. Acupuncture chart of the pig: forelimb (caudal view).

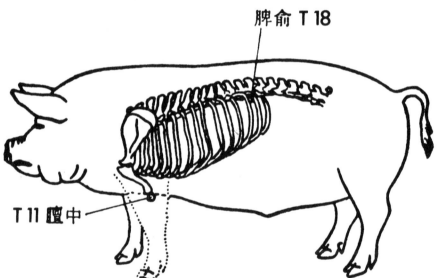

脾俞 **T 18**

T 11 膻中

FIGURE 3–59. Acupuncture chart of the pig (lateral view).

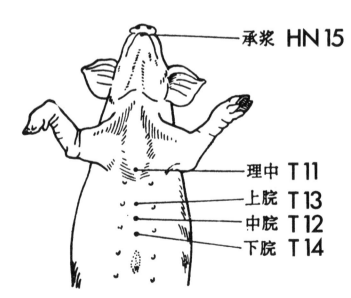

承浆 **HN 15**

理中 **T 11**
上脘 **T 13**
中脘 **T 12**
下脘 **T 14**

FIGURE 3–60. Acupuncture chart of the pig (ventral view).

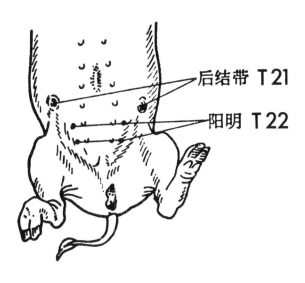

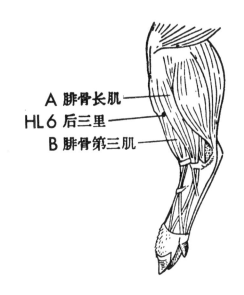

后结带 T 21

阳明 T 22

A 腓骨长肌
HL 6 后三里
B 腓骨第三肌

FIGURE 3–61. (Top, left) Acupuncture chart of the pig (ventral view).

FIGURE 3–62. (Top, right) Acupuncture chart of the pig: hind limb (lateral view).

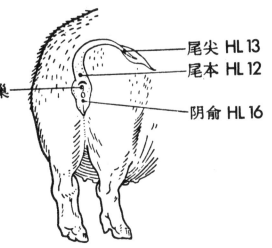

尾尖 HL 13
尾本 HL 12
HL 17 交巢
阴俞 HL 16

FIGURE 3–63. (Middle, right) Acupuncture chart of the pig: caudal view).

FIGURE 3–64. (Bottom, right) Acupuncture chart of the pig: hind limb (lateral view).

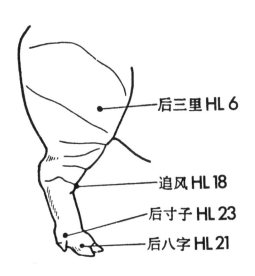

后三里 HL 6
追风 HL 18
后寸子 HL 23
后八字 HL 21

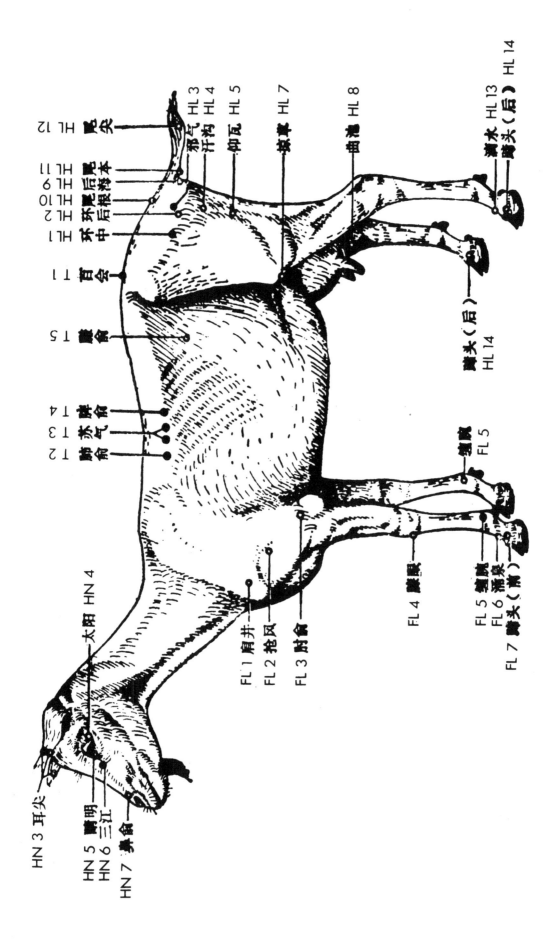

FIGURE 3–65. Acupuncture chart of the goat: (lateral view).

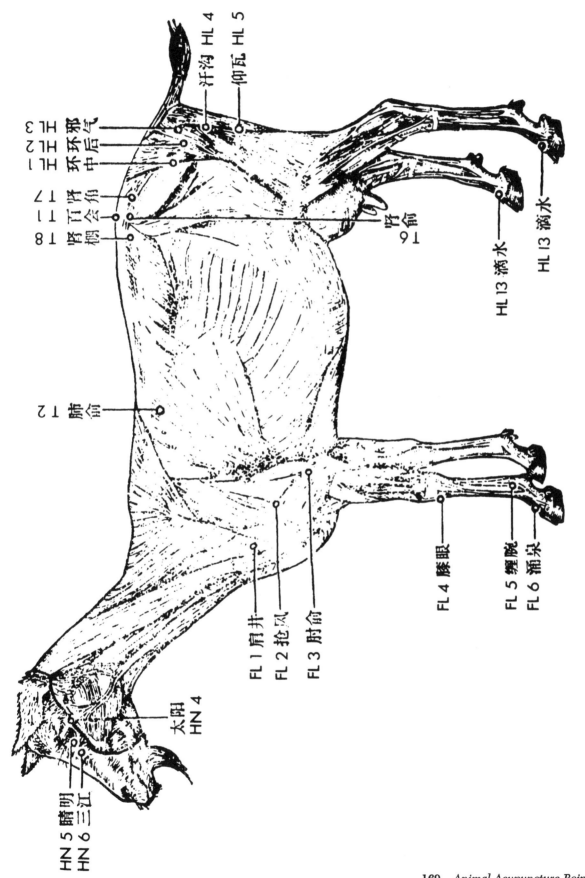

FIGURE 3–66. Acupuncture chart of the goat (lateral view).

汗沟 HL 4
仰瓦 HL 5

正正正
正正正
13 12 11

环环邪
中后气

肾八伯
会伯

TT T
7

肾俞
T6

HL 13 滴水

HL 13 滴水

肺俞
T2

FL 4 膝眼

FL 5 缠腕
FL 6 涌泉

FL 1 肩井
FL 2 抢风
FL 3 肘俞

太阴
HN 4

HN 5 睛明
HN 6 三江

169 *Animal Acupuncture Points*

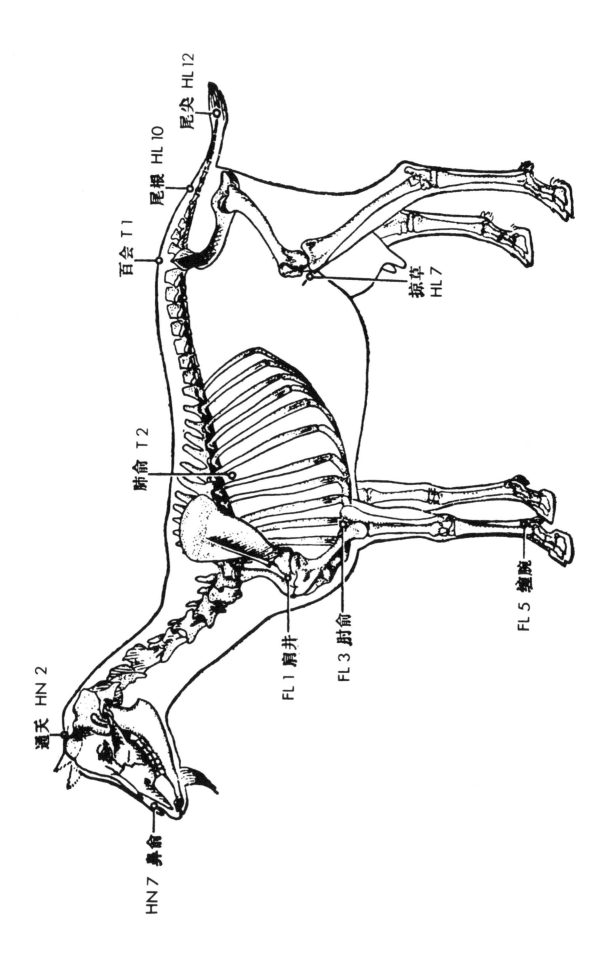

尾尖 HL 12

尾根 HL 10

百会 T 1

髎草 HL 7

肺俞 T 2

FL 5 錢脈

FL 3 肘俞

FL 1 肩井

通天 HN 2

HN 7 鼻俞

FIGURE 3–67. Acupuncture chart of the goat (lateral view).

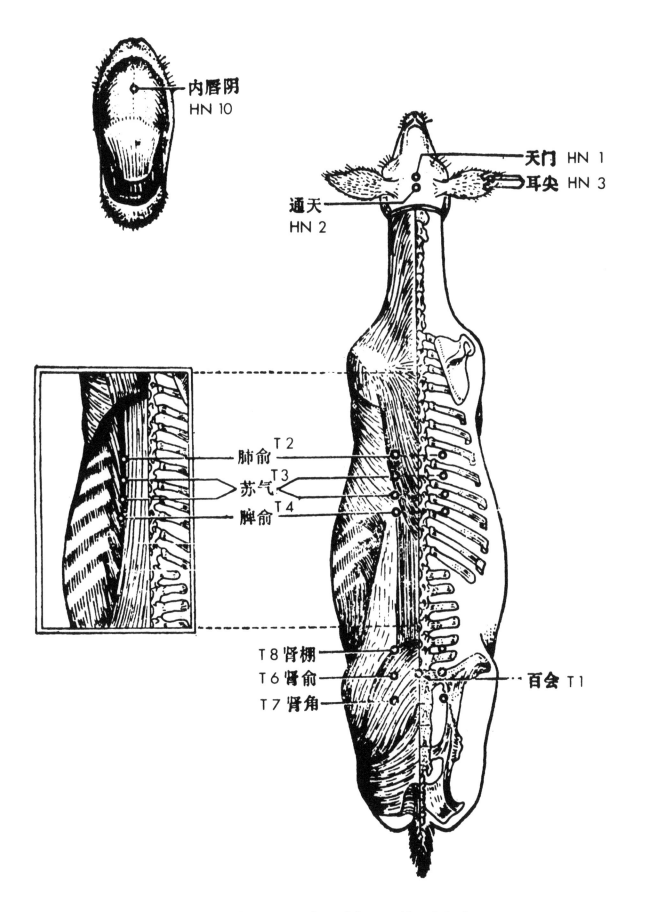

内唇阴
HN 10

天门 HN 1
耳尖 HN 3
通天
HN 2

肺俞　T 2
苏气　T 3
脾俞　T 4

T8 肾棚
T6 肾俞
T7 肾角
百会 T1

FIGURE 3–68. Acupuncture chart of the goat (dorsal view).

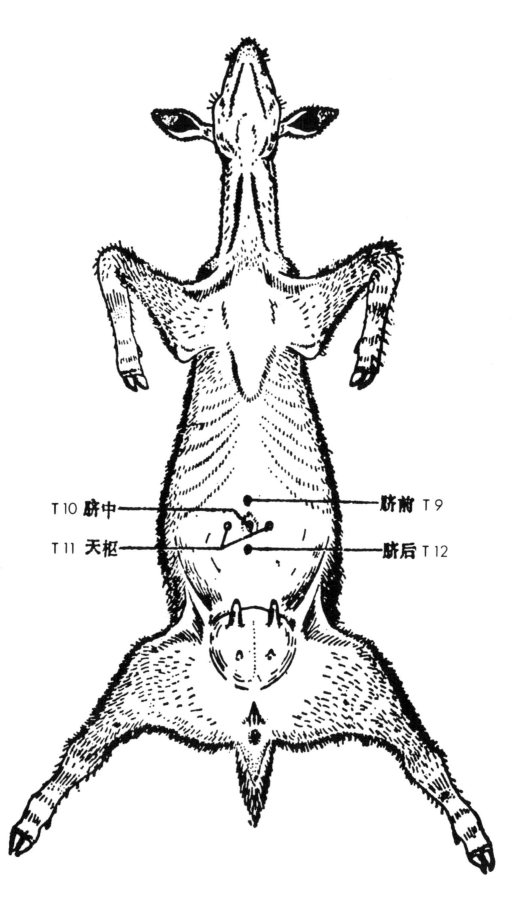

T 10 脐中 ——————— 脐前 T 9

T 11 天枢 ——————— 脐后 T 12

FIGURE 3–69. Acupuncture chart of the goat (ventral view).

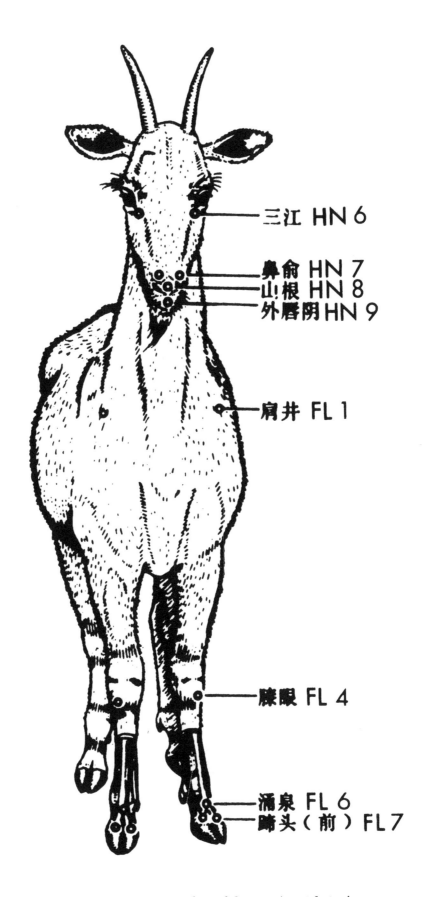

三江 HN 6

鼻俞 HN 7
山根 HN 8
外唇阴 HN 9

肩井 FL 1

膝眼 FL 4

涌泉 FL 6
蹄头（前）FL 7

FIGURE 3–70. Acupuncture chart of the goat (cranial view).

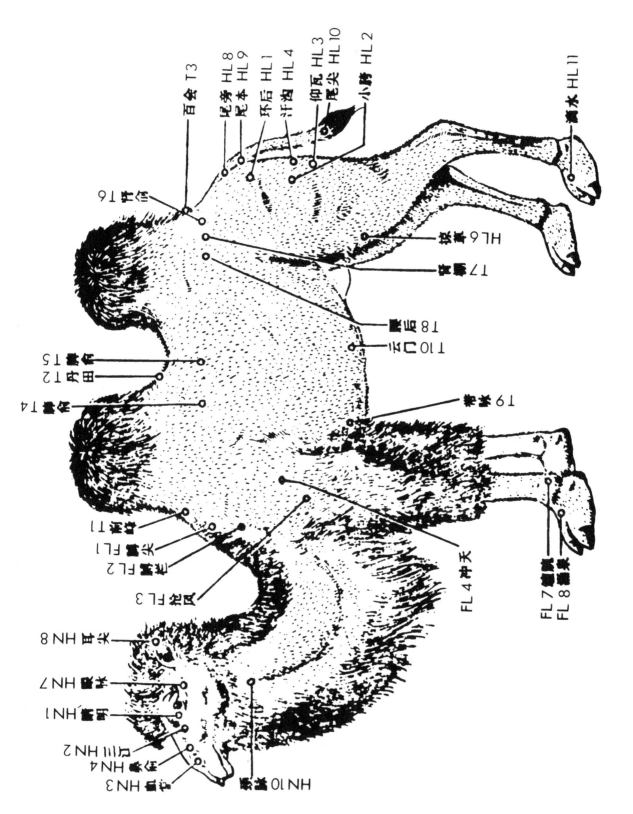

FIGURE 3–71. Acupuncture chart of the camel (lateral view).

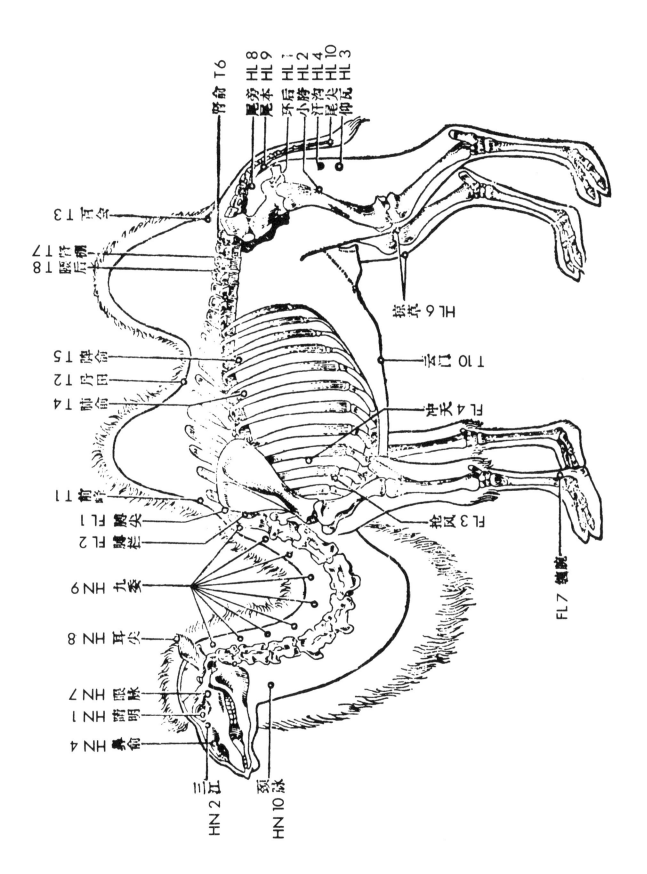

FIGURE 3-72. Acupuncture chart of the camel (lateral view).

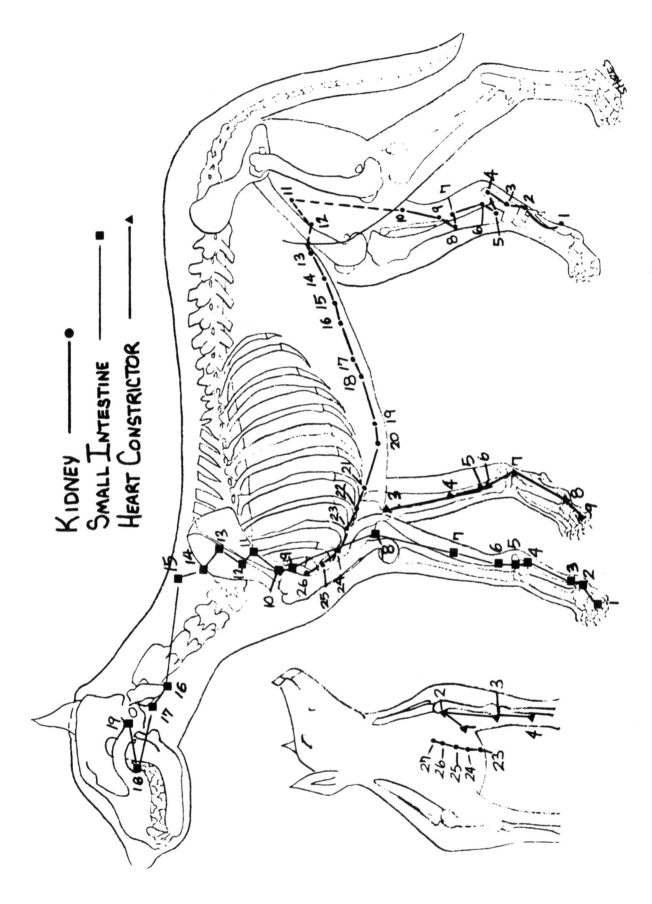

KIDNEY •————

SMALL INTESTINE ■————

HEART CONSTRICTOR ▲————

FIGURE 3–73. Shores' acupuncture chart of the dog: kidney, small intestine, and heart constrictor meridians. (Courtesy of A. Shores.)

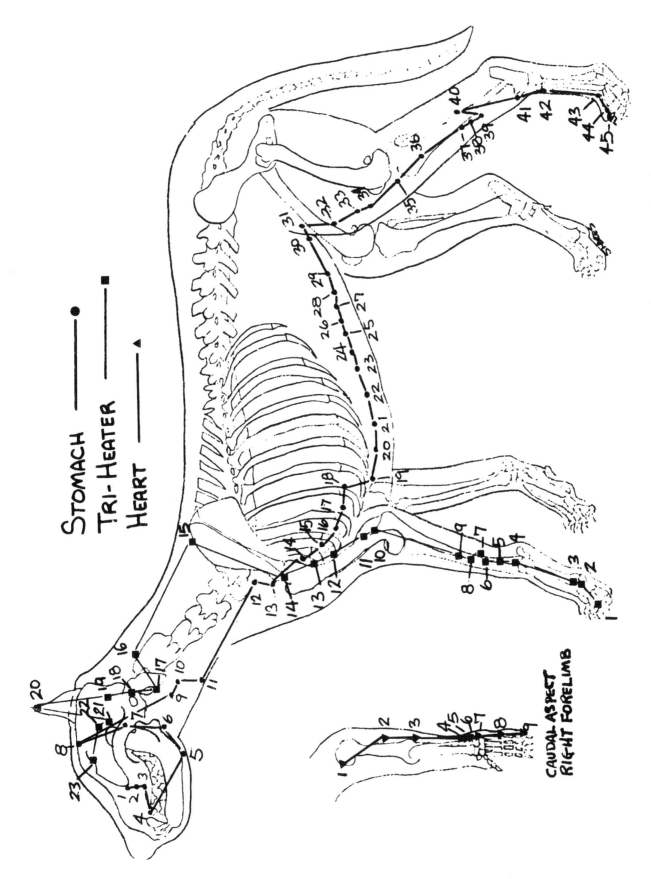

STOMACH •————
TRI-HEATER ■————
HEART ▲————

CAUDAL ASPECT
RIGHT FORELIMB

FIGURE 3-74. Acupuncture chart of the dog: stomach, triple-burner, and heart meridians. (Courtesy of A. Shores.)

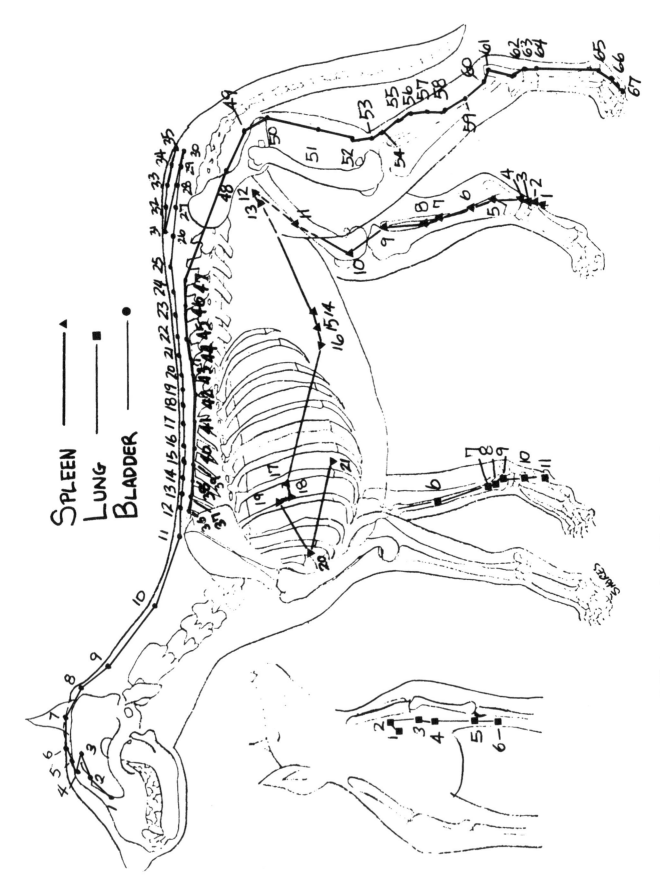

FIGURE 3–75. Acupuncture chart of the dog: spleen, lung, and bladder meridians. (Courtesy of A. Shores.)

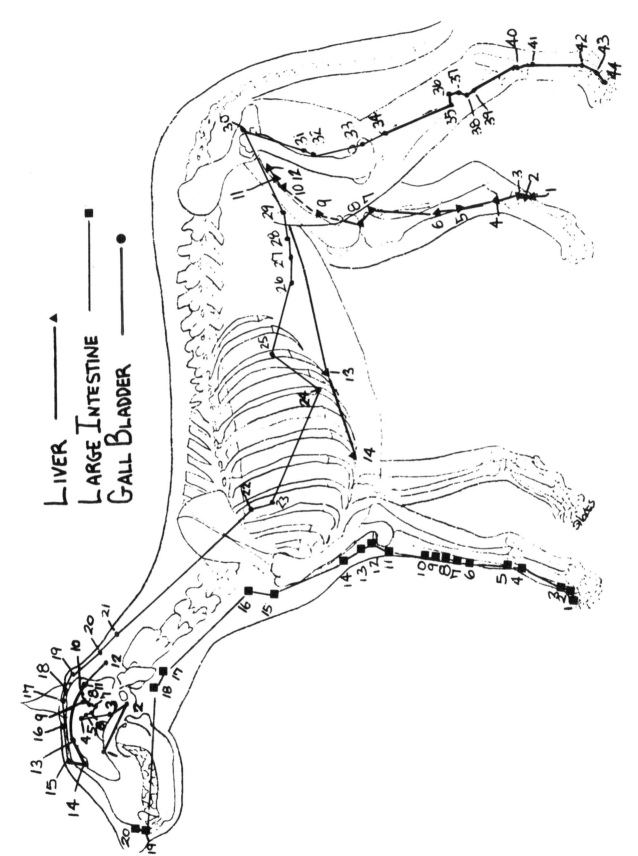

FIGURE 3–76. Acupuncture chart of the dog: liver, large intestine, and gallbladder meridians. (Courtesy of A. Shores.)

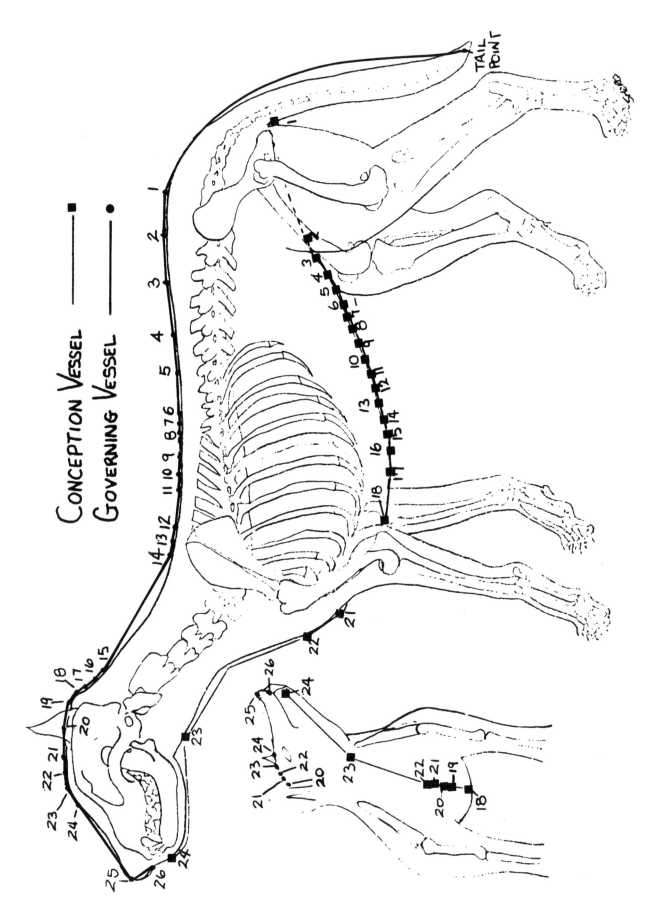

CONCEPTION VESSEL ——■——

GOVERNING VESSEL ——●——

FIGURE 3–77. Acupuncture chart of the dog: conception vessel and governing vessel. (Courtesy of A. Shores.)

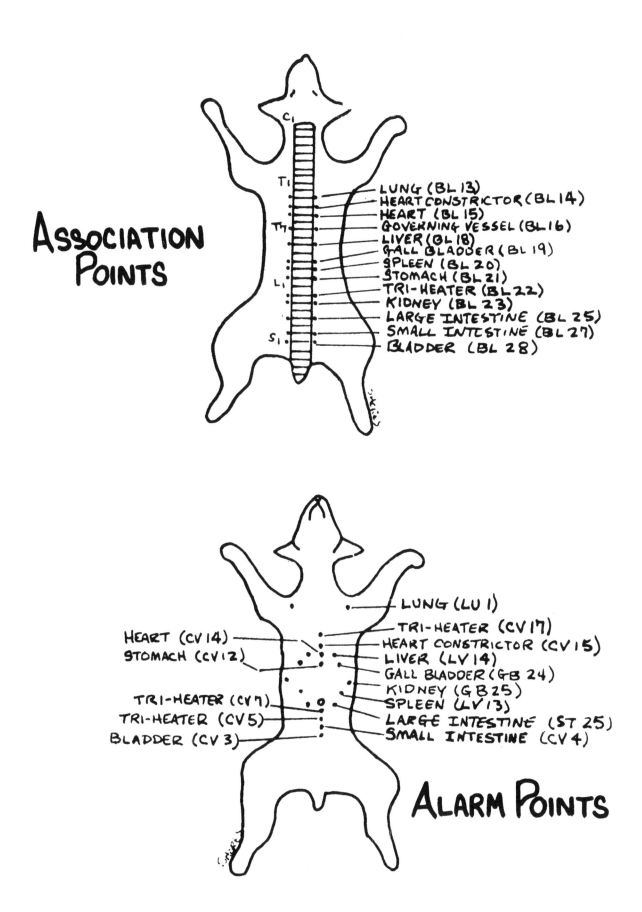

FIGURE 3–78. Acupuncture chart of the dog: association and alarm points. (Courtesy of A. Shores.)

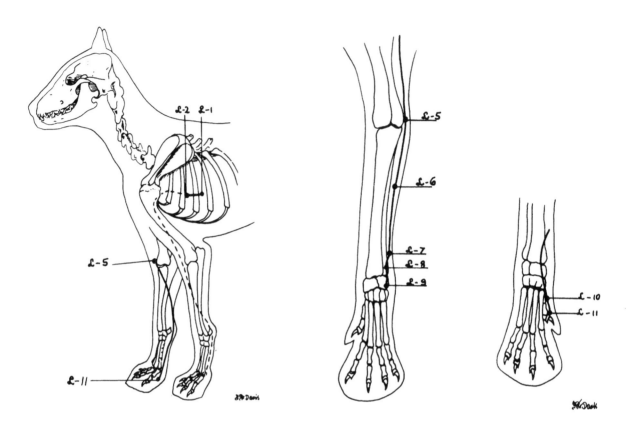

FIGURE 3–79. The Young dog chart: lung meridian. (Courtesy of Dr. H. Grady Young.)

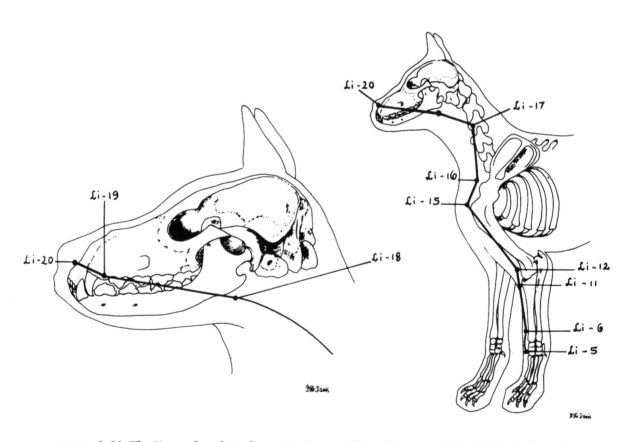

FIGURE 3–80. The Young dog chart: large intestine meridian. (Courtesy of Dr. H. Grady Young.)

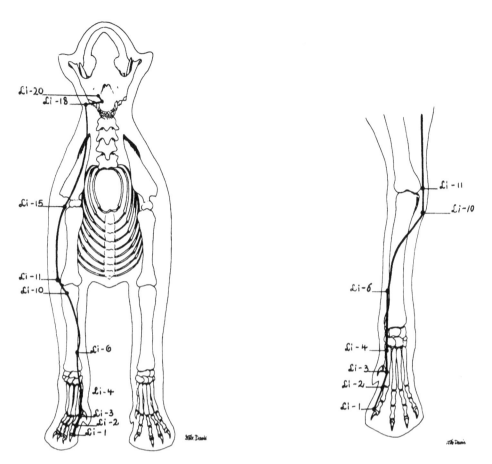

FIGURE 3–81. The Young dog chart: large intestine meridian. (Courtesy of Dr. H. Grady Young.)

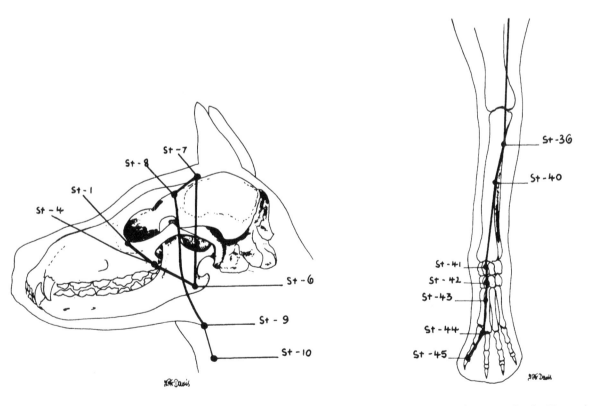

FIGURE 3–82. The Young dog chart: stomach meridian, head, and hindlimb. (Courtesy of Dr. H. Grady Young.)

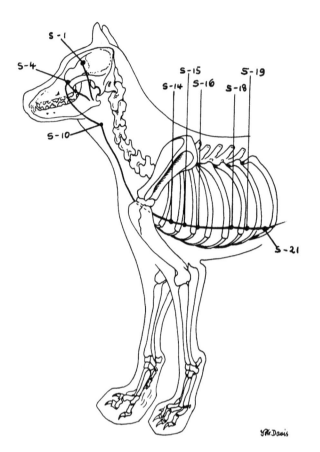

FIGURE 3–83. The Young dog chart: stomach meridian. (Courtesy of Dr. H. Grady Young.)

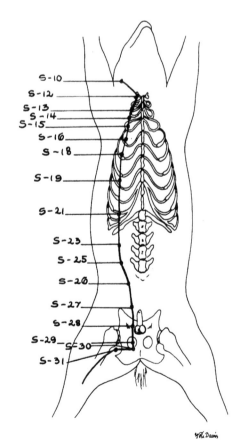

FIGURE 3–84. The Young dog chart: stomach meridian (ventral view). (Courtesy of Dr. H. Grady Young.)

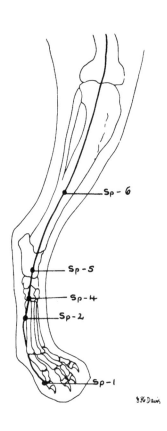

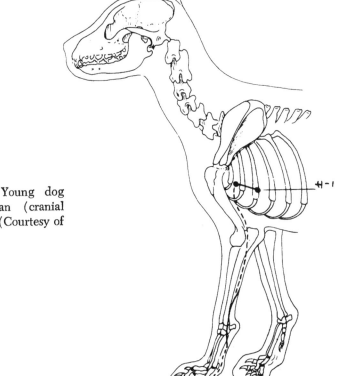

FIGURE 3–85. The Young dog chart: spleen meridian (ventral view and medial view of hindlimb. (Courtesy of Dr. H. Grady Young.)

FIGURE 3–86. The Young dog chart: heart meridian (cranial view of left foreleg). (Courtesy of Dr. H. Grady Young.)

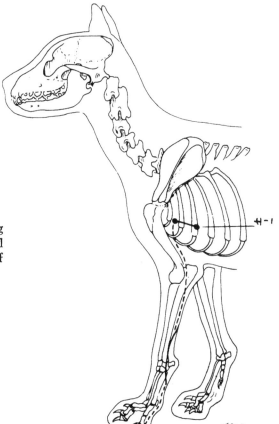

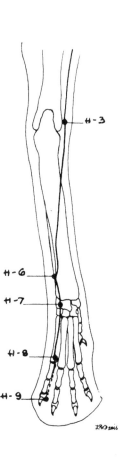

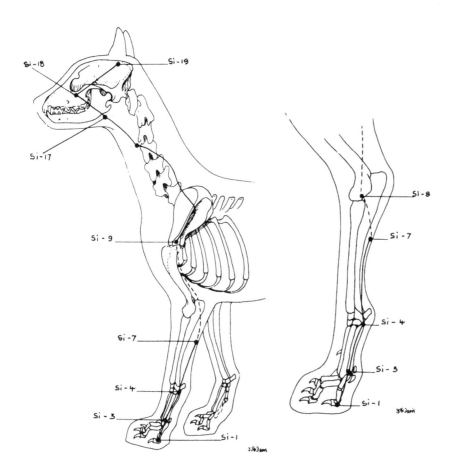

FIGURE 3–87. The Young dog chart: small intestine meridian. (Courtesy of Dr. H. Grady Young.)

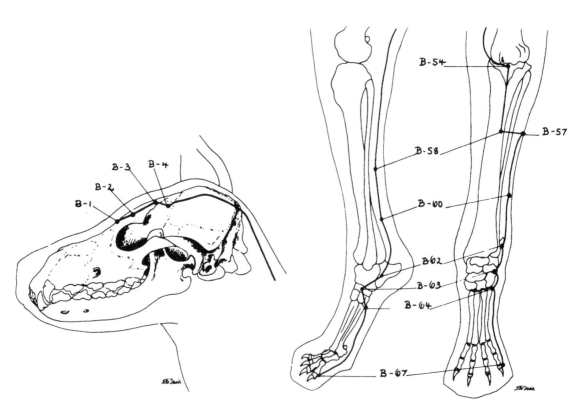

FIGURE 3–88. The Young dog chart: bladder meridian, hind limb (lateral and cranial view). (Courtesy of Dr. H. Grady Young.)

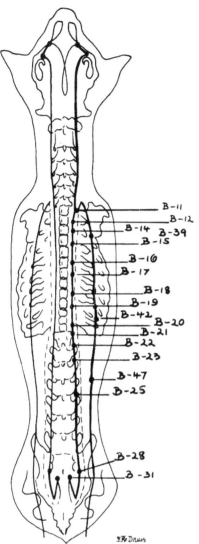

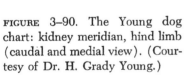

FIGURE 3–89. The Young dog chart: bladder meridian (dorsal view). (Courtesy of Dr. H. Grady Young.)

B–11
B–12
B–14 B–39
B–15
B–16
B–17
B–18
B–19
B–42 B–20
B–21
B–22
3–23
B–47
B–25
B–28
3–31

FIGURE 3–90. The Young dog chart: kidney meridian, hind limb (caudal and medial view). (Courtesy of Dr. H. Grady Young.)

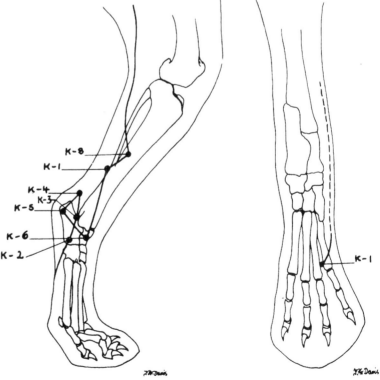

K–8
K–1
K–4
K–3
K–5
K–6
K–2

K–1

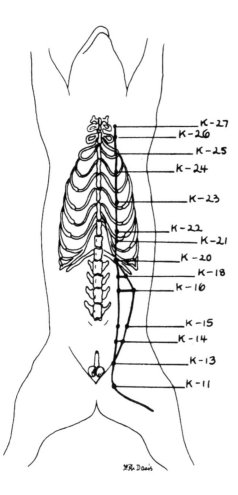

K-27
K-26
K-25
K-24
K-23
K-22
K-21
K-20
K-18
K-16
K-15
K-14
K-13
K-11

FIGURE 3–91. The Young dog chart: kidney meridian (ventral view). (Courtesy of Dr. H. Grady Young.)

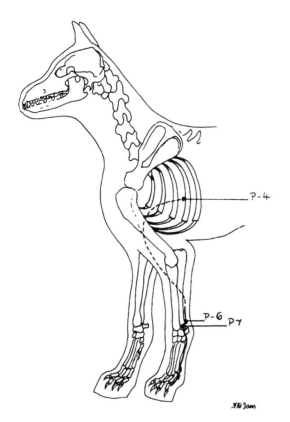

P-4

P-6 P-7

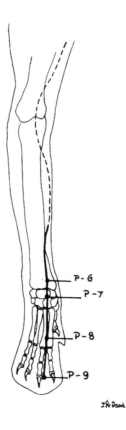

P-6
P-7
P-8
P-9

FIGURE 3–92. The Young dog chart: pericardium meridian. (Courtesy of Dr. H. Grady Young.)

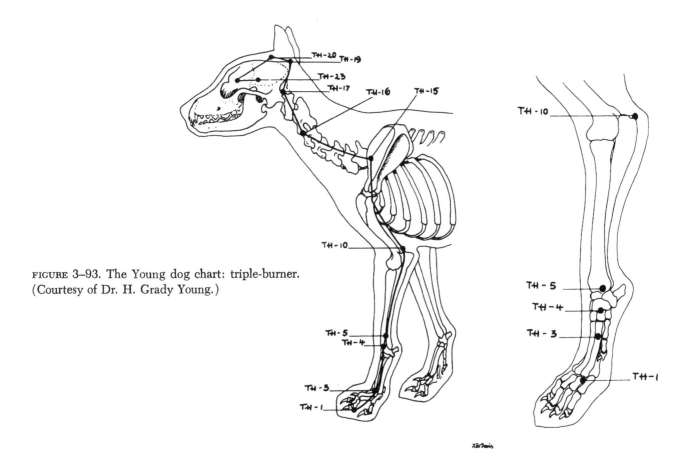

FIGURE 3–93. The Young dog chart: triple-burner. (Courtesy of Dr. H. Grady Young.)

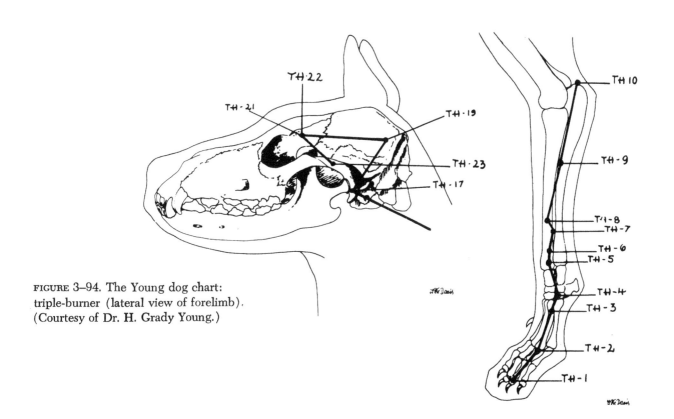

FIGURE 3–94. The Young dog chart: triple-burner (lateral view of forelimb). (Courtesy of Dr. H. Grady Young.)

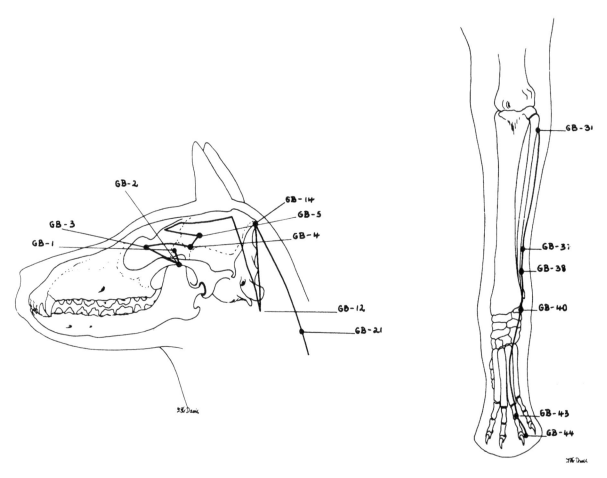

FIGURE 3–95. The Young dog chart: gallbladder meridian (cranial view of left hindlimb). (Courtesy of Dr. H. Grady Young.)

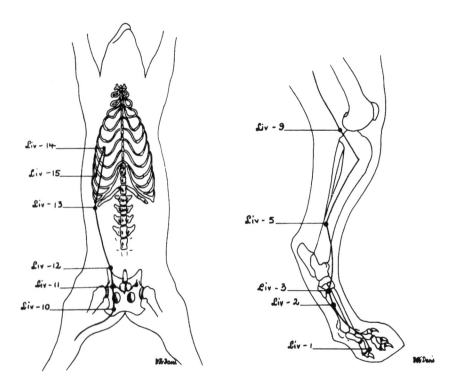

FIGURE 3–96. The Young dog chart: liver meridian (ventral view and medial view of hindlimb). (Courtesy of Dr. H. Grady Young.)

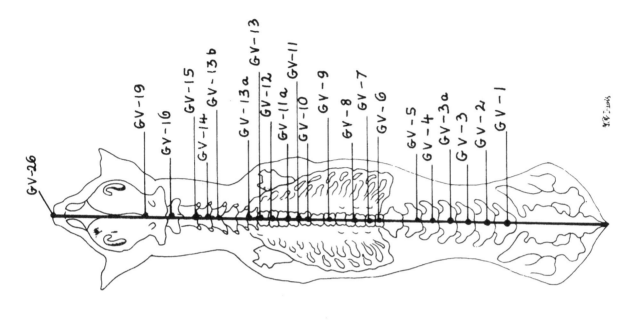

FIGURE 3–98. The Young dog chart: governing vessel (dorsal view). (Courtesy of Dr. H. Grady Young.)

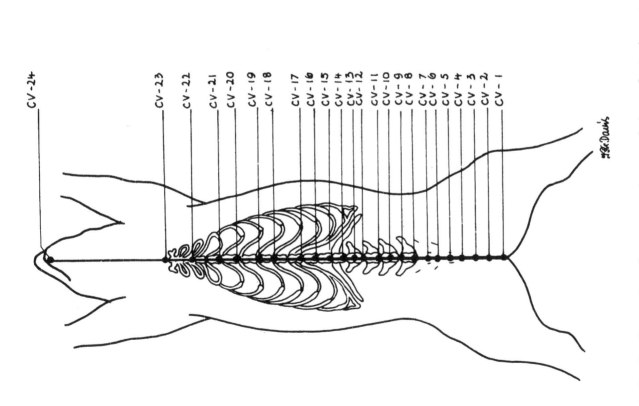

FIGURE 3–97. The Young dog chart: conception vessel (ventral view). (Courtesy of Dr. H. Grady Young.)

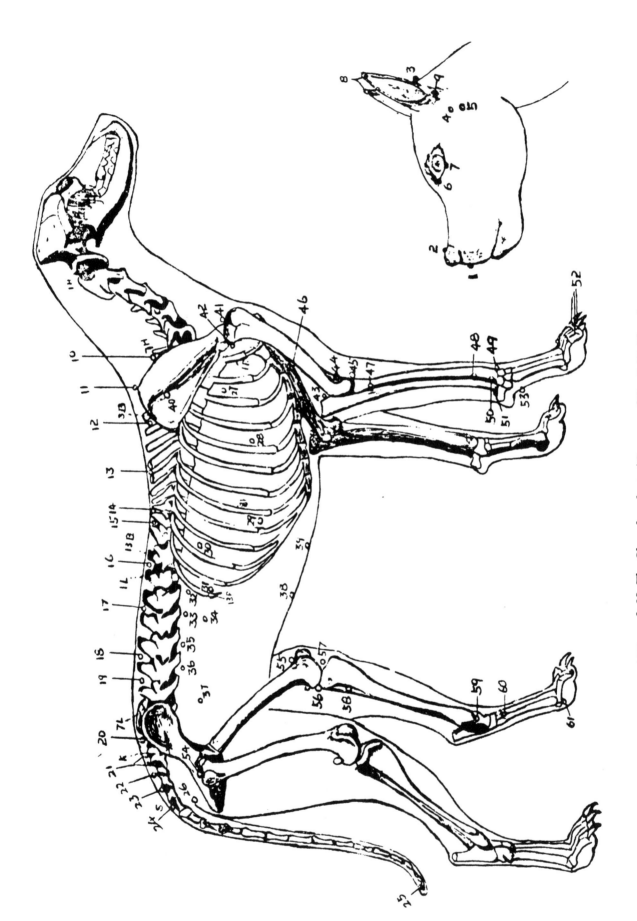

'FIGURE 3–99. The Chen dog chart. (Courtesy of Dr. S. H. Chen.)

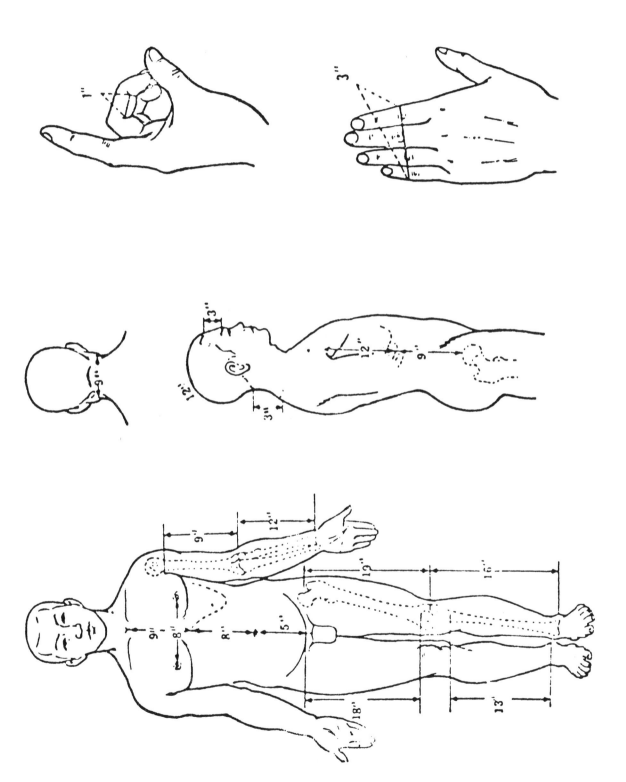

FIGURE 3–100. Acupuncture inch measurement in the human. (Courtesy of E. C. Wong.)

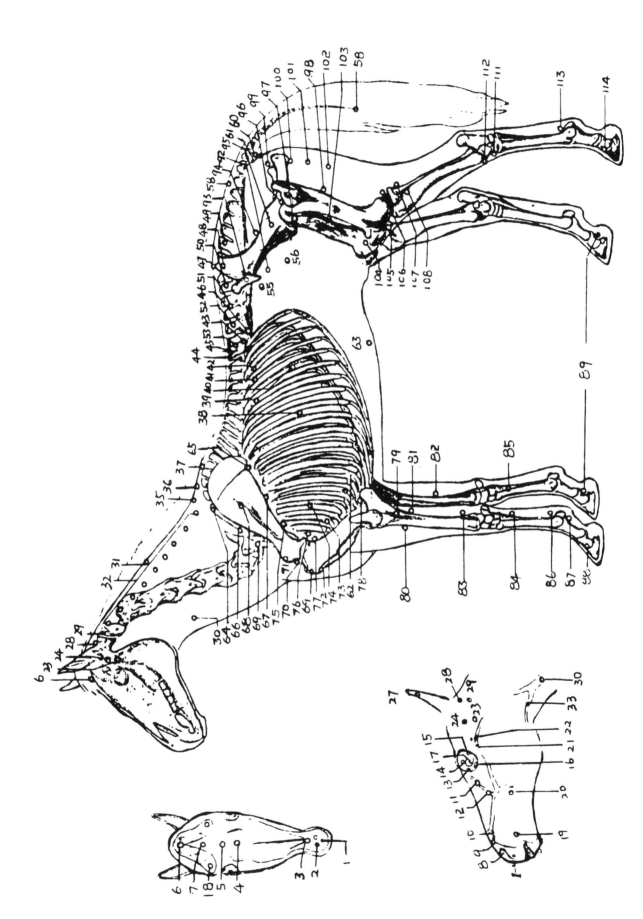

FIGURE 3–101. Chen horse chart: lateral view, skeleton. (Courtesy of Dr. S. H. Chen.)

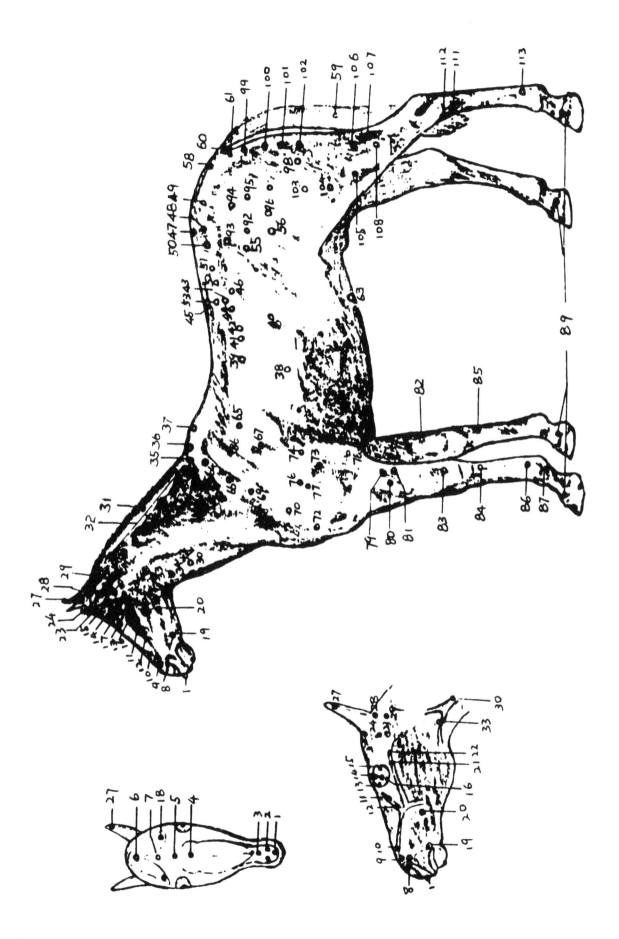

FIGURE 3–102. Chen horse chart: lateral view, skin. (Courtesy of Dr. S. H. Chen.)

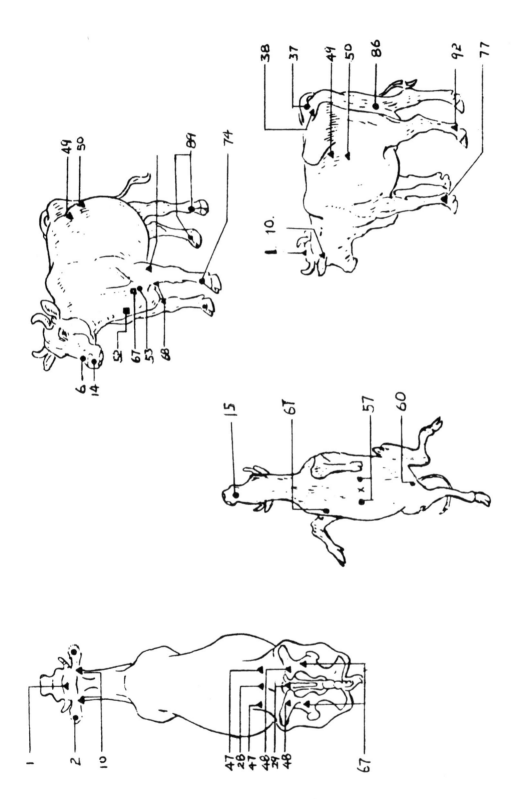

FIGURE 3–103. Chen cattle chart: miscellaneous views. (Courtesy of Dr. S. H. Chen.)

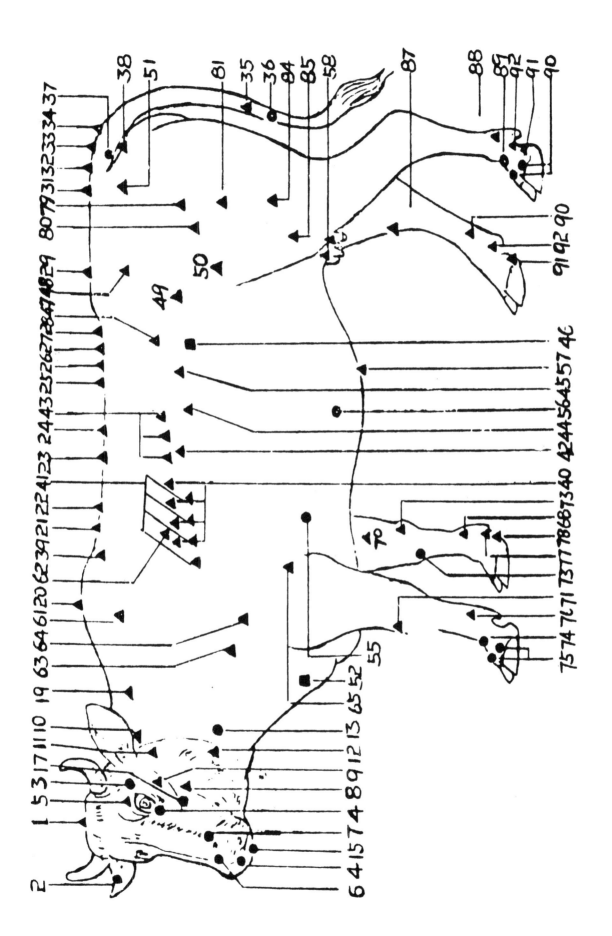

FIGURE 3–104. Chen cattle chart: lateral view, skin. (Courtesy of Dr. S. H. Chen.)

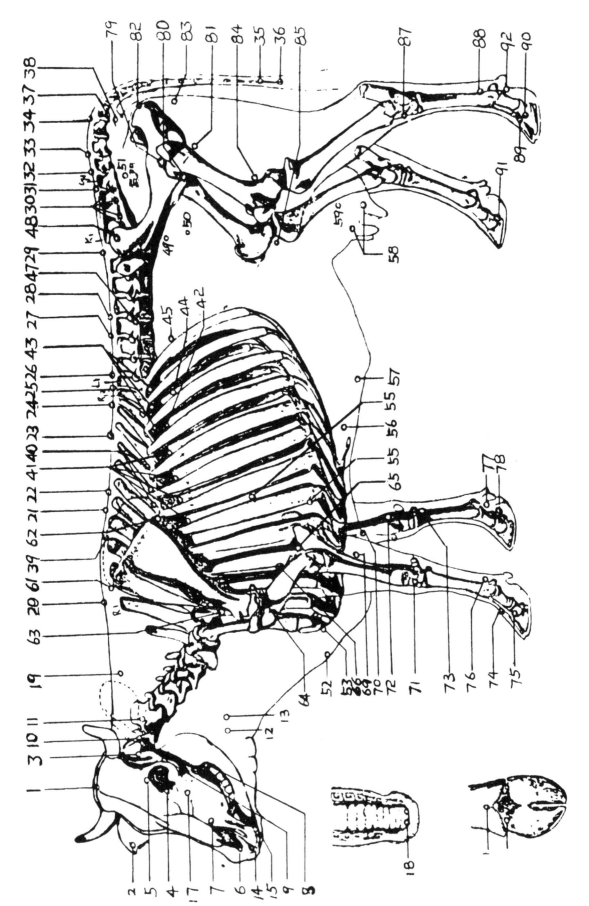

FIGURE 3–105. Chen cattle chart: lateral view, skeleton. (Courtesy of Dr. S. H. Chen.)

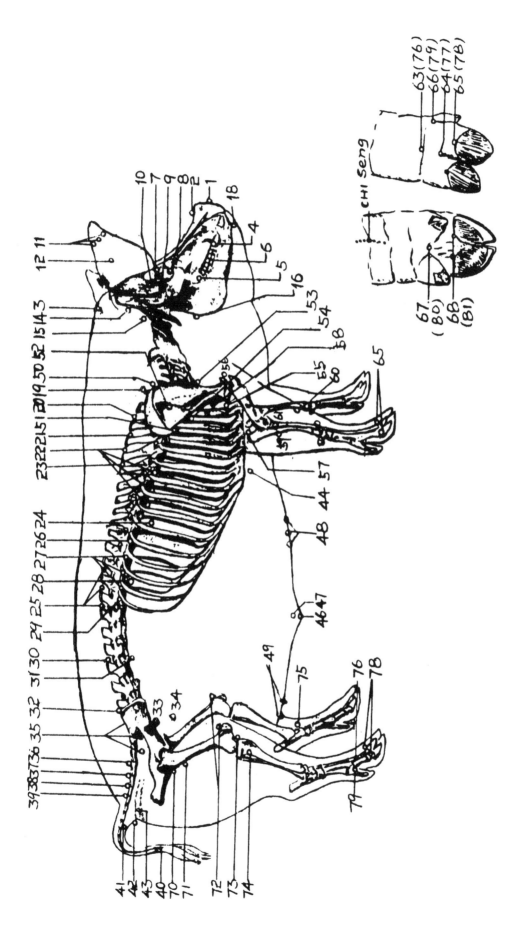

FIGURE 3–106. Chen swine chart: lateral view, skeleton. (Courtesy of Dr. S. H. Chen.)

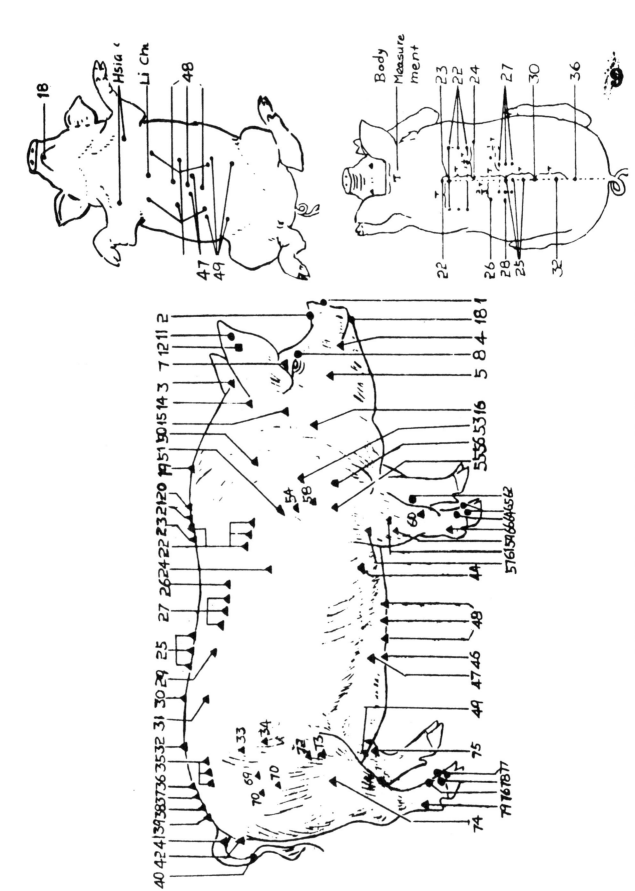

FIGURE 3–107. Chen swine chart: lateral view, skin. (Courtesy of Dr. S. H. Chen.)

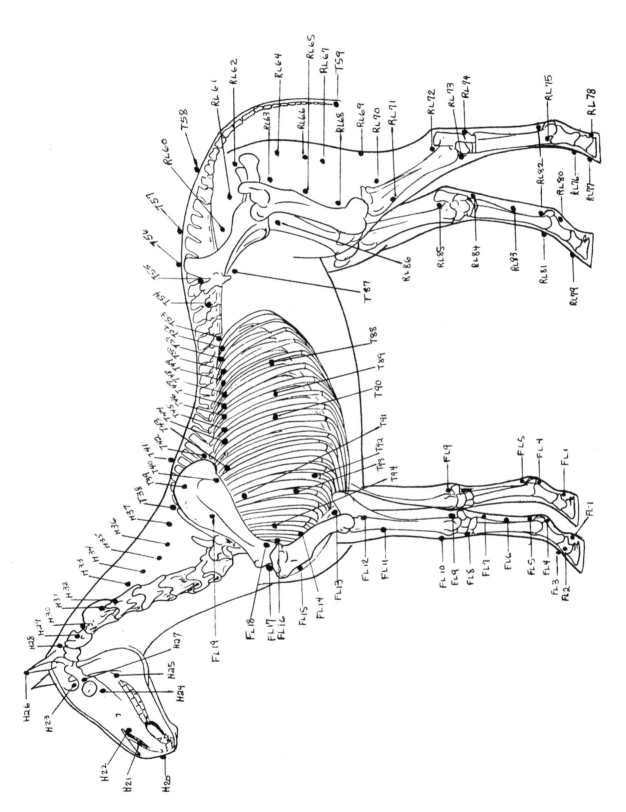

FIGURE 3–108. The Ottaviano Horse Chart: lateral view. (Courtesy of John Ottaviano and NAVA. Copyright © 1975 by NAVA.)

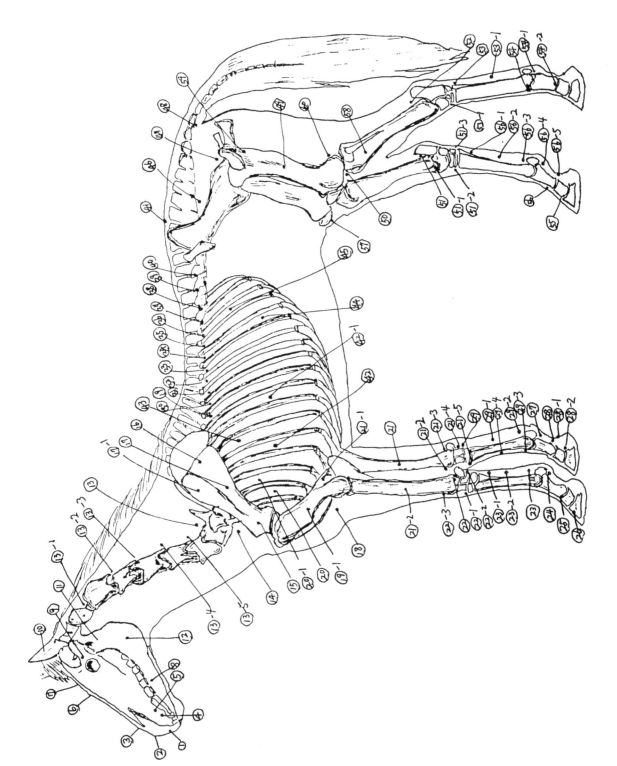

FIGURE 3–109. The Shin Horse Chart: lateral view, skeleton. (Courtesy of Sang H. Shin and NAVA. Copyright © 1975 by NAVA.)

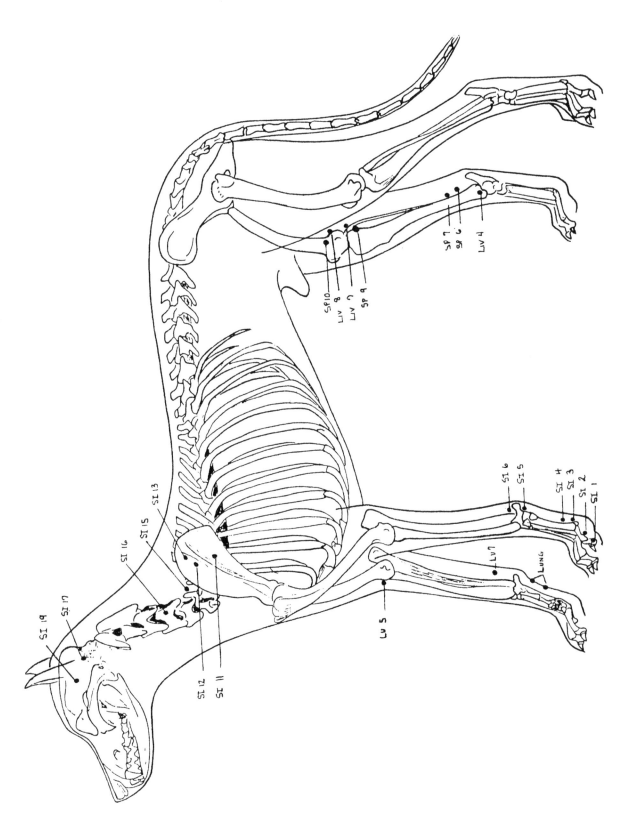

FIGURE 3–110. The Ottaviano Dog Chart: Small Intestine (SI), Lung (LU), Liver (LIV), and Spleen (SP) (lateral view). (Courtesy of John Ottaviano and NAVA. Copyright © 1975 by NAVA.)

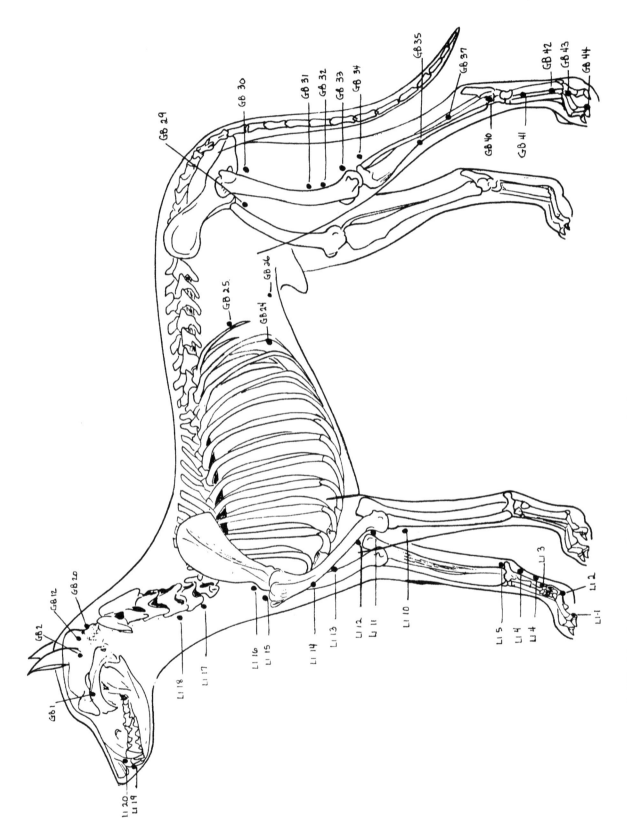

FIGURE 3–111. The Ottaviano Dog Chart: Large Intestine (LI) and Gall Bladder (GB) (lateral view). (Courtesy of John Ottaviano and NAVA. Copyright © 1975 by NAVA.)

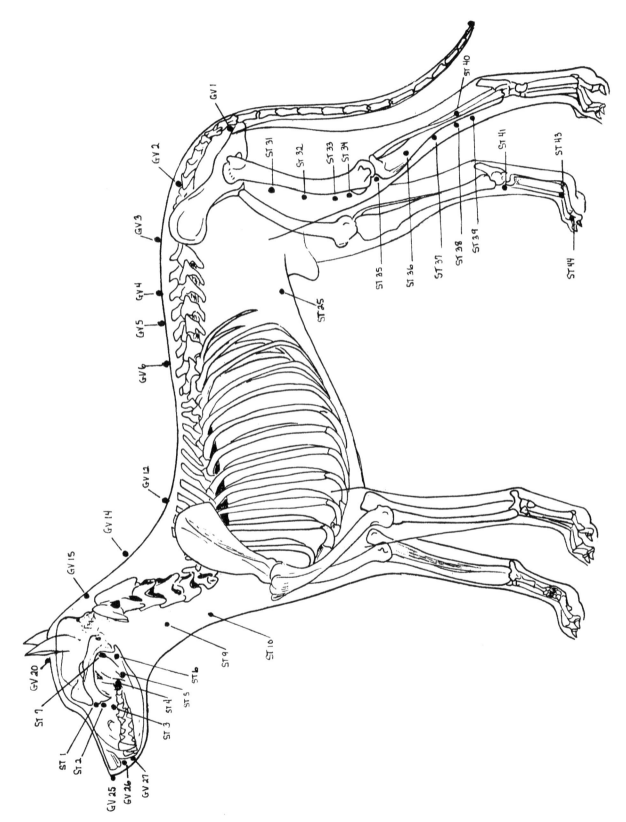

FIGURE 3–112. The Ottaviano Dog Chart: Stomach (ST) and Governing Vessel (GV) (lateral view). (Courtesy of John Ottaviano and NAVA. Copyright © 1975 by NAVA.)

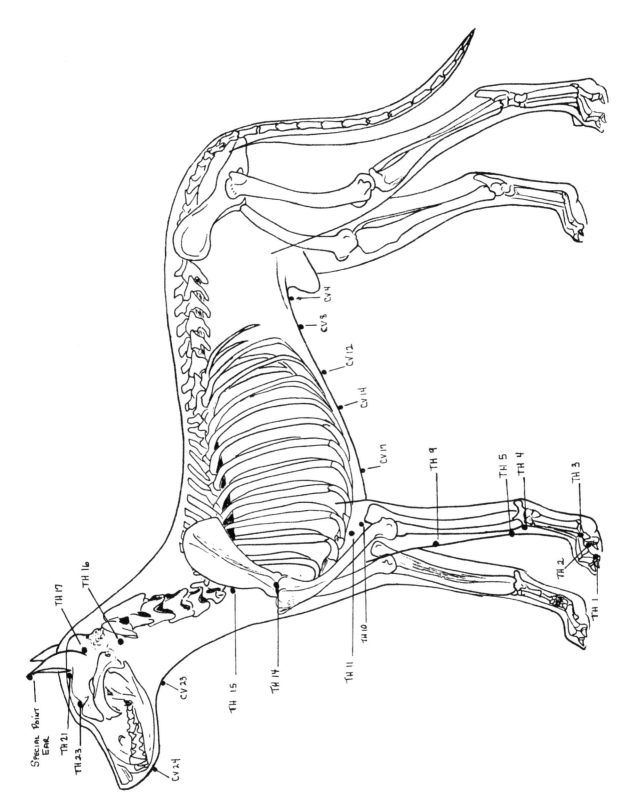

FIGURE 3–113. The Ottaviano Dog Chart: Tri-Heater (TH; same as triple burner) and Conception Vessel (CV) (lateral view). (Courtesy of John Ottaviano and NAVA. Copyright © 1975 by NAVA.)

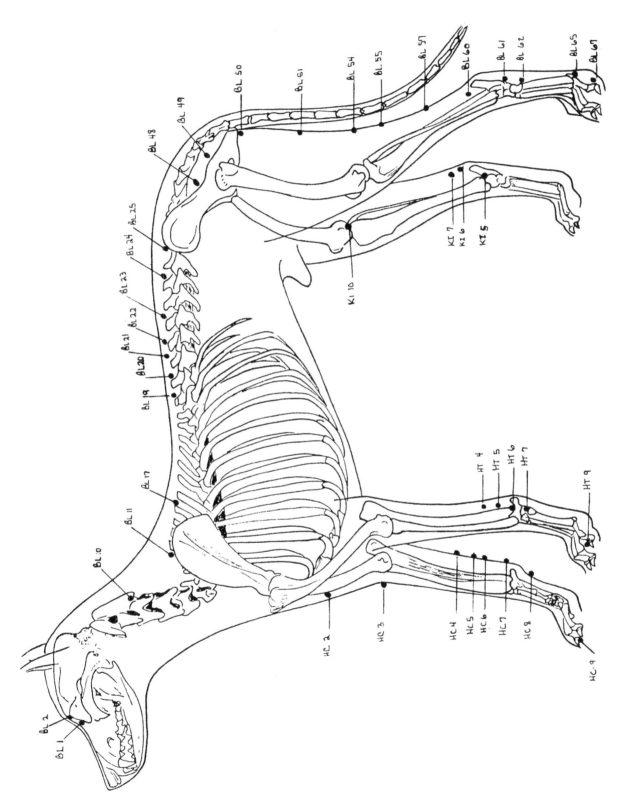

FIGURE 3-114. The Ottaviano Dog Chart: Bladder (B), Kidney (K), Heart Constrictor (HC; same as pericardium) (lateral view). (Courtesy of John Ottaviano and NAVA. Copyright © 1975 by NAVA.)

FORE LIMB

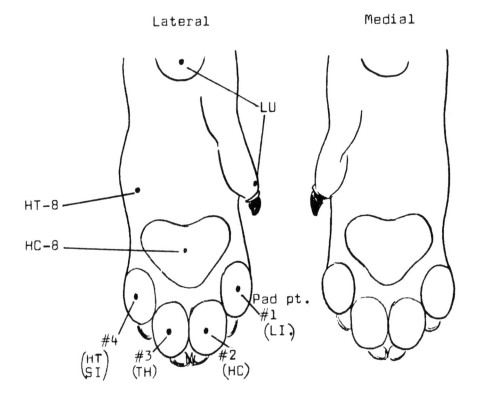

Lateral   Medial

LU

HT-8

HC-8

Pad pt.
#1
(LI)

#4
(HT
SI)

#3
(TH)

#2
(HC)

BL—Bladder
GB—Gall Bladder
HC—Heart Constrictor
HT—Heart
LI—Large Intestine
LIV—Liver
LU—Lung
SI—Small Intestine
SP—Spleen
ST—Stomach
TH—Tri-Heater

HIND LIMB

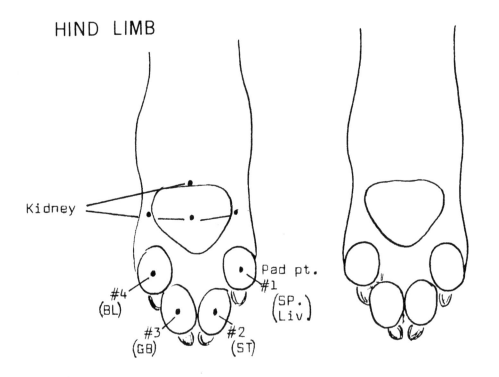

Kidney

Pad pt.
#1
(SP.
Liv)

#4
(BL)

#3
(GB)

#2
(ST)

FIGURE 3–115. The Ottaviano Dog Chart: Ventral View of Paws of hind and forefeet. (Courtesy of John Ottaviano and NAVA. Copyright © 1975 by NAVA.)

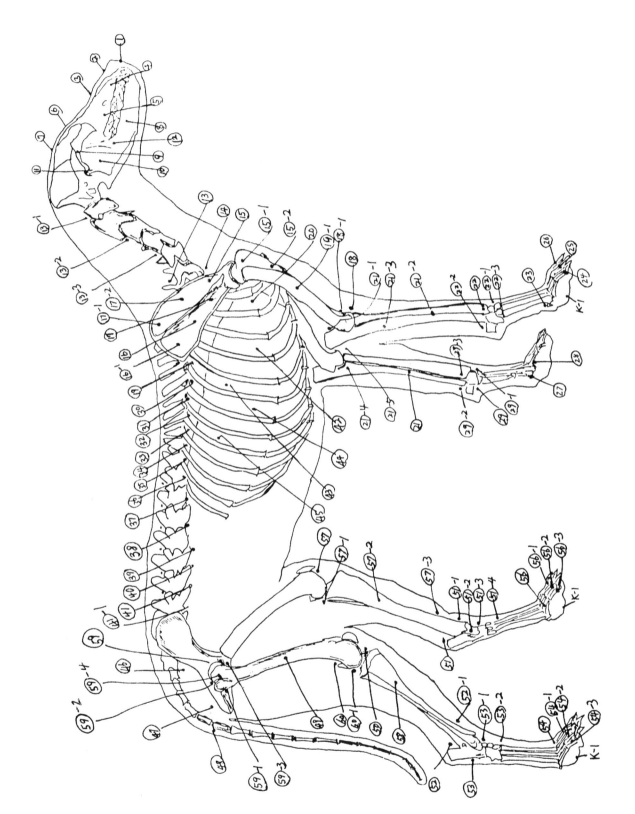

FIGURE 3–116. The Shin Dog Chart: lateral view, skeleton. (Courtesy of Sang H. Shin and NAVA. Copyright © 1975 by NAVA.)

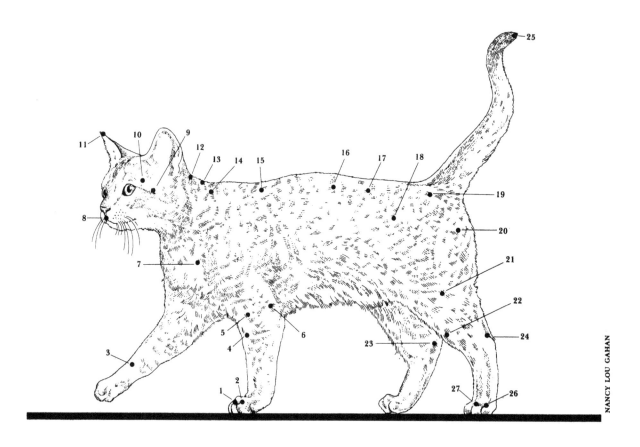

FIGURE 3–117. The Ottaviano Cat Chart. (From *Cat Catalog*, edited by Judy Fireman, copyright © 1976. Workman Publishing, New York, N.Y. Reprinted with permission of the publisher. Illustration by Nancy Lou Gahan.)

4

Acupuncture Therapy

Choosing Points

There are many methods of choosing acupuncture points for treating a specific problem. Each of the methods will produce one or more "prescriptions" of acupuncture points to use. Each of the prescriptions will vary from the other. Some may have many points in common; some may have a few points in common; some may have no points in common. This situation often is distressing to someone just starting to learn about acupuncture.

If one considers more familiar subjects, an analogy might be drawn to clarify the matter. In treating a specific bacterial infection, there are many choices of medication. Some of these drugs have widely different chemical structures and physical characteristics and can be administered by different routes. Yet they serve the same end result—the treatment of a bacterial infection. Another example is the use of different routes to get from point A to point B on a map. One could take many routes, some shorter, some longer, some more or less scenic, but the end result is getting to point B. A third example is stimulating an evoked response in the cerebral cortex. This could be done in many ways—electrical stimulation of a nerve in a foreleg, electrical stimulation of a nerve in a hindleg, electrical stimulation of the face or tail,

pressure on a foreleg, pressure on a hindleg, applying ice to a foreleg, applying ice to a hindleg, and so on.

And so it is with acupuncture therapy and analgesia—there are many ways of achieving a specific result. Of the many ways of arriving at an acupuncture prescription, some are fairly straightforward, and some involve a great deal of traditional Chinese medicine.

LOCAL POINTS

Everyone has had the experience, many times, of injuring himself and responding to that injury by applying gentle pressure in the injured area. This is done because it seems to make the injury less painful. In acupuncture, one can treat a painful condition by finding one or several of the most tender points and treating them. Sometimes these points are so tender initially that treating them is too painful. In that case, the corresponding point or points on the opposite side of the body are treated first. Acupuncture points may also be prescribed very close to yet not on the site of disorders—for example, HN4 (t'ai yang) for conjunctivitis; and HN15 (cheng chiang) for pharyngitis and laryngitis.

Local points, however, do not necessarily have to be painful to be effective. Points treated will include both painful and non-painful.

Sometimes injury or disease of a particular area produces a painful point at a site quite far away from the affected part. This may, in part, be referred pain, but there are also many more of these distant points known in acupuncture. Treatment of these painful distant points is reported to improve the initiating injury or disorder. As with local points, however, distant points may or may not be painful.

An example of a well-known point and a more distant one in the human is appendicitis and the well-known McBurney point. This point in the lower right quadrant of the abdomen becomes tender when the appendix is inflamed, and it is located exactly at the site of the acupuncture point ST25. Another point, called ST36, is located at the proximal lateral surface of the tibia; it is supposed to become painful in appendicitis. If the ST36 point is treated with acupuncture it is supposed to cure the attack of appendicitis.

An example in the cow is a point that can be called B30. There are many conditions in cattle and calves that result in swollen tarsal joints. When this occurs, a point located 3–4 finger widths lateral to the medial sacral crest at the lateral sacral crest in the area of the last dorsal sacral foramen becomes hot and tender, on the ipsilateral side as the tarsal problem. Treatment of this tender point—for example, a local anesthetic—may resolve the hock problem completely, or this therapy may have to be used with another therapy such as antibiotics, in which case the combined therapy usually will aid in a more rapid and complete resolution of the problem than with either alone.[11] This point is also one of those used to produce analgesia off the teat.

An example on the horse is the use of HL6 and FL6 for abdominal pain.

Accurate insertion of the needle is of primary importance in acupuncture therapy to achieve therapeutic efficacy. Bones and muscles are palpated for locating some points—for example, T2 (pai hui) and T9 (pa chiao) in the horse, and T1 (ta chui), T2 (san t'ai), and T3 (su ch'i) in the pig are determined by the location of the spinous process of the vertebrae; T12 (fei shu) and T10 (p'i shu) in the horse and T9 (fei shu), T17 (kan shu), and T18 (p'i shu) in the pig are determined by the location of the ribs.

The skin surface provides such landmarks as skin-folds, depressions, and the outline of the projection of the joints. Some points located in this manner are HN5 (t'ai yang), FL7 (ch'iang feng), FL20 (t'i t'ou), FL21 (t'i men) in the horse and HN6 (ching ming), HN16 (cheng chiang), FL6 (yung chuan), FL6 (t'i shui), and HL21 (pa tzu) in the pig.

Acupuncture Prescriptions

A standard prescription includes a local point or points in combination with a distant point or points.

1. All Species

A. CHEN[9] (FIGS. 3–99, 3–101 TO 3–107)

Disorders of Nerves, Joints, and Muscles

FACIAL PARALYSIS AND TRIGIMINAL NEURALGIA

Rx 1. Points: 19, 20, 23, 24, pao sai (similar to point 9 in the cow).
Method: a. High or low-frequency electric stimulation.
 b. Use 2–3 points daily.
 c. Inject vitamin B₁ (100–200 mg) into pao sai or point 20 or 19 daily.
 d. Use moxibustion on one or two points.
Species: Horse.

Rx 2. Points: 8, 9, shang kuan (similar to horse 24), hsia kuan (similar to horse 23).
Method: See Rx 1.
Species: Cattle.

PARALYSIS OF SHOULDER

Rx 1. Points: 47, 64, 66, 68, 69, 79, 80.
Method: a. Use 2–3 points daily.
 b. Moderate or low-frequency stimulation.
 c. Inject vitamin B₁, 100–200 mg daily.
 d. Use moxibustion on the rest of the points.
 e. Treat for 3–14 days.
Species: Horse.

Rx. 2. Points: 29, 65, 66, 71, 72, 74, 76.
Method: a. Use point 29 daily, and 2–3 of the remaining points.
 b. Other procedures, see Rx 1.
Species: Cattle.

Rx 3. Points: 32, 55, 57, 61, 63, 19.
Method: a. Use point 32 daily, and 2–3 of the remaining points.
 b. Other procedures, see Rx 1.
Species: Swine.

Rx 4. Points: 47, 48, 49, 51, 52, 53.
Method: a. Use 2–3 points daily.
 b. Other procedures, see Rx 1.
Species: Dog.

Rx 1. Points: 71, 73, 76, 77, 79, 83, 84, 88, 47.

Method: a. Use points 47, 73, and 79 first; use 1 or 2 of the remaining points daily.

b. Moderate or low-frequency stimulation for 15–20 min; once daily.

c. Moxibustion and injection treatment are recommended.

d. Duration of treatment: 1–2 weeks.

Species: Horse.

Rx 2. Points: 29, 65, 66, 71, 72, 74, 76.

Method: a. Use 2–3 points daily. Use all points alternately.

b. Other procedures, see *Rx 1*.

Species: Cattle.

Rx 3. Points: 19, 32, 55, 57, 61, 63.

Method: a. Use point 32 daily; other points, use 2–3 daily.

b. Other procedures, see *Rx 1*.

Species: Swine.

Rx 4. Points: 47, 48, 49, 51, 52, 53.

Method: a. Use 2–3 points daily.

b. Other procedures, see *Rx 1*.

Species: Dog.

POSTERIOR PARALYSIS

Rx 1. Points: 47, 48, 49, 50, 57, 94, 96.

Method: a. Points 47 or 57, use one of them once daily. Other points, use 2–3 times daily.

b. Moderate or low-frequency electric stimulation.

c. Moxibustion and injection after each stimulation recommended.

Species: Horse.

Rx 2. Points: 29, 30, 32, 36, 79, 85, 87.

Method: a. Points 29, 30, or 36, use one of them daily.

b. Other procedures, see *Rx 1*.

Species: Cattle.

Rx 3. Points: 20, 21, 23, 25, 54, 56, 57.

Method: a. Points 20, 21, or 25, use one of them daily.

b. Use point 54 daily for 3–4 days.

c. Other procedures, see *Rx 1*.

Species: Dog.

SCIATICA

Rx 1. Points: 47, 57, 94, 96, 98, 108, 111.

Method: a. Use points 47, 57, and 96 for 3 days; then use one of these points once daily. Use 2–3 other points once daily.

b. Strong or high-frequency electric stimu-

lation for 15–30 min, once daily for 3–8 days.

c. Inject vitamin B_1 or steroid.

Species: Horse.

Rx 2. Points: 29, 30, 36, 79, 80, 81, 84, 87, 89.

Method: a. Use points 30, 29, and 36 daily for 2–3 days; then one of these for the next 5–7 days. Use other points alternately, 2–3 at a time.

b. Other procedures, see *Rx 1*.

Species: Cattle.

Rx 3. Points: 20, 21, 22, 52, 54.

Method: a. Use 2–3 points daily for 4–10 days.

b. Other procedures, see *Rx 1*.

Species: Dog.

ARTHRITIS

Rx 1. Points: 47, 48, 57, 69, 73, 79, 80, 96, 105, 112.

Method: a. Fore limbs, use 47, 69, 73, 79, 80. Hind limbs, use 47, 48, 57, 96, 105, 112.

b. Strong or high-frequency electric stimulation for 15–30 min, once daily for 3–7 days.

c. Vitamin B_1 or steroid injection into point or points recommended.

Species: Horse.

Rx 2. Points: 36, 47, 64, 65, 70, 73, 76, 80, 77.

Method: See *Rx 1*.

Indication: Arthritis of shoulder of horse.

Rx 3. Points: 70, 72, 79, 80.

Method: See *Rx 1*.

Indication: Arthritis of elbow of horse.

Rx 4. Points: 80, 83, 84, 85, ah shih (pain spot).

Method: a. Point 85 by bleeding; other points use needle.

b. Other procedures, see *Rx 1*.

Indication: Arthritis of wrist joint of horse.

Rx 5. Points: 47, 48, 49, 57, 96, 97, 98, 100, 106, 108, 111.

Method: a. Points 47, 48, 49, 57; use two of these points once daily; other points use 2–3 times daily.

b. Other procedures, see *Rx 1*.

Indication: Arthritis of hind limbs of horse.

Rx 6. Points: 27, 28, 29, 56, 63, 64, 65, 66, 79, 85, 87.

Method: a. Forelimbs: 29, 63, 64, 65, 66. Hind limbs: 29, 28, 27, 79, 85, 87.

b. Use 2–3 points each treatment, once daily for 2–14 days.

c. Other procedures, see *Rx 1*.
Species: Cattle.

Rx 7. Points: 19, 32, 35, 50, 51, 56, 63, 69, 73, 74, 77.
Method: a. Forelimbs: 19, 32, 50, 51, 56, 63. Hind limbs: 32, 35, 69, 73, 74, 77.
    b. Use 3–4 points for each treatment.
    c. Other procedures, see *Rx 1*.
Indication: Arthritis and neuralgia of swine.

Rx 8. Points: 11, 12, 19, 21, 41, 42, 46, 47, 49, 50, 52, 54, 57, 58, 59.
Method: a. Forelimbs: 19, 12, 11, 41, 42, 46, 47, 49, 50, 52. Hind limbs: 19, 21, 54, 57, 58, 59.
    b. Use 3–4 points for each treatment, once daily for 3–8 days.
    c. Other procedures, see *Rx 1*.
Indication: Arthritis, neuralgia, and posterior paralysis of dog.

SPRAIN

Rx 1. Points: 47, 48, 49, 50, 57, 59, 97, 98.
Method: a. Use 2–3 points for each treatment, once daily for 2–7 days.
    b. Strong or high-frequency electric stimulation for 15–40 min.
    c. Inject steroids into 1–2 points.
    d. Moxibustion or sucking cup treatment recommended.
Indication: Sprain of lumbar region of horse.

Rx 2. Points: 64, 65, 66, 67, 70, 73, 74.
Method: a. Use points 64, 65, and 73 first; then use other points.
    b. Other procedures, see *Rx 1*.
Indication: Sprain of shoulder of horse.

Rx 3. Points: 73, 86, 87.
Method: a. Point 86 by bleeding; points 73 and 87 by needle.
    b. Other procedures, see *Rx 1*.
Indication: Sprain of fetlock joint of horse.

Rx 4. Points: 80, 86, 87, 88, 89.
Method: a. Points 86 and 88 by bleeding; points 80 and 89 by needle.
    b. Other procedures, see *Rx 1*.
Indication: Sprain of digit of horse.

Rx 5. Points: 113, 114, 111, 89 (hind leg).
Method: a. Point 113 by needle, others by bleeding.
    b. Other procedures, see *Rx 1*.
Indication: Sprain of hind fetlock joint of horse.

Rx 6. Points: 66, 71, 72, 73, 74, 76, 79, 85, 87, 88, 89, 92.

Method: a. Forelimbs: 66, 71, 72, 73, 74, 76. Hind limbs: 79, 85, 87, 88, 89, 92.
    b. Points 71, 74, 75, 89, and 92 by bleeding.
    c. Other procedures, see *Rx 1*.
Indication: Sprain of carpus, stifle, or digits of cattle.

Rx 7. Points: 55, 57, 62, 63, 64, 66, 67, 69, 72, 73, 74, 76, 79, 80.
Method: a. Forelimbs: 55, 57, 62, 63, 64, 66, 67. Hind limbs: 69, 72, 73, 74, 76, 79, 80.
    b. Points 63, 64, 66, 76, and 79 by bleeding; others by needle.
    c. Other procedures, see *Rx 1*.
Indication: Sprain of limbs of swine.

Rx 8. Points: 41, 42, 43, 47, 49, 50, 52, 54, 55, 57, 58, 59, 69, 72, 73, 74, 79, 76.
Method: a. Forelimbs: 41, 42, 43, 47, 49, 50, 52. Hind limbs: 54, 55, 57, 58, 59, 52.
    b. For each treatment, use 3–4 points once daily for 3–9 days.
    c. Other procedures, see *Rx 1*.
Indication: Sprain of fore or hind limb of dog.

TENDOVAGINITIS

Rx 1. Points: 84, 85, 86, 87, 88, 89, 98, 111, 112, 113, 114.
Method: a. Forelimbs: 84, 85, 86, 87, 88, 89. Hind limbs: 98, 111, 112, 113, 114.
    b. Points 85, 86, 88, 89, 113, and 114 by bleeding; others by needle.
    c. Steroid injection recommended.
Species: Horse.

Rx 2. Points: 74, 75, 76, 71, 72, 73, 85, 87, 88, 89, 90, 91, 92.
Method: a. Forelimbs: 74, 75, 76, 71, 72, 73. Hind limbs: 85, 87, 88, 89, 90, 91, 92.
    b. Points 74, 75, 89, 90, and 91 by bleeding; others by needle.
    c. Other procedures, see *Rx 1*.
Species: Cattle.

Rx 3. Points: 43, 45, 49, 50, 52, 57, 58, 59.
Method: a. Forelimbs: 43, 45, 49, 50, 52. Hind limbs: 57, 58, 59, 52.
    b. All by needle.
    c. Steroid injections recommended.
Species: Dog.

RHEUMATISM

Rx 1. Points: Cervical region—32.
       Lumbar Region—47, 48, 49, 50, 51, 52, 58, 93.

Forelimbs—64, 65, 66, 67, 73, 74.
Hind limbs—47, 94, 95, 97, 99, 100, 101, 102.

Method: a. Use 3–4 points for each treatment once daily for 4–10 days.
b. Strong or high-frequency electric stimulation for 30–45 min.
c. Moxibustion and injection of vitamin B_1 or steroids recommended.

Species: Horse.

Rx 2. Points: General—27, 28, 47, 59, 86, 87.
Lumbar region—47, 48, 51, 52, 57.
Forelimbs—35, 36, 64, 65, 73, 79, 80, 84.
Hind limbs—93, 96, 97, 98, 105, 108, 111.

Method: See Rx 1.

Species: Horse.

Rx 3. Points: Main points—21, 23, 29, 30.
Accessory points—2, 11, 6, 72, 76.

Method: a. Strong or high-frequency electric stimulation for 15–30 min, daily for 7–10 days.
b. Injection of steroid or vitamin B_1 recommended.

Species: Cattle.

Rx 4. Points: General—11, 20, 29, 36, 51, 75, 79, 87, 6.
Lumbar region—
Group 1. 25, 27, 28, 29.
Group 2. 23, 26, 28, 29, 47, 48, 79.
Forelimbs—20, 21, 61, 62, 29, 40.
Hind limbs—29, 79, 80, 82, 87.

Method: a. Use 3–4 points once daily for 4–10 days.
b. Other procedures, see Rx 1.

Species: Cattle.

Rx 5. Points: Horse—47, 48, 51, 52.
Cattle—25, 27, 28, 29.
Dog—17, 18, 19, 20, 33, 36, 35.

Method: a. All points used alternately. Use 3–4 points once daily for 3–8 days.
b. Other procedures, see Rx 1.

Indication: Rheumatism of lumbar region in horse, cattle, and dog.

MYOTONIA

Rx 1. Points: Main points—3, 32, 19, 20, 21.
Accessory points—47, 48, 49, 50, 60.

Method: a. Facial: 3, 19, 20, 21, 47.
Cervical: 3, 32, 47, 60.
Lumbar: 3, 47, 48, 49, 50, 60, 19, 20, 21.
General: Use main points first; then use 2–3 points daily.
b. Strong or high-frequency electric stimulation for 30–40 min, once or twice daily.

c. Chlorpromazine injection into 1–2 points recommended.

Species: Horse.

Rx 2. Points: 3, 91, 60, 26, 10, shine shau (4 fingerwidths to the cranial border of scapula and 4 fingerwidths ventrally).

Method: a. Point 60 by bleeding; others by needle.
b. Other procedures, see Rx 1.

Species: Horse.

Rx 3. Points: Group 1: 28, 29, 47, 32.
Group 2: 60, 93.
Group 3: 49, 100, 101, 105, 97, 98.

Method: a. Use one group of points once daily. Use each of the three groups alternately.
b. Other procedures, see Rx 1.

Species: Horse.

Rx 4. Points: 2, 3, 11, 19, 29, 47, 48, 31, 37, 82, 83, 85, 79.

Method: a. Points used depends on region of body afflicted.
b. Other procedures, see Rx 1.

Species: Cattle.

LAMINITIS

Rx 1. Points: Forefeet—80, 84, 86, 87, 88, 89.
Hind feet—89, 111, 113, 114.

Method: a. Points 84, 86, 88, 111, 113, and 114 by bleeding; others by needle.
b. Strong or high-frequency stimulation for 30–60 min.
c. Injection of steroid or vitamin B_1 or antibiotics or analgesic drugs recommended.

Species: Horse.

Rx 2. Points: Forefeet—74, 75, 76, 77, 78.
Hind feet—88, 89, 90, 91, 92.

Method: a. Points 74, 75, 89, and 90 by bleeding; others by needle.
b. Other procedures, see Rx 1.

Species: Cattle.

Digestive System Disorders

STOMATITIS

Rx. Points: Horse—25, 26, 11, 12.
Cattle—14, 15, 16, 18.

Method: a. Bleeding once daily for 7 days.
b. Vitamin C injection recommended.

Species: Horse and cattle.

Remarks: From my own experience, the result is not as good as medication.

GLOSSITIS

Rx. Points: Horse—22, 25, 26.

Cattle—14, 16, 17, 18.
Method: a. Bleeding.
      b. Treat once daily for 7 days.
Species: Horse and cattle.
Remarks: Acupuncture treatments help but do not cure.

SALIVATION

Rx. Points: liu ein (at outer surface of upper labia; about 1.5 cm medial to lower commissure of nostril).
Method: a. Oblique needling, 3–4.5 cm depth.
      b. High-frequency electric stimulation for 30 min, once daily.
Species: Horse.

PHARYNGEAL AND ESOPHAGEAL PARALYSIS

Rx. Points: Horse—3, 8, 20, 30, 33, 34, ah shih (pain spot).
      Cattle—9, 12, 13, ah shih.
Method: a. At the ah shih point use low-frequency stimulation for 30–60 min, once daily.
      b. Bleed remaining points.
Species: Horse and cattle.

INTESTINAL BLOAT

Rx. Points: Horse—
      Group 1: 43.
      Group 2: 47, 54, 42, 44, 46.
      Cattle—
        Group 1: kuan yen yu (similar to horse 43).
        Group 2: 18, 44, 45, 46.
Method: a. Use either of the two groups.
      b. Use low-frequency electric stimulation for 30 min, once or twice daily.
Species: Horse and cattle.

GASTROENTERITIS OR ENTERITIS

Rx 1. Points: Horse—39, 42, 61, 63, 108.
      Cattle—38, 57, chung wan (similar to dog 39), hou san li (similar to horse 108).
Method: Strong or high-frequency electric stimulation for 30–40 min, once daily for 6–10 days.
Species: Horse and cattle.

Rx 2. Points: 11, 39, 42, 108, 111, hai men (similar to cattle 57), chung wan (similar to dog 39).
Method: a. Bleed point 11. Needling, high-frequency, or strong stimulation for remaining points.

      b. Vitamin or antibiotic injection recommended.
Species: Horse.

Rx 3. Points: 11, 43, 44, 46, 108.
Method: Bleed point 11; electrical stimulation in remaining points for 15–30 min, once daily for 7–10 days.
Species: Horse.

Rx 4. Points: 14, 32, 43, chung wan (similar to dog 39), hou san li (similar to horse 108).
Method: a. Bleed point 17; needling for remaining points.
      b. 15–30 min. electric stimulation for 7–10 days.
Species: Cattle.

Rx 5. Points: Group 1—28, 42, 44, 78.
      Group 2—2, 11, 25, 27, 32.
      Group 3—11, 25, 30, 32, 37, 40, 65, 78.
      Group 4—2, 7, 11, 17, 28, 32, 42, 74.
Method: a. Use one of the four groups of points daily and alternately.
      b. Other procedures, see Rx 1.
Indication: Swine enteritis.

Rx 6. Points: Group 1—28, 42, 47, 74.
      Group 2—2, 17, 28, 32, 42, 47, 74.
      Group 3—2, 11, 19, 25, 27, 17, 32, 40, 42, 74.
Method: a. Use one of these three groups of points, alternately.
      b. Other procedures, see Rx 1.
Indication: Swine dysentery.

PARALYSIS OF RECTUM

Rx. Points: Horse—47, 61, 57, 59.
      Cattle—30, 32, 37, 38, 48.
      Swine—32, 35, 36, 37, 41, 42.
      Dog—20, 21, 22, 26.
Method: Strong or electric stimulation (low frequency) for 30–60 min, once daily for 4–8 days.
Species: Horse, cattle, swine, and dog.

CONSTIPATION

Rx. Points: Horse—
      Group 1: 43.
      Group 2: 11, 26, 88, 114.
      Cattle—
        Group 1: kuan yen yu (similar to horse 43).
        Group 2: 2, 11, 27, 30, 32, 37, 74.

Method: Use Group 1 first, then use 2–3 points of Group 2. Strong or high-frequency electric stimulation for 30 min.

DIARRHEA

Rx. Points: Horse—
> Group 1: 61, 108.
> Group 2: 39, 42, 43, 44, 46.
> Cattle—
> Group 1: 38, hou san li (similar to horse 108).
> Group 2: 42, 43, 57, chung wan (similar to dog 39).
> Swine—
> Group 1: 42, 47, 74.
> Group 2: 11, 27, 28, 40.
> Dog—
> Group 1: 26, 58.
> Group 2: 38, 39, 26.

Method: a. Use Group 1 first; then use 2–3 from Group 2, daily.
b. Mild hand manipulation or low-frequency electric stimulation for 30 min.

Species: Horse, cattle, swine, and dog.

PROLAPSE OF ANUS

Rx. Points: Horse—tou kan (one point on each side of the anus at the 3 and 9 o'clock positions), 61.
> Cattle—tou kan, 29, 38.
> Swine—tou kan, 32, 42.
> Dog—tou kan, 20, 26.

Method: a. Use tou kan point by cranial and ventral insertion 9 cm deep for horse and cattle, 3–4.5 cm deep for swine and dog.
b. After replacement of anus, use tou kan first; then use in the horse 61, cattle 38, swine 42, dog 26 on first day. Second day onward, use either tou kan or 61 (horse), 38 (cattle), 42 (swine), or 26 (dog) and other points.
c. Mild or low-frequency electric stimulation for 30–60 min, for 7–10 days.

Species: Horse, cattle, swine, and dog.

INDIGESTION

Rx. Points: Horse—
> Group 1: 43.
> Group 2: 39, 42, 43, 40.
> Cattle—
> Group 1: kuan yen yu (similar to horse 43).

> Group 2: 43, 44, chung wan (similar to dog 39).
> Swine—
> Group 1: kuan yen yu (similar to horse 43).
> Group 2: 32, 29, 26, 28, 47.
> Dog—
> Group 1: kuan yen yu (similar to horse 43).
> Group 2: 32, 30, 29, 31, 38, 39.

Method: a. Use Group 1 and 2–3 of the points in Group 2, daily.
b. Mild or low-frequency electric stimulation for 30 min, daily for 7–10 days.

Species: Horse, cattle, swine, and dog.

Respiratory System

EPISTAXIS

Rx. Points: Horse—3, 4, 5, 6, 7, 9, 10, 25, 42.
> Cattle—1, 6, 7, 14, 42, kan yu (similar to horse 40), shine yu (similar to dog 28).
> Dog—2, 3, 28, 29, 32, tong tang (similar to horse 4), tong tien (similar to horse 7).

Method: a. Strong or high-frequency electric stimulation for 30 min.
b. Vitamin K or other coagulating agents recommended.

Species: Horse, cattle, and dog.

LARYNGITIS

Rx. Points: Horse—
> Group 1: 33, 34, 27.
> Group 2: 3, 59, 88, 89.
> Cattle—
> Group 1: 2, 12, 13, 15.
> Group 2: 6, 74, 75, 89, 90.
> Dog—hou yu (similar to horse 34), feng men (similar to horse 28), erh ken (similar to cattle 10), 9.

Method: Strong or high frequency electric stimulation for 15–30 min daily for 7–14 days.

Species: Horse, cattle, and dog.

COMMON COLD AND INFLUENZA

Rx. Points: Horse—2, 6, 28, 44, 46.
> Cattle—
> Group 1:
> Main points: 2, 3, 6, 36.
> Accessory points: 23, 29, 74, 89, ta chui (similar to dog 10).

Group 2: 2, 3, 6, 7, 11, 20, 42, chi chu
(similar to horse 111).
Dog—2, 3, 8, 9, 10, 12, 27, 20.

Method: a. Use 3–4 points daily for 3–7 days.
b. Moderate or low-frequency electric stimulation for 20–30 min.

Species: Horse, cattle, and dog.

BRONCHITIS

Rx. Points: Horse—2, 35, 37, 38, 91.
Cattle—
Group 1:
Main points: 2, 3, 16, 18, 20, 41.
Accessory points: 6, 23, 36, 75, 90.
Group 2: 2, 11, 14, 23, 41, 53.
Dog—see Common Cold.

Method: a. Strong or high-frequency electric stimulation for 30 min.
b. Once daily for 7–10 days.

Species: Horse, cattle, and dog.

PNEUMONIA

Rx. Points: Cattle—14, 16, 23, 29, 36, 41, fei men
(similar to horse 66).
Swine—
Main points: 22, 24, 11, 19.
Accessory points: 2, 40, 65, 78, chi sheng (see Figure 3–106).

Method: a. High-frequency electric stimulation for 30 min, once daily.
b. Vitamin B_1 and antibiotics (kanamycin or dihydrostreotomycin, 50 mg injected into one or two points).

Species: Cattle and Swine.

Remarks: Results uncertain.

PULMONARY EDEMA

Rx. Points: Main points—6, 7, 14, 15, 27, 29.
Accessory points—23, 41, 42.

Method: a. Use main points first; then use 2–3 accessory points daily.
b. Strong or high frequency electric stimulation for 30–60 min.
c. Inject diuretics (Lasix or Diamox) into 1–2 points.

Species: Cattle.

Urogenital and Mammary Disorders

CYSTIC OVARIES AND STERILITY

Rx. Points: Horse—
Main points: 55, 56, 93.
Accessory points: 47, 48, 50, 61.

Cattle—
Main points: 49, 50.
Accessory points: 27, 28, 29, 30.
Swine—
Main points: 33, 34.
Accessory points: 30, 31, 32.
Dog—
Main points: 35, 36.
Accessory points: 18, 19.

Method: a. Use 2 main points and one accesssory point once daily, or once every other day.
b. High-frequency electric stimulation for 30–60 min.
c. Duration of treatment 7–10 days. Two courses of treatment usually necessary.

Species: Horse, cattle, swine, and dog.

CYSTITIS

Rx. Points: Horse—27, 47, 48, 50, 60, 110, hai men
(similar to cattle 57).
Cattle—
Group 1:
Main points: 25, 26, 27, 28, 29, 86.
Accessory points: 2, 57, 77.
Group 2: 27, 28, 29, 86, shen yu (similar to horse 48), pang kung yu (similar to dog 37).
Group 3: 26, 27, 32, 35, 58, 29.

Method: High-frequency electric stimulation for 30 min, once daily for 7–10 days.

Species: Horse, cattle.

Remarks: Results no better than medical treatment.

PURPURAL PARALYSIS

Rx. Points: Horse—
Main points: 48, 49, 50.
Accessory points: 55, 56, 93, 110.
Cattle—
Main points: 21, 23, 27, 29, 86.
Accessory points: 10, 72, 74, 76, 89.
Dog—
Main points: 20, 21, 58.
Accessory points: 17, 33, 19.

Method: a. Use main points first; then 2–3 accessory points once or twice daily.
b. Strong or low-frequency electrical stimulation for 30 min.
c. Vitamin B_1 or steroid injection into 1–2 main points.

Species: Horse, cattle, and dog.

PENILE PARALYSIS

Rx. Points: Horse—yin chin (at penis, about two finger widths from cranial to the scro-

tum), 47, 57, hui yin (between anus and vulva).
Cattle—yin chin, 29, 30, hui yin.
Method: Low-frequency electric stimulation, 30 min daily for 3–7 days.
Species: Horse and cattle.

MASTITIS

Rx. Points: Main points—58, 59, 57.
Accessory points—27, 28, 29, 74, 89, 86.
Method: a. Bleed points 59, 74, 86, and 89. Use needle on remaining points.
b. Strong or high-frequency electrical stimulation for 30–60 min, once daily for 6–10 days.
Species: Cattle.

Physical Conditions

SUNSTROKE

Rx. Points: Horse—
Main points: 27, 30, 59, 91, 110.
Accessory points: 2, 21, 22, 88, 114.
Cattle—Main points: 2, 3, 13, 16, 20, 29.
Accessory points: 36, 75, 86, 90.
Method: a. Bleeding.
b. Use the main point first, then 2–3 accessory points.
Species: Horse and cattle.

FATIGUE

Rx. 1. Points: 2, 9, 10, 26, 30, 47, 59.
Method: Use needle on point 47; remaining points are bled.
Species: Horse.

Rx 2. Points: 45, 47, 48, 59.
Method: Moderate or low-frequency electric stimulation for 30 min, once daily.
Species: Horse.

2. Horse

A. CHINESE VETERINARY HANDBOOK[1] (FIGS. 3–28 TO 3–43)

Each prescription is used daily unless otherwise indicated. The number of daily treatments and length of course of treatment are determined by the course of the disease.

Strain of the Triceps Brachii Muscle

The muscle is strained when it is over-extended because the animal is overloaded, forced to gallop too quickly or fitted with improper horse shoes.

SYMPTOMS

1. The affected limb is extended forward when standing to decrease body weight on the affected limb.
2. Movement is limited when trotting, and stepping is painful when weight is carried.
3. On palpation, there is tenderness over the point FL7 (ch'ang feng). There is pain when the affected limb is moved caudally.
4. Gradually, muscles of the affected limb atrophy.

TREATMENT

1. The hao chen needle is inserted into FL7 (ch'ang feng), FL10 (t'ien tsung), FL8 (ch'ung t'ien), and FL9 (chien cheng). A needle is also inserted into each additional tender spot at the same time. In acute stages, with local tenderness, the blood needle is inserted into FL16 (hsiung t'ang). For chronic or debilitating conditions, the hot needle is applied to FL7 (ch'ang feng) and FL8 (ch'ung t'ien).
2. In addition, the affected area may be rubbed with a 10% camphor, alcohol, or ordinary white-wine solution.

Shoulder Joint Injury

SYMPTOMS

1. The animal uses to the tip of its hoof to touch the ground when standing to reduce the weight on the affected limb. In serious conditions, the whole limb is suspended above the ground, and the joint becomes swollen and warm. Lifting the limb is difficult when running, and movement is limited in abduction. Short steps are taken with the anterior limbs.
On local palpation, there is tenderness in and around the joint. Passive flexion or extension of the joint causes pain.
3. The joint becomes deformed in chronic cases, and the shoulder muscle atrophies.

TREATMENT

1. The acupuncture prescription, using the hao chen and blood needles, is the same as that for treating triceps brachii muscle strain. As an alternative, the hot needle may be inserted into FL7 (ch'ang feng), supplemented by FL11 (chien ching) and FL13 (chien wai yu), if necessary.
2. Cauterization may also be used additionally in chronic or refractory cases.
3. Cold packing may be used additionally in the early stages of the injury when the joint is swollen. After 2 or 3 days, when the swelling has diminished,

a hot pack is used. A 10% camphor, alcohol, or white-wine solution may be used to rub the affected area.

4. In serious cases, herbal medicine is used and may be combined with any of the previous procedures.

Strain of the Biceps Brachii Muscle

SYMPTOMS

1. The joints below the knee are often flexed when standing. Sometimes the tip of the hoof is placed on the ground, slightly caudal to the normal position. Running is difficult, and stepping down causes pain.

2. There are tenderness and pain on palpation, which become more conspicuous if the limb is pulled forward.

TREATMENT

The bleeding of FL16 (hsiung t'ang) with the blood needle is used. In chronic conditions, treatment is similar to the acupuncture prescription for strain of the triceps muscle. Additional supportive therapy such as cold packing may also be used.

Injury to the Elbow Joint

SYMPTOMS

1. The affected joint is usually maintained in a flexed condition when in standing position, and the tip of the hoof touches the ground in order to reduce weight on the affected limb. Difficulty in elbow joint flexion and dragging of the limb in forward movements may be observed in trotting.

2. On palpation, swelling, warmth, and tenderness are felt over and around the joint and tendon. Pulling the limb forward causes severe pain.

TREATMENT

1. In acute cases, FL16 (hsiung t'ang) is bled with the small, wide needle, supplemented with insertion of hao chen into FL7 (ch'ang feng).

2. In chronic cases, the hot needle is used in FL7 (ch'ang feng), FL14 (chou yu), and FL13 (chien wai yu).

3. In addition, cauterization may be used in chronic cases. Additional therapeutic methods are similar to those for shoulder joint injuries.

Paralysis of the Brachial Plexus

SYMPTOMS

1. Total paralysis. There is extension of the shoulder joint and lowering of the knee joint, while standing, and the tip of the hoof touches the ground.

Passive correction of the posture results in a normal standing position, but the slightest movement brings back the pathologic posture. There is difficulty in raising the limb in running, and swinging of the affected limb is frequently observed. Falling is also frequent. On palpation, there is a loss of sensation in the affected area. Very soon after the onset of the disease, the triceps muscle begins to atrophy.

2. Partial paralysis. The tip of the hoof is used to touch the ground to reduce weight on the affected limb. The affected limb is always in a semiflexed position, and the tip of the hoof is always in a semiflexed position, and the tip of the hoof is dragged along. In running, short steps are taken by the anterior limbs.

TREATMENT

1. Hao chen is inserted into FL7 (ch'ang feng), FL10 (tien tsung), FL8 (ch'ung t'ien), and FL9 (chien ching).

2. Insertion into FL10 (ch'ang feng), FL8 (chung tien), and FL12 (chien yu) with the hot needle is an alternative prescription.

3. An 0.1–0.2% strychnine nitrate solution (5–10 cc) is injected into FL7 (ch'ang feng) as an alternative method.

Carpal Joint Injury

SYMPTOMS

1. The carpal and fetlock joints are in flexed position when standing. Steps are short during running or exercise. Pain is felt when the limb is raised or weight is borne.

2. In the beginning, tenderness and warmth are evident when the injured area is palpated. Later, there is induration. There is also limited joint movement. Hypertrophy and hyperplasia of the periosteum are present, causing chronic deformity and inflammation of the carpus.

TREATMENT

1. In acute cases, the blood needle is inserted into the patellar vein at FL18 (hsi mai).

2. In chronic cases, cauterization is used.

3. The injured area may be rubbed with turpentine solution or a 10% camphor or alcohol solution, or a 5% iodine solution as a supportive method of treatment.

Swelling of the Carpus

Swelling frequently occurs between the large and small metacarpal bones. Improper limb posturing, improper hoof shape, or over weight on the medial small metacarpal causes strain on the intercarpal ligament. This will induce periostitis. If inflammation lasts a long time, a tumor (swelling) may form. Similar conditions may be caused by trauma.

SYMPTOMS

1. On palpation of the medial side of the carpal bone, a fingertip-sized tumor will show up.

2. In acute cases, tenderness is felt on palpation. When the disorder becomes chronic, pain is not prominent. In both acute and chronic cases, limping is not obvious. Pain becomes more significant when the animal walks on hard ground or goes downhill. Sometimes it can be aggravated by increased exercise.

TREATMENT

It is essential to correct the shape of the hoof.

1. In the early stages of the disease, the blood needle is inserted into the patellar vein at FL18 (hsi mai) until blood is drawn.

2. In addition, cauterization may be used.

3. For larger, chronic tumors, resection is necessary, and cauterization and pressure bandaging are used to stop the bleeding.

Flexor Tendonitis

The flexor is located on the ventral side of the pedis. Tendonitis includes inflammation of the superficial and deep flexor tendons and their associated structures. The disorder occurs more frequently on the anterior limb of the horse. Poor development, improper posturing, inadequate shoe repair, over-exhaustion, and various traumatic injuries cause this disorder.

SYMPTOMS

1. Superficial tendonitis shows swelling, mostly over the upper third of the metacarpus. The swelling of the deep flexor tendon is located in the middle third and the swelling of the suspensory ligament located in the lower third of the pedis.

2. The affected animal attempts a resting posture when standing. Stepping is heavy and painful. The fetlock joint cannot be lowered, and there is no extension of the flexor tendon.

3. On palpation, warmth, swelling, and tenderness are evident over the affected area. Initially, swelling is mild; later the flexor tendon becomes hypertrophic and indurated.

TREATMENT

1. For acute cases, the blood needle is inserted into the patellar vein at FL18 (hsi mai) until blood is drawn.

2. Procain penicillin may be injected into the inflamed region as a supportive measure or as a major form of therapy.

3. In chronic cases, cauterization is used.

4. Vinegar and alcohol bandages for packing, as well as injection of procaine penicillin, may be used as supportive measures (for local application, 95% mercury paste is used).

Twisted Fetlock Joint

Overflexion or extension of limbs in horses and donkeys during heavy labor often causes twisting of this joint. It happens more frequently to the anterior limbs of horses.

SYMPTOMS

1. The fetlock joint is flexed when the animal is standing and the tip of the hoof touches the ground in order to reduce weight on the affected limb. The associated area is lowering in running. Prominent pain develops when the animal steps forward when carrying a burden.

2. The acutely affected side shows warmth, swelling, and pain. On passive flexion and extension of the joint, there is a prominent painful reaction.

TREATMENT

1. In acute cases, the blood needle is inserted into FL20 (t'i t'ou) or FL19 (ch'an wan) until blood is drawn.

2. In chronic cases, with induration, cauterization alone is used.

Digit Pain

Digit pain occurs in the area on the posterior side of the fetlock joint. When there is excessive galloping, uneven stepping, or knocking of the hindlimbs, this disorder may develop.

SYMPTOMS

1. The tip of the hoof is used to touch the ground and the associated area maintains a standing still position, to reduce weight. Steps are unsure when running. There is instability when placing. Short steps are taken by the posterior limbs.

2. On palpation, the digits show warmth and pain, but swelling is not significant.

TREATMENT

FL22 (ch'ien chiu) should be bled for disorders of the forelimb, and HL25 (hou chiu) for the hindlimb. The blood needle is inserted in both cases.

Pelvic Joint Twist

This joint is also called the pelvic femoral joint. Slipping, collision, and twisting are the causes of pelvic joint twist.

SYMPTOMS

1. The stifle joints of the affected limb are slightly flexed laterally when standing, so that weight-bearing is reduced. Limb-raising and running are difficult. In circumduction, there is pain when stepping with weight. The limping is aggravated by motion, turning, and backing.

2. During passive flexion and extension, abduction and adduction of the pelvic joint are coupled with pain reactions.

TREATMENT

1. Hao chen is inserted into T2 (pai hui), HL3 (yang chu liao), HL4 (huan t'iao), and into associated tender points.

2. In acute cases, HL15 (shen t'eng) is bled with the small, wide needle, or the hot needle is inserted into HL5 (huan chung), HL6 (huan hou), and HL11 (han kou).

3. Herb medicine may be used as a supportive measure, or it can be used alone.

Stifle Joint Twist

SYMPTOMS

1. In acute cases, the stifle joint is flexed when standing. The tip of the hoof touches the ground and is positioned slightly cranial. Warmth and tenderness are evident on palpation. Joint swelling appears in chronic cases.

2. In chronic cases, the cranial wall of the hoof is placed on the ground. A slight upper jerk of the affected limb when stepping is also characteristic. There is a painful reaction when the hoof is placed on the ground. The tip of the hoof touches the ground when the animal first begins to step. Short steps are taken by the posterior limbs. After a while, the posterior hoof begins to be placed flat on the ground.

TREATMENT

1. In acute and inflammatory cases, FL16 (hsiung t'ang) is bled. In chronic cases, the hot needle is inserted into HL14 (lueh ts'ao) as the main point, supplemented by hot-needle insertion into HL11 (han kou).

2. In chronic and acute cases, cauterization may be used as supportive therapy.

3. Herb medicine may be used together with each of the above methods, or alone.

Sciatic Nerve Paralysis

SYMPTOMS

1. The hip and stifle joints are relaxed when standing. The fetlock joint curves, and the hind part of the hoof touches the ground. The animal cannot bear weight. When running, there is difficulty in the affected limb. The hip and stifle joints are passively extended. The area below the fetlock joint is curved and dragged along. Backing is very difficult, and the animal is unable to rise without aid to a standing position after lying down.

2. There is a loss of sensation in the affected area coupled with muscle atrophy.

TREATMENT

1. The hao chen or hot needle is inserted into T2 (pai hui), HL10 (hui yang), HL11 (hsieh ch'i), HL12 (yu wa), HL13 (ch'ien shen), HL5 (huan chung) and HL6 (huan hou).

2. 5–10 cc of a 0.1–0.2% strychnine nitrate solution is injected into the deep tissues of HL9 (hsieh ch'i) and HL11 (hui yang) as an alternative.

Hypertrophy of the Tarsal Joint

The tarsal joint is formed by many small bones and is composed of the tarsal tibial joint, the intertarsal joint, and the calcaneal tarsal joint with the associated tendons. Poor structure, improper posture, poor development, and any traumatic injury or excessive strain from hard labor cause hyperplasia of bony tissue, which gives rise to hyperplasia of the joint.

SYMPTOMS

1. When standing, the animal places the hoof on the ground, slightly anterior to the normal position. Sometimes, the anterior wall of the hoof is placed on the ground. The affected limb drops immediately after raising, and limping is more severe when the animal begins to run. There is difficulty in limb-raising, owing to incomplete flexion of the tarsal joint. There is pain when stepping on the ground, and short steps are taken by the posterior limbs. There is significant movement of the thigh. Limping is aggravated after rest.

2. Palpation of the medial posterior margin of the joint shows hyperplasia of the bony tissue, forming an induration without warmth or tenderness. There is also joint deformity. However, after vigorous exercise, some warmth with hypersensitivity appears in the affected area.

3. To test for hyperplasia of the tarsal joint, the affected part is raised and flexed for 3 to 5 min, and the animal is then permitted to run fast. If limping is prominent, or if the animal runs using three limbs only, the diagnosis is confirmed.

TREATMENT

Cauterization or local packing with 5% Mercurochrome paste is used.

Swelling of the Tarsal Joint

This is a common disorder in horses. When pressure is exerted from the bursae of the Achilles tendon over to the bursae on both sides, the swelling is prominent. It is mainly caused by traumatic injury, excessive labor, or long-term, irregular motion. An inadequate hoof surface or irregular horseshoe surface causes the disease, especially when there is lateral twisting of the tarsal joint when weight is borne.

SYMPTOMS

1. In acute cases, the joint swells. On palpation, the joint is soft and wavy, with pain and tenderness. There is difficulty in moving forward or bearing weight.

2. In chronic cases, the animal limps, and the inflammatory symptoms are reduced.

3. In both cases, there is reduced sensitivity on palpation, limitations in movement, and low and short steps.

TREATMENT

1. In acute cases, HL16 (chu ch'ih) is bled.

2. In chronic cases, cauterization is used.

3. Initially, the shape of the hoof must be corrected. After shaving and sterilizing the swollen area, a No. 16 hyperdermic needle is used to draw fluid. A pressure bandage is then applied.

Rheumatism

This common systemic disease usually occurs in the limbs, the lumbar muscles, and the joints. The etiology of the disease is still not known. However, poor nutrition, general weakness, or excessive sweating in windy or cold weather easily gives rise to the disease.

SYMPTOMS

There is sudden illness, often associated with high fever, general weakness, and loss of appetite.

2. The affected area is not limited to one limb, but is often migratory. Mostly, it affects the hindlimbs,

creating a prominent sign of stiff neck. There is pain and tenderness in the affected muscles, which are hard and tense on palpation. There is swelling if the joint is involved.

3. The gait is limping, and steps are short and stiff. This is most evident in the beginning of motion, and is less evident after motion is initiated.

TREATMENT

1. For rheumatism of the neck, the hao chen or hot needle is inserted into HN20 (chiu wei), supplemented by insertion into other tender points.

2. For rheumatism of the front limb, the hao chen is inserted into FL7 (ch'ang feng), FL8 (ch'ung t'ien), and FL9 (chien cheng), supplemented with needle insertion into the tender spots. One hao chen should be inserted through two of the four points. Or the hot needle may be inserted into the FL7 Point (ch'ang feng), supplemented by insertion into FL8 (ch'ung t'ien), FL11 (chien ching), and FL13 (chien wai yu).

3. For rheumatism of the hindlimb, the hao chen is inserted into T2 (pai hui), HL10 (hui yang), HL3 (chu liao), and HL4 (huan T'iao). This is supplemented with insertion into the tender points. The hot needle is then inserted into HL5 (huan chung), HL6 (huan hou), and HL11 (han hou). This is supplemented by insertion into HL1 (pa shan), HL9 (hsieh ch'i), HL12 (yi wa), and HL13 (ch'ien shen).

4. For rheumatism of the knee joint, the hao chen is inserted into HL14 (lueh t'ao) as the principal acupuncture point. In addition, hao chen must be inserted into HL11 (han kou) and HL13 (ch'ien shen), or into HL7 (ta k'ua) and HL8 (hsiao k'ua).

5. For rheumatism of the lumbar region, the hao chen is inserted into T2 (pai hui), T7 (sahng chiao), or T9 (tzu chiao) through T8 (yao ch'ien). Sometimes, HL18 (wei ken) is also used. The hot needle is also inserted into T2 (pai hui), T3 (shen yu), T4 (shen chiao), and T5 (shen cha). Sometimes, T8 (yao ch'ien), T7 (yao chung), and T6 (yao hou) are used. For the shen and yao points, one needle is inserted through both points at the time time.

6. Oral intake of 60 gm of salicylate and 60 gm of sodium bicarbonate is used. Intravenous injections of 250 mg of hydrocortisone or 150 mg of hydrocortisone over the points once daily may be a supportive or independent method of treatment.

Facial Nerve Palsy

SYMPTOMS

1. Unilateral facial nerve palsy is most frequently

manifested in the sag of the ears. The upper eyelid and the lower lip fall downward. The upper lip falls toward the affected side. There is depression of the nostrils. The tip of the nose and the upper lip are tilted to the right or the left, depending on the side where the palsy occurs. Eating and drinking are difficult. Also food is retained in the mouth.

2. In bilateral facial nerve palsy, there is no tilting of the lips, but they droop downward. Respiration is difficult, and eating and drinking are seriously affected.

TREATMENT

1. Hao chen is inserted into HN12 (so k'ou), HN15 (k'ai kuan), HN1 (shang kuan), and HN2 (hsia kuan).

2. Electroacupuncture or injection of strychnine nitrate may be used as substitutes.

3. Into the loose connective tissue surrounding the ganglion of the horse (located over the region of the buccinator nerve) or trigeminal nerve or infraorbital nerve, 8–10 cc of 0.2%, strychnine nitrate is injected. When the upper lip is tilted to the left, the injection is in the right side and vice versa. If both lips drop downward, both sides are injected. This may be used as an independent method of therapy.

Colic

This disease is caused by intestinal stimulation by cold. There is an acute spasmodic contraction of the intestine. This disease has several etiologies. Some occur in early spring and late fall when there is a sudden change in weather; others occur after excessive drinking of cold water or eating of frozen food. Others occur after exposure to rain or frost.

SYMPTOMS

1. Any cold stimulation should be noted in taking the case history.

2. The spasm occurs initially within 1–3 hours after eating or drinking. Abdominal pain is severe; the animal then doubles up and rolls over from discomfort. Later, the pain becomes intestinal. Exacerbation and remission occur every 10–15 min.

3. The ear and nose become cold. Other symptoms include pallor of mouth, smooth tongue surface, drooling, weak pulse, and abnormal body temperature.

4. There is an increase in bowel sound and watery diarrhea.

5. Rectal examination shows no fecal retention and a collapsed stomach.

TREATMENT

1. The hao chen is inserted into HN4 (san chiang), HN11 (fen shui), HN7 (chiang ya), and HN17 (erh chien).

2. Antispasmodic and analgesic drugs may be used as supportive or independent methods of treatment.

B. SHIN[20] (FIG. 3—109)

Allergy

HYPERSENSITIVITY (ANAPHYLAXIS FROM FOREIGN PROTEIN MATERIAL)
Rx. Points: 26, 44, 13-1, 30.
Method: Bilateral, 25 min, 2 times/week.

ALLERGY OF THE RESPIRATORY TRACT (POLLEN, LACRIMATION, SNEEZING)
Rx. Points: 14, 42, 42-1, 45.
Method: Bilateral, 25 min, 2 times/week.

ALLERGY OF SKIN (UTICARIA, ECZEMATOUS DERMATITIS, CONTACT DERMATITIS)
Rx. Points: 26, 44, 13-1, 29, 22, and local points with multiple needles.
Method: Bilateral, 15 min, 3 times/week.

ALLERGY OF DIGESTIVE TRACT (GASTROINTESTINAL DISTRESS)
Rx. Points: 20-1, 44, 45, 23, 14.
Method: One side each time, 15 min, 3 times/week.

Shock
Rx. Points: 44, 45, 20-1, 8.
Method: Bilateral, 5 min, 5 times/week.

Anorexia
Rx. Points: 44, 45, 20, 8.
Method: Bilateral, 30 min, 1 time/week.

Glossoplegia
Rx. Points: 6, 12, 5, 46.
Method: Bilateral, 25 min, 2 times/week.

Colic
Rx. Points: Formula 1. 44, 45, 20-1.
Formula 2. 31, 23, 18.
Formula 3. 48, 19, 20-1, 41.
Formula 4. 19, 13, 8, 18, 33, 39.
Method: Each formula for 1 time. Bilateral, 5 min, 3 times/day.

Obesity
Rx. Points: 1, 44, 45, 20-1.
Method: Bilateral, 30 min, 1 time/week.

Lameness

SHOULDER LAMENESS

Rx. Points: 15, 17, 19, 21-2.
Method: One side each time, 25 min, 2 times/week.

ELBOW LAMENESS

Rx. Points: 19-1, 18, 20, 39.
Method: One side each time, 25 min, 2 times/week.

CARPAL LAMENESS

Rx. Points: 22, 29, 21, 21-3, 37.
Method: One side each time, 25 min, 2 times/week.

HIP LAMENESS

Rx. Points: 49, 59, 46, 58.
Method: One side each time, 25 min, 2 times/week.

STIFLE LAMENESS

Rx. Points: 49, 50, 60, 33, 57.
Method: One side each time, 25 min, 2 times/week.

HOCK LAMENESS

Rx. Points: 51, 51-1, 51-3, 52.
Method: One side each time, 25 min, 2 times/week.

Bucked Shin

Rx. Points: 27, 24, 23, 40, 18.
Method: Bilateral, 25 min, 2 times/week.

Laminitis

ACUTE LAMINITIS

Rx. Points: *Formula 1.* 46, 44, 33, 39, 18.
　　　　　Formula 2. 18, 46, 23, 21-2.
Method: Bilateral, 25 min, 3 times/week.

CHRONIC LAMINITIS

Rx. Points: *Formula 1.* 15, 20, 42, 44.
　　　　　Formula 2. 19-1, 8, 21-2, 22, 23, 24, 25.
Method: One side each time, 35 min, 2 times/week.

Navicular Disease

ACUTE NAVICULAR DISEASE

Rx. Points: *Formula 1.* 18, 44, 33, 21-2.
　　　　　Formula 2. 17, 15, 41, 33.
Method: One side each time, 25 min, 2 times/week.

CHRONIC NAVICULAR DISEASE

Rx. Points: *Formula 1.* 27, 28, 24, 23, 29-2.
　　　　　Formula 2. 28-1, 29, 23-2, 29-1.
Method: One side each time, 20 min, 3 times/week.

Osteoarthritis

Rx. Points: Local tender points, 33, 35, 37, 39, 44.

PATELLA LUXATION (UPWARD FIXATION)

Rx. Method: a. Push patella into original place.
　　　　　　b. Insert needle into patella ligaments, first above the patella then below.
　　　　　　c. Turn both needles in the direction that the patella needs to go.
　　　　　　d. One side only, 15 min, 2 times/week.

Myositis

Rx. Points: 44, 33, 39, 40, and local tender points.
Method: Bilateral, 25 min, 2 times/week.

Facial Paralysis

Rx. Points: *Formula 1.* 33, 1, 3, 7, 9.
　　　　　Formula 2. 13, 9, 11, 33.
　　　　　Formula 3. 20, 1, 2, 3, 12.
Method: One side each time, 15 min, 3 times/week.

Muscle Spasm

Rx. Method: a. Find main pain point (local) with careful palpation of tender area.
　　　　　　b. Insert main point needle perpendicularly.
　　　　　　c. Find secondary pain point with palpation and pressing with thumb.
　　　　　　d. Insert secondary pain point needle perpendicularly.
　　　　　　e. Rotate main pain point needle clockwise and secondary pain point needle counterclockwise at the same time for about 5–7 min.
　　　　　　f. Use moxibustion on both points for 2 min.
　　　　　　g. Remove both needles.
　　　　　　h. Watch for 30 min to determine if there is still a spasm.
　　　　　　i. If there is still a spasm, repeat the above treatment once. At this time, the main and secondary pain points are not necessarily the same points that were used in the first treatment. Generally, they are not.

3. Pig

A. CHINESE VETERINARY HANDBOOK[1] (FIGS. 3–49 TO 3–64)

Each prescription is used daily unless otherwise indicated. The number of daily treatments and length of course of treatment are determined by the course of the disease.

Pig Epidemic (Cholera in pigs, or plague)

Each of the prescriptions should be used independently. The hao chen needle is used.

1. The main points are as follows: T4 (pai hui), HL13 (wei chien), HN8 (shan ken), HN2 (erh chien), FL6 (yung chuan), T1 (ta chui). Two of the following supplementary points should also be used to ensure maximum effect: HN10 (yu t'ang), HN1 (t'ien men), T10 (liu mai), HL11 (wei ken), T10 (t'i men), HL21 (hou pa tzu), HL12 (wei pen), HL21 (chien pa tzu). The following points are also used, if specific signs are also present: asthma, T8 (fei shu) and T3 (su ch'i); diarrhea, HL17 (chiao ch'ao).

2. This prescription is used in combination with treatment using streptomycin to reinforce the effect of the drug: HN8 (shan ken), HN9 (pi chung), HN10 (yu t'ang), HN2 (erh chien), T4 (pai hui), HL13 (wei chien), HL17 (chiao ch'ao), and HL21 (pa tzu).

Lung Epidemic Hemorrhagic Disease (Pig Bacillus Disease)

Each of the following prescriptions is used independently. The hao chen needle is used.

1. The main points are as follows: T3 (su ch'i), T9 (fei shu), T18 (tuan hsueh), HL13 (wei chien), HN2 (erh chien), HN4 (erh ken). The supplementary points are: HN8 (shan ken), HN10 (yu t'ang), HL21 (pa tzu).

2. The main points are: T11 (t'an chung), T9 (fei shu), FL6 (yung chuan), FL6 (t'i shui). The supplementary points are: HN10 (yu t'ang), HN9 (pi chung), T18 (p'i shu), HL13 (wei chien), and HL6 (hou san li).

3. The main points are: HN8 (shan ken), HN2 (erh chien), T9 (fei shu), HN17 (so hou), HL13 (wei chien). The supplementary points are: HN10 (yu t'ang), T10 (liu mai), HL14 (wei chieh), HL12 (wei pen), and HL6 (hou san li).

Viral Pneumonia, or Pig Asthma

Each of the following prescriptions is used independently. A treatment session is 7 days. Daily treatment is administered for 3 days and every other day for 4 days. There is a 3-day interval between each 7-day treatment session. Hao chen is used.

1. The main points are: T3 (su ch'i), T9 (fei shu), T11 (t'an chung), and FL4 (ch'i hsing). The supplementary points are HL13 (erh chien) and HN8 (shan ken).

2. The main points are: HN8 (shan ken), T3 (su ch'i), T9 (fei shu), and HL13 (wei chien). The

supplementary points are: HL21 (pai tzu), T10 (liu mai), HL13 (hou san li), and moxibustion for T11 (t'an chung).

For prescriptions 3 and 4, a treatment session is 6 daily treatments, and there is a 3-day interval between each treatment.

3. The main points are: T3 (su ch'i), T9 (fei shu), FL11 (fei men), HL6 (hou san li). The supplementary points are: HN9 (pi chung), HN8 (shan ken), HN2 (erh chien), T10 (liu mai), HL21 (pa tzu), T11 (t'an chung), and HL13 (wei chien).

4. The main points are: HN9 (pi chung), HN2 (erh chien), T3 (su ch'i), T9 (fei shu), and HL13 (wei chien). The supplementary points are HN10 (yu t'ang), HN8 (shan ken), T10 (liu mai), and HL21 (pa tzu).

Diarrhea of Baby Pigs

Each prescription may be used independently. Prescriptions 1 and 2 may be used alternately in successive treatment sessions, which is daily treatments for 7 days. Prescription 3 may be used as a supplement when the indicated conditions exist.

1. The main points are: HN2 (erh chien), HN4 (t'ai yang), HN9 (pi chung), and HL13 (wei chien). The supplementary points are: HL6 (hou san li) and HN8 (shan ken).

2. The main points are: HL17 (chiao ch'ao) and HL6 (hou san li). The supplementary point is: T4 (pai hui) or T18 (p'i shu).

3. If the stool is creamy white or pale white, T8 (kai feng) is used. If the stool is yellowish, HL17 (chiao ch'ao) and HL6 (hou san li) are used.

Pig Influenza

The following prescriptions are used independently. Hao chen is used.

1. The main points are: HN8 (erh chung), HL13 (wei chien), HN20 (erh ken), T3 (su ch'i), and FL4 (ch'i hsing). The supplementary points are: HN10 (yu t'ang) and HL21 (pa tzu). This prescription is used at late stages of the disease.

2. The main points are: HN4 (t'ai yang), HN9 (pi chung), HL13 (wei chien), HN20 (erh ken), T4 (pai hui), and HN2 (erh chien). The supplementary points are: HN8 (shan ken), HN10 (yu t'ang), and T9 (fei shu).

3. The main points are: HN8 (shan ken), HN10 (yu t'ang), T3 (su ch'i), and HL13 (wei chien).

4. The main points are: HN5 (nao shu), HN4 (t'ai yang), HN6 (ching ming), HN2 (erh chien) and HL13 (wei chien). The supplementary points are: HN9 (pi chung), HN10 (yu t'ang), and HN21 (pa

tzu). This prescription is used at the initial stage of the disease.

Pig Mouth-and-Hoof Disease

Acupuncture is used to supplement the use of drugs. A quick diagnosis and isolation of the sick animal are essential if there is an outbreak of mouth-and-hoof disease.

1. Hao chen is used. The main points are: HN10 (yu t'ang), HN15 (cheng chiang), T1 (ta chui), and FL6 (yung chuan). The supplementary points are: T17 (kan shu), HL10 (ti men), HN8 (shan ken), and T4 (pai hui).

Stomatitis

1. Hao chen is used. The main points are: HN15 (cheng chiang), HN10 (yu t'ang), and HN17 (so hou). The supplementary points are: T18 (p'i shu), T17 (ken shu), T10 (liu mai), and H113 (wei chien).

Pharyngitis

Hao chen is used: HN17 (so hou), HN15 (cheng chiang), HN8 (shan ken), T3 (su ch'i), HN2 (erh chien), and HL13 (wei chien). The supplementary points are: T4 (pai hui), HN10 (yu t'ang), HL6 (hou san li), and T10 (liu mai).

Laryngitis

Hao chen is used. The main points are: HN17 (so hou), HN15 (cheng chiang), and T9 (fei shu). The supplementary points are: T3 (su ch'i), HN10 (yu t'ang), HN8 (shan ken), and T10 (liu mai).

Gastroenteritis

Each prescription is used independently. Hao chen is used for the first three prescriptions.

1. The main points are: HN10 (yu t'ang), T18 (p'i shu), HL6 (hou san li), HL13 (wei chien), and HN2 (erh chien). The supplementary points are: HN8 (shan ken) and T4 (pai hui).

2. The main points are: HN8 (shan ken), HN10 (yu t'ang), HN9 (pi chung), T18 (p'i shu), and HL6 (hou san li). The supplementary points are: HN2 (erh chien), HL13 (wei chien), and HL17 (chiao ch'ao).

3. The main points are: HN8 (shan ken), HL6 (hou san li), T1 (ta chui), T10 (liu mai), and T8 (kai feng). The supplementary points are: HN20 (wei ken), HL17 (chiao ch'ao), and T9 (fei shu).

4. Hao chen is inserted at HL12 (wei pen). A hot needle is inserted at T18 (p'i shu), and moxibustion is administered at the following points: T12 (chung wan), T13 (shang wan), and T14 (hsia wan).

Indigestion

Prescriptions 1 and 2 are used independently. Prescription 3 is used as a supplement for the indicated condition. Hao chen is used.

1. The main points are: HN10 (yu t'ang), T9 (fei shu), and HL6 (hou san li). The supplementary points are: HN8 (shan ken), HN9 (pi chung), and HL21 (pa tzu).

2. The main points are: HN9 (pi chung), HN10 (yu t'ang), T10 (liu mai), and HL6 (hou san li). The supplementary points are: T17 (kan shu), HL13 (wei chien), and HL15 (wei kan).

3. Supplementary points are used for the following conditions: constipation, HL17 (chiao ch'ao) and T21 (hou ger dai); diarrhea, HL17 (chiao ch'ao); slight elevation of temperature, HL12 (wei pen); and cold of the extremities and ears, FL5 (ch'an wan).

Pneumonia

Each prescription is used independently. Hao chen is used.

1. The main points are: HN2 (erh chien), HL13 (wei chien), T3 (su ch'i), and T9 (fei shu). The supplementary points are: FL4 (ch'i hsing), T4 (pai hui), and T18 (p'i shu).

2. The main point is: T3 (su ch'i). The supplementary points are: HN10 (yu t'ang), FL6 (yung chuan), FL11 (fei men), and FL12 (fei p'an).

Bronchitis

Hao chen is used. Each prescription is used independently.

1. The main points are: T9 (fei shu), FL11 (fei men), FL12 (fei p'an), T3 (su ch'i), HN2 (erh chien), and HL13 (wei chien). The supplementary points are: HN9 (pi chung), HN8 (shan ken), T4 (pai hui), T12 (ta chui), T10 (liu mai), T18 (p'i shu), FL8 (shen chu), and HN10 (yu t'ang).

2. The main points are: T3 (su ch'i), T9 (fei shu), FL4 (ch'i hsing), HL13 (wei chien), and HN2 (erh chien). The supplementary points are: HN10 (yu t'ang), HN8 (shan ken), HL21 (pa tzu), and T4 (pai hui).

3. The main points are: HN2 (erh chien), FL8 (shen chu), T11 (t'an chung), and T9 (fei shu). The supplementary points are: T3 (su ch'i), T1 (ta chui), and HN10 (yu t'ang).

Nephritis

Hao chen is used. Each prescription is used independently. Two supplementary points are used for each treatment.

1. The main points are: HL16 (yu shu) and T14 (t'ien shu). The supplementary points are: HN10 (yu t'ang), HL13 (wei chien), and T4 (pai hui).

2. The main points are: T4 (pai hui), HL13 (wei chien), and T22 (yang ming). The supplementary points are: T1 (ta chui), T6 (kai feng), HN10 (yu t'ang), HN8 (shan ken), HL6 (hou san li), and HN13 (wei chien).

Urinary Tract Infection

Each prescription is used independently. Hao chen is used.

1. The main points are: T4 (pai hui), T20 (shen men), T14 (t'ien shu), and T22 (yang ming). The supplementary points are: FL6 (yung chuan) and T1 (ta chui).

2. The main points are: T20 (shen men), T14 (t'ien shu), and HL16 (yin shu). The supplementary point is T4 (pai hui).

Constipation

Each prescription is used independently. Hao chen is used. Only two of the supplementary points are used when indicated.

1. The main points are: HN10 (yu t'ang), HL17 (chiao ch'ao), FL4 (ch'i hsing), and T21 (hou ger dai). The supplementary points are: T3 (su ch'i), T4 (pai hui), HN8 (shen ken), and HL21 (pa tzu).

2. The main points are: T10 (liu mai), HL14 (wei chieh), HL15 (wei kan), HL13 (wei chien), and HL17 (chiao ch'ao). The supplementary points are: HN8 (shan ken), HN10 (yu t'ang), T20 (shen men), T4 (pai hui), and HL6 (hou san li).

3. HN10 (yu t'ang), HL13 (wei chien), T4 (pai hui), HL11 (wei ken), HL17 (chiao ch'ao), and HL6 (hou san li).

4. HN10 (yu t'ang), T18 (p'i shu), HL17 (chiao ch'ao), T21 (hou ger dai), and HL21 (ch'i hsing).

Vitamin A Deficiency

Hao chen is used for insertion. Two of the supplementary points are used for each prescription. The main points are: FL4 (t'ien men) and HL18 (tsui feng). The supplementary points are: HN2 (erh chien), HL13 (wei chien), HN10 (yu t'ang), and HL21 (pa tzu).

Anemia

Hao chen is used. The main points are: T17 (p'i shu), T17 (kan shu), HL6 (hou san li), T10 (liu mai), FL6 (yung chuan), and T1 (ta chui). The supplementary points are: HL8 (shan ken), HN10 (yu t'ang), and FL5 (ch'an wan).

Sunstroke

Each prescription is used independently. Hao chen is used. Two of the supplementary points are used for each treatment.

1. The main points are: HN1 (t'ien men), HN2 (erh chien), HN20 (erh ken), and HL12 (wei pen). The supplementary points are: FL6 (yung chuan), T1 (ta chui), HL21 (pa tzu), and HN9 (pi chung).

2. The main points are: HN1 (t'ien men), HN5 (nao shu), HN2 (erh chien), and HN4 (tai yang). The supplementary points are: HN18 (erh men) and HN12 (k'ai kuan).

3. The main points are: HN9 (pi chung), HL8 (shan ken), HN6 (ching ming), HN2 (erh chien), T8 (pai hui), HL13 (wei chien), HL6 (hou san li), T1 (ta chui), FL6 (yung chuan), and HL21 (pa tzu).

Rickets

Hao chen is used. Two of the supplementary points are used for treatments. The main points are: FL6 (yuon chuan), T1 (ta chui), HN10 (yu t'ang), HL6 (hou san li), and T18 (p'i shu). The supplementary points are: HL8 (shan ken), T4 (pai hui), HL13 (wei chien), FL5 (ch'an wan), T9 (liu mai), and T16 (kan shu).

Rheumatism of Muscles

This disease is usually seen when pigs are exposed to extreme cold and humidity. The onset is usually acute.

SYMPTOMS

1. There is a muscle spasm with pain and edema, initially in the hindlegs of the affected animal.

2. The lesion may migrate to the forelimbs or hindlimbs.

3. There are limping, small steps or total immobilization.

TREATMENT

Each treatment is used independently.

1. The hot needle is used for the main points: T4 (pai hui), T20 (shen men), T2 (san t'ai), and T15 (ling t'ai). The supplementary points are: FL5 (ch'an wan), FL1 (ch'ang feng), HL6 (hou san li), FL6 (yung chuan), and T1 (ta chui).

2. Hao chen is inserted into FL5 (ch'an wan), FL6 (yung chuan), and T1 (ta chui). The supplementary points are: HL8 (shan ken), HL18 (tsui feng), and T4 (pai hui).

Arthritis

Traumatic arthritis is commonly due to injury of the cartilage and ligaments of the joints. Bacterial infection and other inflammations are common causes of rheumatoid arthritis.

SYMPTOMS

1. In traumatic arthritis, there are limited movement, edema, and tenderness of the joints.

2. Rheumatoid arthritis is usually associated with high fever and multiple migratory involvement of the joints.

3. Alternate remission and exacerbation occur.

TREATMENT

Hao chen is used. Each prescription is used independently for daily treatment.

1. The main points are: FL6 (yung chuan), T1 (ta chui), FL1 (ch'ang feng), and HL6 (hou san li). The supplementary points are: T2 (san t'ai), T4 (pai hui), and FL4 (ch'i hsing).

2. For forelimb arthritis, the main points are: HL18 (tsui feng), HL21 (pa tzu), FL5 (hou ch'an wan), T4 (pai hui), and HL7 (ta k'ua). For hindlimb arthritis, the main points are: FL6 (yung chuan), FL4 (ch'i hsing), FL5 (chien ch'an wan), and HL21 (chien pa tzu). The supplementary points are: HN10 (yu t'ang) and T17 (p'i shu).

Contusion

Contusion includes all soft tissue injury secondary to trauma on the four limbs. Hao chen is used. The main points are: FL6 (yung chuan), T1 (ta chui), FL1 (ch'ang feng), and HL6 (hou san li). The supplementary points are: T2 (san t'ai), T4 (pai hui), and FL4 (ch'i hsing).

Conjunctivitis

Hao chen is used. The main points are: HN6 (ching ming), HN4 (t'ai yang), and T16 (ken shu). The supplementary points are: HN2 (erh chien) and T4 (pai hui).

Prepartum and Postpartum Paralysis

Weakness in the muscles or total paralysis of the extremities can be found perinatally when the mother pig has a deficiency in calcium and phosphorus. It can also be caused by trauma to the birth canal, or injury to the pelvic nerve secondary to the delivery. Each prescription is used independently. Hao chen is used for insertion.

1. Moxibustion is used for 15 min on each of the following acupuncture points: T4 (pai hui), FL6 (t'i shui), T19 (shen men), and HL18 (tsui feng).

2. The main points are: FL6 (yung chuan), T1 (ta chui), T4 (pai hui), HL7 (kai feng), and HL8 (shiao k'ua). The supplementary points are: HL11

(wei ken), HL13 (wei chien), HL9 (liu mai), FL1 (ch'ang feng), and HL8 (tsui feng).

3. For the paralysis of hindlimbs only, the main points are: HL7 (ta k'uo), HL6 (hou san li), HL21 (hou pa tzu), and HL18 (hou feng men). The supplementary points are: T4 (pai hui) and FL5 (hou ch'un wan).

4. The main points are: HL5 (tzu ta feng men), HL19 (t'i ch'a), FL6 (yung chuan), T1 (ta chui), HN10 (tsui t'ang), and FL5 (ch'an wan).

5. The main points are: T20 (shen men) for hao chen insertion; and T4 (pai hui), T6 (kai feng), HL7 (ta k'ua), HL8 (shiao k'ua), FL4 (ch'i hsing), FL5 (chien ch'an wan), and T1 (ta chui) for hot-needle insertion. Hao chen is used to insert the supplementary points: HN10 (yu t'ang), T10 (liu mai), HL13 (wei chien), and HL6 (hou san li).

6. Hao chen is inserted into T4 (pai hui) (or HL7—ta k'ua), or HL8 (shiao k'ua). Heat treatment is then applied to the acupuncture points for 20 min. One treatment session comprises four to five treatments. In severe cases, two treatment sessions are indicated, with 2 days' interval between sessions.

4. Dog

A. MILIN[18, 19]

The points cited below indicate human points anatomically transposed to the dog.

Amenorrhea

(1) "Empty amenorrhea," which is always accompanied by digestive disorders: B20, B21, CV12, CV6, ST36, B43, B18, CV4, SP6.

(2) "Full amenorrhea" without digestive troubles, but with congestive, hypertense manifestations: B25, CV4, LI11, SP6, SP10, LIV2. Add: B23 (if kidney troubles exist at the same time), P5 (when circulatory troubles require it), LIV8, LIV4 (in the case of lumbar pains and difficulties of urination).

Dysmenorrhea

(1) Early menstruation, with very red blood, congestive state, rapid pulse. H5, LIV2, SP6.

With pale blood and in small quantity, sensitivity in the lumbar region, it will be necessary to tone: LIV3, LIV8, K3, K7.

(2) Late menstruation, with pale blood, in small quantity, pale mucous, small, rapid pulse, vertigo, tone: SP2, LIV3, LIV8.

With abdominal pains, whitish tongue indicating digestive trouble: LIV3, LIV8, K3, K7, B23, B18.

With very bright blood, asthenia, anorexia, digestive troubles, tone: LIV1, SP6, CV6, CV4, CV3, GV4.

With dark-rosy blood, polydipsia, yellowish layer on the tongue, rapid and slipping pulse, tone: LIV1, SP6, CV6, CV4, and disperse LIV3, ST30.

False Pregnancy

Disperse in all cases: CV17, CV4, CV6, ST36; and tone: ST30, ST13.

Finally, tone SP6 if the menstruation that preceded was abundant or separated from the previous one by a less than normal interval; disperse in the opposite case.

General Points for Treatment of Rheumatism

TB15: silver needle, calm the pain of the shoulder and the arm, the contracture of the neck. When the pains or local contractures are improved by the silver needle, then use the gold needle for its general action upon rheumatism. B60: (often called the Chinese aspirin because of its secondary role upon the adrenal gland). In pain of the tarsus, of contractures located in this area, lumbar and coccygeal neuralgias, sciatica, this point will be first punctured with the silver needle, then gold after the disappearance of the painful signs. LI4: acts with the silver needle upon all the contractures and pains of the cranial part of the animal.

Silver needle: GB30, indicated in al lameness of the hind limb, weakness of leg and stifle, pains of the loins and hind limb. Particularly indicated in case of coexistence of cutaneous problems. Silver needle: TB5, B58, indicated in rheumatism in the joints with sharp pain. Silver needle: SI7, will calm muscle spasms while tonifying the heart; indicated in spasmodic pain and rheumatismal neuralgias. Silver needle: LU1, particularly indicated in the pains of shoulder and arm.

Puncture with a silver needle all the points which are definitely painful under pressure, even if they don't correspond to Chinese points.

Arthritis of the Shoulder

Gold needle: TB15; silver needle: LI15. When the pains of the shoulder worsened by the movement, use silver needle LI4 and SI 10.

Humeroradio Cubital Arthritis

Gold needle: LI4; silver needle: LI10 (active upon neuralgias and contractures of the arm); silver needle: S18; silver needle: TB10 also acts upon the muscular pains located along the spinal column).

Arthritis of the Carpus

Gold needle: LI10; silver needle: P6, LI4, TB5, LI6.

Coxofemoral Arthritis

Gold needle: GB30; silver needle: B60, GB26 (also acts for lumbar pain), GB28, ST30 (also for lumbar pain), LIV12 (active upon all contractures and painful spasms of the hind limb and lumbar pain).

Arthritis of the Stifle

Gold needle: LIV9, B60; silver needle: K2 (also active upon lumbar pain and foot pain), ST36 (limb edema), GB34 (for arthritic pain of the stifle and for cramps).

Arthritis of the Tarsus

Gold needle: B58, K6 (active upon all mobility troubles of the hind leg and upon chronic nephritis); silver needle: SP5 (acts particularly upon osseous pain, also upon constipation), B60.

For arthrosis of these joints, switch the needles (gold instead of silver, and vice versa) during the last session.

Vertebral Arthritis

The important thing in the treatment of vertebral arthritis with acupuncture is to calm down the muscular contractures. First, use the main points of contractures: GB40 (also for pain in the hind leg), B62, B56, B57. One can also add the following antispasmodic points: LIV2 (indicated for lumbar pain, articular pain, cramps), LIV3 (indicated for lumbar pain). To suppress the abdominal contractures which often go with the meningeal pain: CV12 (indicated in case of hard and tight abdomen). Finally, put the silver needle on both sides of the spinosus processsus of the vertebrae, at the level of the painful joint, on the meridian of the bladder.

Temporomaxillary Arthritis

L14. Gold needle: ST2, ST3, TB23. All these points are also the points to use in atrophic myositis of the masseters with the needles indicated here. As long as there are contractures, switch gold and silver needles to tonify muscles or what remains of them.

Paralysis in Dogs Caused by Age

Gold needle: GV19, GB34, GB37.

Chronic Cough in the Dog

Gold needle: B13, LU9; silver needle: K25, P6.

B. SHIN[20] (FIG. 3–116)

Allergy

HYPERSENSITIVITY (BY FOREIGN PROTEIN MATERIAL)

Rx. Points: 26, 44, 13-1, 30.

Method: Bilateral, 15 min, 2 times/week.

ALLERGY OF RESPIRATORY TRACT (FROM POLLEN)

Rx. Points: 14, 42, 45, 33, 33C (interspinous space T10-T11).
Method: Bilateral, 15 min, 2 times/week.

ALLERGY OF THE SKIN

Rx. Points: 26, 44, 13-1, 29, 22, 52.
Method: Bilateral, 15 min, 2 times/week.

ALLERGY OF DIGESTIVE TRACTS

Rx. Points: 20, 44, 45, 14.
Method: Bilateral, 15 min, 2 times/week.

Hip Dysplasia

UNILATERAL MALFORMATION

Rx. Points: 37, 37C, 41, 41C, 59 (other side only).
Method: Bilateral, k5 min, 3 times/week.

BILATERAL MALFORMATION

Rx. Points: 38, 38C, 40, 40C, 59-2, 59-1, 46.
Method: Bilateral once, then left side once, then right side once. 20 min, 3 times/week.

HIP DYSPLASIA WITH DISC SYNDROMES

Rx. Points: 37, 37C, 38C, 40, 40C, 41C, 59.
Method: Bilateral, 20 min, 3 times/week.

Epilepsy

Rx. Points: 13, 19-1, 18, 12.
Method: Bilateral, 15 min, 2 times/week.

Facial Paralysis

Rx. Points: 13-1, 11, 8, 44, 12 (other side only).
Method: Bilateral, 15 min, 2 times/week.

Chorea

Rx. Points: 26, 25, 22, 12.
Method: Bilateral, 15 min, 2 times/week.

Intervertebral Disc Syndromes

Rx. Points: Contingent upon disc afflicted.
Method: a. Locate the disc that is abnormal (for example, T13-L1).
    b. Use the points one above and one below (for example, 36, 38, and pain points).
    c. Rotate point 36 needle clockwise and point 38 needle counterclockwise.
    d. Do not touch 36 pain point and 38 pain point after insertion.
    e. Mild moxibustion on points 36 and 38 for 5 min.
    f. Bilateral, 20 min, 2 times/week.

Quotations, Abstracts, and Case Reports

Unless keyed to a specific figure in this book, points cited are human equivalent.

LARGE ANIMALS

Quotations and Abstract

"When other treatments have been ineffective for treating overworked or debilitated horses, I have used acupuncture occasionally, and in a few cases, it seemed to be beneficial."[10]

"In Tokyo, where there are about 1000 race horses in residence, equine acupuncture is an important medical specialty. Masayashi Kirisawa DVM, treats about 50 patients a day, doing fine needle acupuncture primarily for inflammation and rigidity of muscles in the neck and shoulders. Another technique, done with bigger, knife-like needles, recalls ancient blood-letting. These are inserted to purge "bad blood", in a process which is said to restore health to exhausted horses."[3]

"Talking about a 10-year-old gelding jumper—three-quarters thorobred and one-quarter Arabian—who had developed osteoarthritis in the left outside hock, Feinman said, 'We knew it was calcification or bone spurs; the horse had been treated with all the standard methods, so we asked Dr. Becker to use acupuncture.

" 'The results were incredible . . . he inserted one acupuncture needle in the hip, by hand. The horse didn't flinch.' Immediately after insertion, the horse put his weight on the leg he had been favoring, stood square, and became tranquil. The needle remained affixed for about a minute and then was removed easily.

"The horse was then immediately trotted in hand, showing only the slightest indication of discomfort. 'Dr. Becker advised me to exercise the horse.'

"Becker's records indicate that the gelding, treated with acupuncture twice a week over a three week period, was jumping five-foot courses in three weeks.

"Another horse treated with acupuncture responded even more dramatically. Suffering from inflammation so severe he could not stand, the swelling was extreme from shoulder to hoof. Becker needled the horse, who walked immediately after treatment. The inflammation, reduced within four hours, required only one treatment."[5]

"Upon entering the stall, the boar was lying down and would not get up until prodded and given support at the hindquarter and at the tail. This caused the animal a great deal of pain, and it cried out during the whole examination. There was, however, no evidence of temperature rise or bone fracture, so, on that basis, I thought that the animal could have been suffering from something like lumbago. Actually, the affliction was of a traumatic genesis, so, at first, it was treated with cortisone, antihistamines and injections from a *pyrazol* derivative.

"On the next day, the animal's condition had not noticeably improved.

"I decided to try acupuncture . . . with some needles that I had made before, for work on larger animals, . . . from piano wire.

"With these needles, I then pierced the dorsal and lumbar regions on the boar in the area of the bladder meridian.

"These slight, probing needle pricks directed into the hyperalgesic zones of the animal produced loud cries of pain, and even an occasional short spasm as well. . . . Because of the thickness of the boar hide, I was only able to force the needles in just a few millimeters.

"After piercing five or six very painful points in the lumbar region, I brought the animal out of its stall and walked it around. At first, the boar took very small, halting steps and was quite stiff; but after about 20 meters, the animal's gait became much freer and easier.

"After about 100 meters, we came upon the boar's herd of sows. From these sows, he had selected one two days ago, and she was still in heat. After a short period of time, the boar approached her and began foreplay with her; about five minutes after this, the boar mounted the sow and achieved sexual climax. A few minutes later, the same thing occurred."[13]

"In a mare, lumbar pain had been present for six weeks and grew worse despite the usual treatment. The examination revealed a painful zone along the spine with a maximum in the left lumbar region. The day after the first treatment, there was an improvement. The pace was less stiff and the paravertebral zone less painful. After four treatments within 12 days, there remained just a slight stiffness, after the fifth treatment the cure was complete. Exercising was started again and after a short while, it was able to cover a long distance."[14]

"Reports of past work stimulated me to try to use acupuncture in daily practice. . . . Of course, I used modern antibiotics and sera in infectious diseases of bacterial origin, since their value is without doubt. But I still want to point out . . . that according to my opinion acupuncture increases the effect of other medication.

"I would like to mention the case of a seven-year old Berber horse (used by its owner for walks in the woods) that had bilateral spavin and osteoarthritis of the tarsal joint. This disease led to complete uselessness of the hind extremities, so that the horse was not able to run anymore. Local therapy was used, but it did not bring any improvement. The owner had already made up his mind to get the animal killed. I had been asked to come for that reason.

"In this condition, I used acupuncture twice and chose the following points: B60 (gold needle), SP5 (silver needle), K9, and BL58.

"If it would have been a case of acute arthritis of the tarsal joint, I would have chosen silver needles instead of golden ones, I want to point out.

"After these treatments, the horse gained back its usual mobility while the changes in the bones remained.

"Two years later, I saw the horse again in very good condition."[17]

"Eddie, the arthritic giraffe at Windsor Safari Park outside London, is moving around with ease after two acupuncture treatments. Park director Gary Smart said that he and park veterinarian David Taylor visited China earlier this year to study animal husbandry and zoo management. While there, they also saw how the Chinese use acupuncture to treat arthritic cows. 'Dr. Taylor was so impressed,' Smart said, 'that we thought we'd try it on Eddie the giraffe.' Apparently, it's working—Eddie now walks without a limp."[4]

Chan[8] has reported on the treatment of colic using acupuncture:

Horses of mixed breeding were used. The age of affected horses ranged from 1 to 11 years. Of the 21 cases, 6 were spasmodic colic, 2 were engorgement colic, 8 were impaction colic, and 5 were flatulent colic. Three kinds of needles were used for colic treatment: (1) Hao chen needles, which usually are used for stimulation of points, but in this study chiefly for blood-letting; (2) prism needles, used for letting small amounts of blood on insertion into blood vessels; and (3) wide needles, used when larger quantities of blood are let (a scalpel may be used instead, but care must be taken not to cut up the blood vessel or cut too deeply).

Many acupuncture points are prescribed in treating colic, but through the result of his past research work, blood-letting at points HN4 (san chiang), FL20 (chien ti tou), and HL22 (hou ti tou) has proved most effective and has been used throughout this present study. (Figs. 3–28, 3–32, 3–34b, 3–37).

The treatment of colic by acupuncture gives satisfactory results. Generally, in colic cases, peristalsis of the intestines is slight or absent and abdominal pain is severe. However, approximately 15 min after bloodletting at the specific points, peristalsis can be detected, and pain gradually subsides. The intervals between periodic spells of pain lengthen (spasmodic colic), and within 1–2 hours symptoms of colic disappear and conditions return to normal. The efficacy rate for both spasmodic and engorgement colic was 100%; of the other two types of colic, pain was relieved in one case of flatulent colic, but pulse and appetite did not become normal until 24 hours later. Two cases of impaction colic did not give favorable results because treatment was given too late after complications had already set in. Thus, the average efficacy rate for the three types of colic besides spasmodic colic was 80–90%.

Based on experience, acupuncture treatment of colic in horses is most likely to be successful when undertaken early in the course of illness. Improvement of dietary management and new medical drugs may be helpful in eradicating colic altogether, but in out-of-the-way places where medicine is not available, prompt treatment with acupuncture in emergency cases can be life-saving. Acupuncture has proved effective, convenient, and economical, and it has been used and recorded as a practical therapy for equine colic for more than a thousand years in China.

Points used for the treatment of colic in horses are: HN17 (erh chien), HN4 (san ching), HN11 (fen shui), HN9 (chiang ya), Sobin 64 (wei shu), T10 (pi shu), Sobin 69 (ta chang shu), FL20 (chien ti tou), HL22 (hou ti tou), HL17 (hou hai), HL19 (wei pen), and HL20 (wei chien) (Figs. 3–28, 3–29, 3–31, 3–32, 3–34b, 3–35a, 3–37, 3–43).

Prescriptions for different types of colic are: (1) Spasmodic colic: HN17, HN4, HN11, HN9, FL20, HL22, Sobin 69, and HL20. (2) Engorgement colic: HN4, HN11, HN9, FL20, HL22, T10, and Sobin 64. (3) Impaction colic: HN11, HN9, FL20, HL22, Sobin 69, T10, HL17, and HL19. (4) Flatulent colic: HN4, HN11, FL20, HL22, Sobin 69, T10, and HL17.

Case Reports

These are some of the case reports submitted to the International Veterinary Acupuncture Society by members of that society and distributed in the newsletter of the society.

1. *Equine 6-year-old, standardbred, gelding, trotter.* This horse had an old fracture in his left carpus. The horse was so lame that he could hardly walk, much less race. I treated the knee with acupuncture and in 1 hour the horse was much improved and raced 2 days later 100% sound. Butazoldin® was also given to the horse before the race, but he had not been sound with cortisone alone before acupuncture. The points used were: eyes of ken—the 2 points in front of the knee and in the intercarpal joint, TH3 and TH5, LU4, LI1 (Figs. 3–13 to 3–18). The needles were twirled fast and left in 10–15 min to achieve sedation. The beneficial effects on this lameness last 3–7 days, and the horse was treated 1–2 days before every race.

2. *Equine, American saddlebred, 12-year-old gelding.* Chronic pulmonary emphysema of 2 years' duration. Treatment: left side, Shin's lung point, 5 min; Shin's liver point, 12 min; Shin's stomach point, 12 min daily for six treatments (4/26/75–5/1/75). One week later, owner reported more heaving. I repeated acupuncture treatment on right side. Placed animal on daily choline chloride and vitamin A supplement. Symptoms have not yet recurred as of 6/4/75. This animal was known by me to have a respiratory problem for more than 2 years. It seems at this time that acupuncture treatment alone is effecting a cure.

3. *Equine, appaloosa, 4-year-old stallion.* Equine influenza with heaves. Clinical signs: temp. 104.6, resp. rate 18–25, running nose, running eyes, catarrh, cough, rales, emphysema, pumping of flanks, history of combiotic for 3 days and getting worse. Treatment: IV sulfa dimethoxine, 50 cc; 20 cc Flucorticin® IM; 10 cc antihistamine; 10 cc camphorated oil, 5 cc vitamin ADE. Thirty-six hours later, he was brought to equine hospital and continued ½ dose IV sulfa, Flucorticin® and camphor oil daily for 4 more days; plus, Shin's lung point, 5 min; Shin's liver point, 15 min; Shin's stomach point, 15 min (all daily for 4 days). (See pp. 122–214 and Fig. 3–109) On fourth day when needles were removed, sites were all injected with 3 cc camphor oil. Animal was released on fifth day. Temperature is normal and practically no heaves but still has cough; eats well. Combining western medicine with eastern looks promising.

4. *Equine, American saddlebred, 7-year-old gelding.* Horse coughs in stall and in exercise and heaving breathing at rest. Treated with different medication with no results. Bronchial sedative powder (F–D), etc. Diagnosis: chronic emphysema. Treatment: Okada points SI6, BL13, BL17, BL40, LI8, LI9, LI10; treated manually once weekly for 3 weeks bilateral (Figs. 3–13 to 3–18). Stopped coughing at exercise and in stall, and breathing at rest was almost normal. Horse sold, and I could not follow results.

5. *Equine, Shetland pony, 13-year-old mare.* Foundered several years ago, and pony recovered under medication. However, suffered acute relapse after turned out on grass in spring after hay diet all winter. Pony could not move, lay down constantly, hooves were hot, strong digital pulse. Treated with Azium® and Butazolidin® daily. Pony responded to medication; however, as soon as medication was stopped, symptoms reappeared. Diagnosis: chronic laminitis. Treatment: Treated Okada points TH4, SI2, LU8, LI1, TH1 manually daily for 12 days and then periodically once every 3 or 4 weeks for five treatments (Figs. 3–13 to 3–18). Pony recovered completely with no relapse after 6 months.

6. *Equine, Thoroughbred, gelding.* Chronic carpitis of 18 months' duration, with extensive bony proliferation of radial intermediate and third carpal bones. Also much proliferation or anterior radius on each side of common extensor tendon. Treatment: Previous treatment had been draining the synovial fluid from carpus and extensor sheath and injecting 80 mg of Depo-Medrol. This was done twice about 6 weeks apart. No steroids were given 2 months prior to acupuncture treatments. 5/6/75: (Fig. 3–109) points 22, 29, 46, 38; needles were put in place, then moxibustion applied to each point for approximately 2 min. Needles were left in place 30 min. At this time, the horse was stiff and could hardly flex his carpal area. He did so with aggravation. The horse seemed to enjoy this treatment, especially after the moxa was used. At this time, however, there was no improvement of gait or swelling. 5/10/75: The same treatment was given. 5/11/75: The swelling was beginning to subside, synovial fluid only, not bone. 5/14/75: Used points 22, 29, 38, 44, and two local points on each side of common extensor tendon about 2 cm apart. Lower needles were 3 cm above carpus. Moxa was used on all points. Needles were left in place about 30 min. 5/17/75: All synovial swelling was gone. Horse could flex knee about 75% with no resisting, and the owner started light riding. Also, his spirit or desire to go seemed much better than before starting the treatments.

I have given no further treatments at this time. The horse has remained the same and has not been worse or better. I am waiting to see how long these effects last. I don't believe that we can help the bone proliferation, but the acupuncture surely has improved his gait, reduced the swelling, and seemingly provided an increased desire to use the leg.

7. *Equine, paint, long yearling, colt.* Swelling and pain following administration of intramuscular bio-logical. The colt was being prepared for showing in the Paint Horse Association. The owner administered Equine Encephalomyelitis vaccine (Eastern and Western) with tetanus toxoid, intramuscularly in the right cervical region. Within 2 hours, the neck was held rigidly with swelling and pain involving an area approximately 20 cm in diameter. Acupuncture was suggested and its use agreed upon. The most sensitive locus was determined to be 2 cm from the injection site. A needle was inserted into this point 3 cm deep. Four additional needles were inserted 1 cm deep surrounding the central needle at the margins of the sensitive area and resembling the points of a compass. Sedation manipulation was administered to the central needle and tonification to the balance for 30 min. Twenty hours later, the colt could nibble hay off the ground with difficulty. Three most sensitive points were ascertained, and needles were placed in them 2 cm deep. Sedation manipulation was administered, and needles were left in place 30 min. The owner reported that within 7 hours of the second treatment, the colt was using its head and neck in a normal fashion. Four days after treatment, all actions appeared normal.

8. *Equine, 18-month-old Morgan filly.* A wobbler, x-rayed at the University of Pennsylvania. A subluxation between C2 and C3 was diagnosed as the cause of the Wobbling. The filly was hospitalized for 2 weeks, at which time she received 10 treatments of acupuncture using the points and techniques as follows. First treatment: Shin points, bilateral, 13, 11, 17, 30, 40-1, 32, 10, spleen point, liver point (Fig. 3–109). All points except 10, which was just pricked, were treated for 30 min with moxa applied to each needle twice for 15–30 sec. Depth: 11–¼ in., 17–1 in., 30–1 in., 40–½ in., 32–1 in., 13–4 in., spleen point–½ in., liver point–½ in. Turning of needles was not done. Second treatment: Same Shin points used as in first treatment except I eliminated the spleen point and liver point. I added another point bilaterally on the neck at the level of the 3rd cervical vertebra, otherwise treatment was the same. Third to tenth treatments: same points and technique as used in second treatment. After each treatment, a spring-loaded tei shin was used to stimulate the area lateral to the spine for 10 min. The filly seemed to enjoy the moxabustion, especially on the cervical points. When moxa was used, time was determined by the filly's reaction. I applied moxa to hair (not skin) and base of needle. Blistering did not occur. However, some swelling was evident around the points at various times during therapy.

Improvement was noticed the day after the second acupuncture treatment. The filly appeared stronger, and movement of the front legs was improved. This improvement was evident by her picking her legs up higher and stumbling was reduced. She kept improving but seemed to be worse immediately after each treatment. However, on the day after treatment, her condition would be much improved. The filly was released to her owner. Three days after her return home, the owner called to say she was very pleased and excited for she felt that the filly was dramatically improved.

9. *Equine, eight-year-old thoroughbred gelding.* Fractured shaft of ilium on right side 2 years ago during a race. Fracture healed, but horse could not be put back into training because of lumbar and sacral pain. Various drugs (hormones and anti-inflammatory) and exercise programs (such as swimming) did not change the condition, and the animal still could not be worked. The gluteals on the right side began to decrease in size. Acupuncture treatment was started, utilizing the points and numbers of the Sobin chemical horse model. The needles were put in place, left for 20 min and gently twirled a few times. The horse had been treated 10 times. The first seven treatments used points 82, 79, 80, 78, and 86 on the right; 79, and 78 on the left, and 81. The next three treatments utilized just 78 on the right and 81. The horse is back in training, gallops 1–2 miles a day and jumps 3½ ft fences. Treatment was only done when the horse became uncomfortable, about every 3 weeks, and was continued for six months.

10. *Equine, bay gelding quarter horse, 13 years old.* Intermittent lameness becoming progressively worse for 4 to 6 months in the right front leg. Radiographs indicated navicular changes, early ringbone, and early osselet changes. Diagnostic nerve blocks were tried, and the horse did not become sound until given a volar nerve block above the fetlock. Corrective shoeing was instituted using neoprene pads and rolling the toes. This was unsuccessful. The period from the onset of the lameness until acupuncture was about 6 months. Treatment: (Figs. 3–13 to 3–18) SI1, LI1, TH1, HC3, B34, BL54, SI2 (all points treated bilaterally). Main point for navicular disease in fossa above the bulbs of the heel, and any trigger points along the bladder meridian (6 treatments). At this point the owner feels the horse is 80% better. I have not treated the horse since because the owner moved to another state.

11. *Equine, gray gelding quarter horse, cutting horse, 7 years old.* Intermittent lameness between the front and rear legs. The horse was taken to the university for diagnosis. Radiographs showed pedal osteitis. It was then also believed that he had early bone spavin in the rear legs, with the right leg being more severe. The horse was shod with neoprene pads and put on powdered azium for 10 days. At the end of this period, the horse was sound and put back in use. Within 3 weeks, he was lame again. At this time, the university re-radiographed him, and it was determined that he also had navicular disease with no advancement in the pedal osteitis. There was also a lateral spur formation of the navicular bone and a small osteoporetic cyst. At this time, a 3-degree wedged neoprene pad was used, and the horse was placed on Butazolidin for 7 days. From this point on, the horse has been lame off and on. Ten months after the onset, he was completely lame and totally unusable.

Treatment: Corrective shoeing for 2 months was unsuccessful. Acupuncture was suggested instead of a neurectomy. To help correct the spavin in the back feet, the angle of the foot was increased 3 degrees with flat plate shoes. This took care of the spavin, but he was still lame in the front. Acupuncture treatment: (Figs. 3–13 to 3–18) Treatment 1, needles only. Main point in depression above the bulbs of the heels, bilateral on both front legs; also TH5 bilateral; BL17 and BL34 were both trigger points on palpation. Duration of time was 10 min. Treatment 2, same as 1. Treatments 3, 4, and 5 were the same, adding electrical stimulation: time, 10 min. Results: 50% remission of lameness after five additional treatments. The horse is back in training and at this point shows no signs of lameness with hard work.

12. *Equine, palamino gelding, 7-year-old quarter horse.* Illness began in December, 1973. The horse had labored breathing and a dry, hacking cough. On ascultation, there were increased lung sounds. Temperature and CBC were normal. At this point, there was a double exhilatory lift. Treatment: IV Liquamiacin and antiphrene. The horse responded for 1 month, then relapsed.

The owners then took the horse to the University of Missouri. A CBC showed a slight increase in the white blood cell count (1500 over normal). An EKG showed no heart damage. Their diagnosis was chronic bronchitis. At this point IV sulfa therapy was instituted along with oral isoniazid. The horse responded for approximately 8 days.

The horse was then brought home, and within 4 days relapsed. I then gave the horse IV sulfa and oral isoniazid. This treatment was unsuccessful. Eight months later the horse was treated with acupuncture. Treatment: (Figs. 3–13 to 3–18) bilateral LI4, LU6, BL17, and all trigger points along the BL meridian. After six treatments, all signs regressed. The last treatment was 14 months ago, and the horse is now showing again.

13. *Equine, standardbred, 3-year-old gelding.* Left shoulder lameness; nods on each step and not sensitive on any palpation or examination at feet, ankles, or knees. Treatment: acupuncture and ultrasound to bladder meridian points, (Figs. 3–13 to 3–18) LIV3, L14, B23, B25, B27, GB7 (point 44 on Fig. 109). This horse was sore when it trotted, also sore on the bladder meridian. After treatment, he handled hindquarters better and improved and smoothed out his gait when driving. To date, horse moves sound on leg.

14. *Equine, quarter horse, 3-year-old stallion.* Sore on front shoulders; walked peg-legged on both sides. Acupuncture points used were LI2 and LI11 sedate; B65 sedate; GB65 and GB43 tonify (Figs. 3–13 to 3–18). This horse was treated on Saturday afternoon, then again on Sunday morning. Same points as above plus some ultrasound over its shoulders. The animal was then taken to the track and raced in the afternoon of the same day. He won his race.

15. *Equine, standardbred, 2-year-old stallion.* Low, bowed tendon, very tender on palpation with heat in local area. Insertion of needles in bowed area on each side just above the ankle. Sedated for 20 min. One needle at posterior part of bow stimulated for 5 min. Three treatments; ultrasound used for the last treatment. This horse walked soundly on affected leg after treatment and was not sore on palpation or extreme pressure to the superficial or deep digital flexor tendons.

16. *Equine, standardbred, 5-year-old gelding.* Nods head when trotting or pacing. Had qualified at race track in 2:08 but finished lame. Treatment: acupuncture and ultrasound. Right front shoulder treated with 21-1, 21-2, 18, 15, and 17. Treated four times (Fig. 3–109). The horse was box-stalled 2 days before going home. He showed no lameness in a trot or pace. He was feeling very good and hard to hold when he left the clinic.

17. *Equine, standardbred, 8-year-old mare.* Sore in hindquarter, with short, choppy steps. Raced but not finishing strong and sore after racing. Acupuncture and ultrasound on bladder meridian, BL23, BL25, BL27 (Figs. 3–13 to 3–18), point 44 (Fig. 109). Treated five times in 5 days. When mare was brought to clinic, she was very doggy and walked with her head down and slow to lead. When the mare left the clinic, she was eating and feeling good, wanting to play and jump. She was full of spirit when led.

18. *Equine, thoroughbred, 15-year-old gelding.* Myositis of longissimus dorsi muscles, tenderness, was not flexing over fences, elevated SGOT. E-Se-steroids, heat, etc.; SGOT reduced but not jumping well. Injected 1–2 cc McKay's® into points 30, 38, 39, and 44 bilaterally (Fig. 3–109). One week later the horse was jumping and using his back much better. I have used this drug along or near the bladder meridian for years and have seen apparent improvement.

19. *Equine, 5-year-old thoroughbred gelding.* Subluxation and luxation of off stifle; showed swinging leg lameness plus occasional complete luxation with "locking" of joint. Suggested surgery, but trainer refused because horse had to be shown in about 10 days. Injected McKay's® in SP6, B1, B54, ST36, and around joint (Figs. 3–13 to 3–18). Repeated in 5 days. Horse not completely sound, but was able to be shown on phenylbutazone, and was second-year green working hunter champion at the show. Has been treated once since then and seems to have recovered.

20. *Equine, standardbred, 6 years old.* Laminitis and navicular disease. This horse was treated six times every other day. These treatments consisted of needling the coronary band, heel points, bleeding, electricity, and moxa. After six treatments, no improvement was noted. The owner called in another veterinarian and routine medical treatment is now being pursued.

21. *Equine, Tennessee walking horse, 8-year-old gelding.* Animal had history of emphysema for past 2 years, could not be used because any exertion triggered heavy abdominal breathing and coughing. The horse coughed persistently and regularly. Treatment of wetting hay, antihistamines, and steroids were ineffective. Treatment: FL19, FL1, FL2, FL3, and T31 were used (Figs. 3–13 to 3–18). The animal responded well after first treatment, but was still unable to be ridden; also did some erratic coughing. Treated about 2 weeks later using Shin's 4 points for

emphysema. The horse is being used and has shown no abnormal or unusual breathing after riding.

22. *Equine, Morgan, 8-year-old mare.* Laminitis. This animal had been purchased by a blacksmith about 8 months previous to being seen. The blacksmith felt that by corrective shoeing the animal could be brought back to functional use. The animal was severely lame on the front feet, but showed no pathologic changes of the hoof and sole. Treatment: bleeding with a stylet, 3 point at the coronet 1. Medial 2. Lateral 3. Anterior. Animal examined 3 days later and appeared more comfortable. Retreated at the same points. The animal exercised about 1 week later and was moving soundly. After 6 months, the animal is being shown with no signs of former problems.

23. *Equine, 5-year-old standardbred mare, trotter.* This mare had a chronic thoracolumbar myositis lasting 6 months. The back muscles had been injected with Sarapin® and steroids a number of times and later with an internal blister, all to no permanent relief. Treatment: 10 bladder points on the back where the points were sore, starting from the B21 clear back to B31 (Figs. 3–13 to 3–18), five needles were inserted in points and stimulated strongly (sedation) with a DC stimulator from Japan to cause a rippling effect on the muscles. This was done for 3 min, and the five posterior points were then done in the same way. I repeated the procedure on the opposite side. This mare was so sore before treatment that you could run your hand with slight pressure down the back longissimus dorsi muscle and the mare would nearly drop to the ground. Ten minutes after treatment, I could not make the mare flinch. She raced 2 days later and finished third in her best time of the year. In fact, she had been making breaks for the last five races.

24. *Equine, 8-year-old standardbred, gelding.* This horse was diagnosed as having navicular disease. Radiographically, nerve blocks and hoof testers substantiated this diagnosis. The horse had been lame for 2 months. I used the three points around the coronary band. 1. In front and anterior medial and lateral points. 2. HT6 (Figs. 3–13 to 3–18) or point at area where navicular bursa is blocked. 3. The two points above the bulbs of the heels. After the first treatment, the horse was definitely improved and trained 3 days later very well. I have treated this horse several times, usually 1–2 days before every race. Treatment appears to relieve the pain dramatically for 4–7 days. Lameness then recurs.

25. *Equine, 7-year-old quarter horse type mare.* Very muscular, heavy body, 1300 lb, and small feet. This mare became crippled with laminitis in both front feet 3 years before present treatment. Gross rotation of the 3rd phalanx occurred at that time with resultant dropped sole. Conscientious corrective trimming and shoeing had achieved near-normal alignment of the 3rd phalanx with the hoof wall after 3 years. However, radiographically, a pedal osteitis existed on the cranial surface of the coffin bone. The heels were contracted and thrushy, and the toes were seedy. The digital pulse was continuously very strong, and the mare was grossly lame at a walk and very reluctant to trot. High levels of Butazolidin had previously been used without successfully achieving a functionally sound animal. In addition to the laminitis, the mare had a history of navicular arthritis. The entire surface of the foot was sensitive when examined with the hoof testers.

Acupuncture therapy was begun using points for treating laminitis. The Acuflex dual model CZ 110 was used for electrical stimulation. Modulation setting was at 100, rate setting at 100 Hz, voltage setting between 7.5 and 10 (depending on the mare's level of discomfort). I use a total of 16 leads at one time; the meter indicates approximately 5–10 microamps.

Treatment was given daily except on weekends for 2 weeks. The mare was not exercised during this time. No improvement was noticed until after the sixth treatment. She was still lame in both front feet but not as reluctant to move out. By the 10th treatment, she was completely sound in the left front, but pain persisted in the right front and was manifested by a nodding head lameness. After the first 2 weeks, the mare was treated once or twice a week. Light riding exercise was provided thereafter to get the mare off the cement floors of the stall. After the third week, the mare was still lame in the right front and a lameness re-evaluation was made. One cubic centimeter of 2% lidocaine was deposited over the posterior digital nerve at the level of the apex of the collateral cartilage of the third phalanx. This enabled the mare to travel 100% sound. Treatments thereafter included additional points for navicular arthritis. Within another 2 weeks, the mare was completely sound. The digital pulse had even subsided in its intensity. Two weeks later, the mare was at the Quarter Horse Congress and took 2nd Place in the Amateur Western Pleasure and 3rd in the Senior Western Pleasure Classes. In two shows, she has qualified to go to the World Finals in Kentucky.

Points used: The points used don't exactly correspond to the charted points but may be the same—(Figs. 3–13 to 3–18) HT6, both feet; BL14, both sides; LI7, both sides; medical—HC4, LU6, HC3, LU8, LU5, and LU2; lateral—HT7, SI1, SI2, LI1, SI3, TH3, and LI5.

26. *Porcine, Duroc 450-lb boar, herd sire*. This boar hog had been down in his loins approximately 1 week. The owner had applied poultices and other decongestants to the loin area, but he still continued to lie on the ham and drag himself around with his legs extended behind him. I placed a snare on his nose and used an 18-gauge, ½ in. needle on a 12-cc syringe. I administered 2 cc of vitamin B₁ solution, 100 mg/cc posterior to the transverse processes bilaterally. I instructed the owner to report the following Monday. I failed to hear from her on Monday, but she returned to my office on Tuesday. She stated that the hog was up on his feet the next day and on Sunday was chasing around the paddock looking for food, and he served a sow on the 29th. No further treatment was administered other than the injection of the vitamin B₁ solution into the bladder meridian points B21, B22, B23, B24, and B25. I am confident that if I had not used the vitamin B₁ solution, camphorated oil injected 1 cc in each site would have done equally as well. This is very gratifying in that in years gone by I have seen farmers take such animals to the packing house and dispose of them for tankage. They have always regarded such cases as a total loss. In this case, acupuncture works fast and very effectively.

SMALL ANIMALS

Quotations

1. "My acupuncture treatment [for sudden paralysis in the dachshund] is quite simple and consists of inserting silver needles into the painful or sensitive paravertebral points that belong to the bladder meridian. I also puncture the two points LIV2 and LIV3 with silver needles to influence the muscles and the vessel stricture. As compensation, I puncture B60 with a gold needle. In certain cases, this point is replaced by B58 or B67; for instance, if the sick animal starts to walk again, but still drags its hind paw.

"If I don't see an improvement after three treatments, I chose the "wonder vessel", either Conception Vessel or Governing Vessel if pain and spasms exist, with the following points: TB5 (gold needle), GB41 (silver needle), B60 (gold needle), SI3. Of course, you can only expect success in vago-sympa-

thetic tonus disturbances, but not in spinal cord compressions or infections. I also would like to point to paralyses in dogs caused by age that are punctured according to Dr. de la Fuye in the paralysis points with a gold needle. The point combination is: GV19, GB34, GB37.

"I often also had failures, in part because my knowledge of acupuncture was not good, in part because of irreparable damage, especially when concerning the central nervous system. There are still a lot of unclear questions in the field of veterinary acupuncture."[17]

2. "In my practice, I have often come across cases of apparent myalgia in dogs, which is a well-known malady to all doctors. I will now discuss such a case:

"The dog was standing on the examination table, and for purposes of general examination and anamnesis, the dog was touched very slightly with a very thin needle . . . on the skin in the areas near the neck, the shoulder and the back, the muscle region in question was readily identifiable because of the more or less strong contractions in the cutaneous muscles. This zone is then touched with another needle in the same way, thus determining the Locus dolendi. It is in that place that the steel needle is then inserted, all the way up to the grip or the finger, where, according to the muscle mass, it can remain inserted anywhere from a few seconds up to a few minutes.

"After completing this first phase (treatment of hyperalgetic skin points), we then have to look for the proper "bladder points", which are located on the sides of the vertebral column, and which must be transferred mentally from the illustrations from a textbook on human anatomy onto the animal's body.

"For the most part, we can treat corresponding body parts wherever Loci dolendi are found on animals and humans in much the same way. . . .

"Well over one hundred dogs have been treated in this way, and there have been very few relapses.

"By using the above-described acupuncture treatment, the length of treatment was able to be drastically reduced—in most cases, only one session was necessary. If, after this treatment, there is no significant change in the sick animal's condition, then a re-examination of the diagnosis would be advisable."[12]

3. "On April 14, 1955, a five-year old boxer was sent to me by the Surgery Department of the Veterinary School of Alfort, suffering from osteoarthritis of the right knee joint. It had been treated for three months the usual way without success. The report showed a

deformed puffed up swelling in the affected knee, and walking was almost impossible. I used a point combination that Mr. de la Fuye had advised me for cases of that kind: LIV9 (gold needle). The dog has to be kept standing, another position immediately changes the topography because of the extreme flexibility of the skin. This golden needle is combined with a puncture on GB34 with a silver needle. B60 is combined with a puncture on K2 with a silver needle.

"The dog was presented again on April 21, and there was an obvious improvement in standing and in walking. The deformity of the knee remained, but the functional disturbance was resolved by four treatments. . . .

"An 8-year-old spaniel had a sudden attack of lumbago because of cold weather. Examination revealed a very painful and pressure-sensitive point that corresponds to Triple Burner 15. In the lumbar region, two painful pressure points could be palpated that were punctured with two silver needles.

"TB15 was punctured with a gold needle.

"The silver needles, 2 centimeters deep, stayed for 5 minutes, the gold needles for 10. After removal of the needles, the dog was able to walk, and the next day, his signs were gone.

"Acupuncture is a method for cure that every veterinarian should know about, no matter whether he treats small or large animals. Acupuncture is of great value to him. Often it cures alone, or it makes treatment easier by combination with other methods, influencing the constitution. It would be desirable if needle treatment would become a common treatment in veterinary medicine."[16]

4. "One case concerned a five-year-old short-haired dachshund which had been suffering from bronchial asthma for three years. All medications and treatments had failed to alleviate the condition until it reached the point where the dog suffered daily attacks and would have surely ended up by being put to sleep. The owner, a former client, brought the dog to me for this condition.

"I selected the following points, piercing them with small, thin needles: K27, K26, GV1, B12, and B13. The dog was treated in this way at first twice a week, and then once a week with progressive recovery. Each time, the needles were inserted for about 10 minutes. In total, the treatment was given six times. After this, since the dog did not have another attack, and since the attacks had been occurring on a daily basis before treatment, the acupuncture was con-

sidered successful. And, in support of this, according to the dog's owner, the animal has been free of all trouble since the acupuncture."[6]

5. "I can now also report about the success of acupuncture with dogs with cases of catarrh or sinusitis (SI3, LI4, LI20, B2, B10, LU19, 23a (P.d.M), ST10, ST40, GV23), of lumbago (local "Ju-" and LU-points, eventually combining with a B54 and B60), of the syndrome which occurs in the cervical segment of the vertebral column (local points on the bladder meridian, TB15, LU13, etc.), of gingivitis (SI3, LI4, LI20, ST6–8, LU25, LU1, LIV13, for example), of bladder incontinence (B64, B65, SP5, SP6, SP9, K2, K6, K7, local GV-, ST- and K-points, as well as B31 and B28 for example), of stomach and intestinal afflictions (GV15, GV13, GV12, GV4, ST21, ST25, L13, LI4, SP4, for example), of thunder nerves, which are caused in dogs by explosions and thunder, etc. (LU19, GB20, B10, GB3, B13, GV15, for example). Naturally, not all points are pierced at the same time. In general, I have had no trouble inserting needles in dogs. In most cases, the needles only fall out when a dog is unruly or will not stand or lie still for a few minutes. In these instances, the needles have to be re-inserted until the animal remains calm enough so that they do not fall out."[7]

6. "All together, I treated 150 animals, mostly dogs. Of 150 observations, I finally decided to report on 86, since the rest of them after a closer look had to be eliminated because of an unclear diagnosis, other therapeutic treatments, or because of self-cure. Among these 86 cases, 35 showed a very good result, 30 were medium successful, and 31 without success.

"Treating 17 arthropathies, I achieved very good results in 7 cases, good results in 3, and failures in 7. Some of them were very unclear in their etiology; others showed a strong blockage; others, because of tumors, were not likely to be successful. . . .

"Acupuncture is very good in treating pain, neuralgies, myalgies, and paralyses with some spectacular results. The etiology of the paralyses often is unclear and mostly slight arthrosis, sprain or myalgias. . . .

Lumbalgias were treated quite successfully. In 5 cases, improvement occurred immediately after acupuncture treatment.

"There are still a lot of trials and observations necessary to decide on the topography of the Chinese points. Up to date, I transferred human topography to the animal and often the transfer was extremely difficult or even impossible especially for the distal extremities. A lot of points that are important in man proved worthless in the animal. That is also the reason why I don't mention any of the points used by me. I only would be able to mention the points along the spine and especially in the lumbar and sacral regions that seem to me to be of great importance in pain and lumbalgias in these areas; also in neuralgias of the hind extremities and in paralyses.

"I don't want to make a precise statement of the points as it also could be an effective zone and not just one single point."[14]

7. "We have applied acupuncture to residual coughing in canine filariasis, modeling current acupuncturists' treatment of cardiac asthma by acupuncturing ST9 (Jen Ying) and CV22 (Tien Tu). Instances of such acupuncture are few, but their effects are apparent; the following is a report on these instances, and it is hoped that the readers will follow up on them with further experiments. Case No. 1: A six-year-old cross-bred male underwent trimelarsan treatment for filariasis, residual coughing persisted despite the administration of various drugs, coughing eased after acupuncture of Stomach 9 and Conception Vessel 22, coughing stopped upon a second acupuncture session administered seven days after the first; one and a half years have since passed, without any recurrence of coughing. Case No. 3: A five-year-old female underwent three acupuncture sessions at one-day intervals; coughing ceased with no further changes for the next ten months. Case No. 4: A five-year-old female underwent four acupuncture sessions at one-day intervals; as in Case No. 3, coughing stopped without recurrence in the ten months that has since passed."[20]

Case Reports

These are some of the case reports submitted to the International Veterinary Acupuncture Society by members of that society and distributed in the newsletter of the society.

Convulsive Diseases

1. *Canine, 5-year-old female Irish Setter.* Had her first epileptic seizure in December 1975; Rx: Dilantin®, 1½ gr TID. 12/2/75: Convulsions increasing; acupuncture with steel beads; points treated were GV-20, GB13, 15, TH18, and SP16. 2/17/75: Had another convulsion, patient had not had any convulsions since treatment 12/2/74; repeated treatment with more steel beads. Points used were GV20, GB13, 15, TH18, and SP16. 3/28/75: Had another convulsion, very

mild. Got very upset and nervous for about 45 min. She has had no convulsions since 2/17/75. 6/5/75: The owner reported that the dog's convulsions since her first acupuncture treatment had been very mild and also that her disposition was much better.

2. *Canine, 3-year-old white female Poodle.* 11/14/74: Patient was having epileptic seizures three or four times daily. Had been on Dilantin®, 1½ gr. BID, for several years. 11/14/74: Acupuncture with steel beads; points used were GV20, GC13, GC15, TH18, and SP16. 6/5/75: Owner reports dog's seizures are very mild, about one every 3 days. Still on Dilantin® 1½ gr. BID.

3. *Canine, 6-year-old male Welsh Corgi.* Grand mal seizures started on September 1973 with increasing frequency. In spite of increased doses of Primidone® then Phelantin®, Dilantin® and phenobarbital and Valium®, seizures occurred every 2–3 weeks. Seizures were sustained, and control was effected only after IV pentobarbital sodium. Implantation of steel beads was done on May 5, 1975, at GV20, GB13, GB15, TH18, and SP16. Dog was taken off all medication. Dog was normal until morning of May 18, when it came into hospital after many sustained seizures. Anesthetized with Nembutal®. X-rayed head to check the positions of beads; found two beads missing. Reimplanted missing beads. Dog has remained normal to 6/4/75.

4. *Feline, 4-year-old male Domestic Shorthair.* Incoordination and periodic spastic seizures since owners have owned cat. Cat was on Mebroin®, which reduced the spastic seizures, but only when the cat was doped up by the pills. Acupuncture treatment was granted by the owners, and injection with camphorated oil was done on the following points: LI4, B54, GV20, GV15, and GB20. The treatment was performed under Surital anesthesia. The cat had several seizures during the following week and then had none for more than 1 month.

5. *Canine, 8-week-old female Poodle.* One week after my partner's sister-in-law bought a new puppy, it came down with distemper. In 2 weeks, the puppy was having 4–7 grand mal seizures daily, and a request for euthanasia was made. Permission was granted to try acupuncture and injection with 1 minim of camphorated oil was performed on the following points: LI4, B54, GV20, GB7, and 20 bilaterally. The dog was under Surital anesthesia and whimpered and jerked when each point was injected.

One day later the dog had three convulsions, and the second day had one convulsion. Since then, the dog has had no more seizures to anyone's knowledge.

6. *Canine, 8-year-old female Poodle.* Epilepsy uncontrolled with medication. Versa Clips® implanted in GB20, GV8, GV9, GV10, and GV20. All medication removed. Convulsions after 10 days; therefore, placed on 100 mg Dilantin®, which controlled seizures without oversedation. Without acupuncture the medication was not successful.

7. *Canine, 8-week-old male Mixed Cocker.* The dog was presented to the hospital with a temperature of 104. Eyes and nose were runny, and dog was not eating. Dog was having a typical chewing-gum fit when presented. In addition to distemper, the dog also had hookworm. The dog was given DNP® for the worms and antibiotics and supportive therapy including Primidone® for the distemper. After 4 days' treatment, the patient was much better and eating, but still was having repeated chewing-gum fits. On the 5th day, we started acupuncture treatments. The dog was only observed to have two additional light fits after the first treatment with acupuncture. We used points GB13, 14, 15; B1, 20, 67; LI4; GV1, 20, and 27. In all cases, we treated each of the points for 7 sec each day. We used a needle injector attached to our LC/ Meter® with the voltage set at 12 and the microamps at 200. The dog was treated on days 5, 6, 7, and 10 with acupuncture and released. Forty-five days later, the owner reported the dog normal with no seizures at home since released.

8. *Canine, 5-year-old male Poodle.* Treated 3 years for epileptic seizures. Convulsions were never stopped but were semicontrolled with Dilantin® and Primidone®. Although dog was being given maximum daily dosage, it began to have continuous seizures and was presented for euthanasia. The dog was anesthetized and Versa Clips® were inserted through a stab incision at points bilateral GB20, GV20, GV8, GV9, GV10; CV14, CV15, CV17. Dog was taken off all medication, and seizure-free for 2 weeks, at which time a "mild" seizure was observed. The dog was readmitted, and a Versa Clip® was inserted unilaterally on the left side at GB30 and ST36. The dog has remained seizure-free for 1 month. Another veterinarian briefly mentioned that in one of his cases he used points GV20, GV21, GV22, GV23, GV24, and GB13, GB14, GB15, and GB2. The effects of acupuncture lead to reduction in the dosage of medication for epileptiform seizures rather than being successful as the sole treatment modality.

9. *Canine, 8-year-old female Samoyed.* Dog presented on 2/6/75 with postdistemper chorea, which had rendered the dog immobile for 1½ years. Owners had been carrying the dog in and out of the house and caring for it as a total invalid. Prognosis of this case was considered impossible; but at the owners' insistence acupuncture therapy was initiated. Dog was hospitalized until 2/13. Treatment was given daily with Acustat 2® at 150 V., the frequency exceeding the chorea pattern. B54, ST36, GB20, and B25 were used bilaterally, as well as LI4, GV20, and GV4. Dog treated on 3/6/75. Was attempting to stand. Now capable of maintaining a sitting position. Dog hospitalized on 3/13 and treated every 3rd day. On 3/28/75 dog was dismissed, walking, a slight tremor still persisted in temporal area, but limbs were chorea-free.

10. *Canine, 6-year-old female Beagle.* Postdistemper convulsions and chorea. 5/23/75: Owner reported convulsion-like activities, and a twitch in the right front leg. She was sent home on Myelepsin® tablets (one a day). For the next 4 years, she had numerous convulsions in spite of Myelepsin® and later Dilantin®. Sometimes a combination of both was given. The convulsive activity was never completely suppressed. 4/2/75: Versa Clip® implants were made at GB20, GB21 and GV23, GV21, GV13, and the animal was taken off medication. 4/16/75: No convulsions and owner reported the twitch that had been in the right front leg for 4 years was gone. 4/21/75: Had a mild convulsion (2 min), according to owner. 5/7/75: Doing fine. 5/20/75: Had a series of severe convulsions, nature according to owner. At this time it is impossible to evaluate the long-range effects of metal implants on this animal. It is hoped that if they do not completely eliminate the convulsions, they will at lease modify and soften their severity.

11. *Canine, 2-year-old male Norwegian elkhound.* Grand mal convulsions of unknown origin. 12/18/75: Owner reported one convulsion. The dog appeared normal. 4/10/75: Owner reported a series of convulsions. 4/11/75: Acupuncture surgery was undertaken and implants of Versa Clips® were made subcutaneously at GB20, GB21, and GB13. 4/14/75: The dog exhibited slight frothing at the mouth, and was hyperkinetic and very hungry. 5/31/75: The animal has been free of symptoms to date. Although it is too early to draw conclusions, it looks as though metal implants over the proper acupuncture points will modify or eliminate convulsive activity.

12. *Canine, 5-year-old male Mixed Breed.* 3/24/75: Dog treated for epilepsy but it could not be controlled. Acupuncture therapy decided upon with consent of owner. Dog was on 3 Primidone® daily, but did not stop epileptiform seizures. Versa Clips® implanted at GV20, GV21, GV22, GV23, GV24; GB13, GB14, GB15; and X2. Medication was slowly withdrawn over a 5-day period and no convulsions have occurred since that time. 4/20/75: Convulsing again; had to put dog on Primidone®, 3/day. Primidone® therapy now controls seizures whereas prior to Versa Clip® implantation this dosage was ineffective.

13. *Canine, 4-year-old male Poodle.* Dog had history of epileptic seizures; started about 2 years ago. Spells were controlled by Dilantin® and phenobarbital for about 1½ years. Seizures recurred, and other anticonvulsants were ineffective. Gomenol® was injected at suggested points, B5–10, GB13, GB14, and GB15. Seizures appeared to be stopped for about 1 week, but recurred. Insistence on euthanasia; no conclusion determined in this case.

14. *Canine, 8-year-old female Mixed Dachshund.* Brought to our clinic March 28, 1975, convulsing approximately every hour with complete unawareness of surroundings. History of convulsing for 2 years, and had been on Mebroin® medication. 3/28/75: Versa-Clips® inserted into GB13, GB15, and GB20 bilaterally under general anesthesia. 3/29/75: No convulsions, but not completely aware of surroundings. 3/30/75: Dog acted perfectly normal and was discharged. 4/2/75: Dog readmitted to hospital with slight convulsions. Versa Clips® inserted into GB34 bilaterally and CV15. Died the next day. Autopsy revealed brain tumor lateral to right ventricle.

15. *Canine, 3-month-old male Basset Hound.* Distemper leading to chorea and posterior paresis. September 25, 1975: The pup presented for treatment. He had bloody diarrhea, pus from a crusted nose, purulent conjunctivitis, increased vesicular sounds over the lung field, fever, and cough. He had been adopted from an animal shelter almost 2 weeks previously and had had no vaccinations. Distemper was diagnosed. He received an injection of Flocillin®, prednisolone, and B vitamins with iron. He went home on Entrocalm® and Tetrachel® (weight, 9 lb). October 15, 1975: Dog came in with chorea of the ears and shoulders, first noted 3 days earlier. Novin® tablets were dispensed for the patient. A prognosis

of "very poor" was given when the signs became worse (weight, 12 lb). October 22, 1975: Dog presented for euthanasia because his condition had worsened; he could no longer walk because of complete posterior paresis. Euthanasia was delayed, and I implanted Hemoclips® under the skin at GV20, and bilaterally at TH18, SP16, and in the GB13–15 area. The clips had been autoclaved, the sites clipped and disinfected. Incision was made through the skin with a hooked-blade scapel, and the clips inserted. One stainless-steel suture was needed at SP 16. October 23, 1975: The dog ran and played about the hospital. He was normal to all outward appearances.

16. *Canine, 6-month-old female Doberman.* The dog contracted distemper 11 weeks before presentation and had been treated for distemper. However, the owner elected not to complete the course of treatment for the dog, and the dog in the meantime changed ownership. The diagnosis was based on the history and clinical signs and a report of the symptoms occurring just subsequent to the distemper infection and persisting since that time. Treatment was by acupuncture, and the only medication was the initial antibiotic B-complex therapy. The dog's diet was improved and the owner instructed in the use of a general physiotherapeutic regimen.

Acupuncture needling techniques and electroacupuncture were the main methods of treatment. The following points were used: GV20, LI4 bilateral, LIV3 bilateral, ST40, and GB34 (both unilateral and alternated at subsequent visits). Needles were left in place 15–30 min and turned periodically. The needles were removed when they became loose in the tissues and frequently some of them fell out after 20 min.

The dog was treated twice a week. In the second week of treatment, GV20 was treated by direct current using the positive pole of the Neurometer® for 10 sec (6 volts and 200 milliamps). After 2 weeks for no particular reason other than intuition, GV20 alone was used for 3 further weeks on a once weekly/twice weekly alternating schedule. A tei shin was used on the bladder meridian on each treatment session. Four days after treatment, the owner reported definite improvement. This was confirmed on the third visit. The dog was stronger, though still uncoordinated, more alert, and less depressed. She could walk 10–12 steps and go up 2–3 steps on a staircase without falling. She'd invariably fall on turns and when trying to trot.

Eight days after treatment, improvement was marked. The dog could walk and run without falling except on sharp turns. She could take four ascending staircase steps, but could not descend. She was just about normally alert to surroundings, but still appeared to be deaf. The right ear remained dropped. The dog was somewhat restless initially on treatment, but consistently became relaxed and contented during treatment.

In the fourth week of therapy, an approach was taken to treat the paralyzed right ear and deafness. It appeared from the animal's behavior that she had some hearing to higher pitched sounds in the left ear. Acupuncture loci in the neighborhood of the ear were treated concurrently with the aforementioned points. The following additional points were used: TH21, SI19, and GB2. Ten days later, the owner thought her hearing was improved, but this became apparent only on examination 2 weeks later.

Three weeks later, the dog's hearing appeared to have returned. Also overnight, toward the end of the third week, the dog's right ear returned to the erect position. This appears to be a case in which acupuncture can be conjectured to have had some beneficial effects given the long-standing history of symptoms that had shown no change until therapy was begun.

17. *Canine, 3½-year-old male Pomeranian.* Epilepsy. Versa Clips® were implanted in the following: GV20, GV21, GV8, GV9, GV10, and GB20. All medication was removed. Dog had one convulsion on the tenth day after implantation. Was put back on medication for 2 weeks. Since, has had no convulsions and no medication. Before acupuncture, 300 mg/day would not control the seizures.

Spinal Cord Diseases

1. *Canine, 6-year-old female Beagle.* March 13, 1975: referred in front leg rigidity, total absence of rear sensory or motor toe pad reflex. Rear legs extended under dog stiff and rigid. No bladder or bowel control. Radiograph indicated disc lesions at T12, T13, L1, and L2. Dog had been paraplegic 4 weeks and had been given steroids and Butazolidin®. Hospitalized. Needles were used in pad points and ST36, BL54 bilaterally. Ultrasound was used along course of bladder meridian including all association points. Toe pinch was evident after second treatment. Treatment every other day. Bladder control reestablished after 8th treatment. CV1 was used along with aforementioned points to avoid necessity of giving enema. Bowel control established after 12th treatment. Dog walked and was dismissed on 5/5/75. Gait was

stilted, but improvement in locomotion has continued without further treatment.

2. *Canine, 5-year-old male German Shepherd.* Day 1: Posterior paralysis, hindlegs in extension. Animal was given Butazolidin® IV and taken in the hospital for radiographs and compartment rest. The radiographs were negative. Day 3: Acupuncture treatments were started on the governing vessel, between the lumbar vertebrae 1–2, 2–3, 3–4, and 4–5. These treatments were carried out daily, inserting the needles at 90-degree angles and leaving them in for 15-min intervals. Day 6: There had been no change in the animal, so a new treatment was instituted. All rear toe pad points and the tail point were punctured for 15-min periods, once a day at 90-degree angles until Day 12 with no results. Day 13: The animal was sent to the University, where he was destroyed. Postmortem diagnosis: degenerative myelopathy. To date, degenerative myelopathy has not responded to any form of treatment. In this case, acupuncture also failed, as administered by my hands.

3. *Canine, 9-year-old female Mixed Breed.* Day 1: Examination. Pronounced arching of back, crying, restlessness, slight posterior ataxia more pronounced in left rear leg. A tentative diagnosis of IV disc syndrome was made and radiographs scheduled for the next morning. Day 2: The dog's condition had progressed to posterior paralysis with complete loss of voluntary motor control in rear legs and bladder function but retention of sensory or cortical reflexes. Radiographs revealed calcification of all lumbar and more than 50% of thoracic discs. Treatment: 10 cc mannitol IV, OD; 2 cc Flucort® IV, OD; 1½ cc Butazolidin® IV, BID; 0.5 cc Acepromazine® IV, OD. Day 3: No change in motor control and bladder function. Sensory or cortical reflexes extremely depressed. Treatment: 1 cc Butazolidin® IV, OD; 1 cc Depo-Medrol® IM. Acupuncture therapy begun: Needling only (stainless steel), rapid turning of the needles, 15 min. Points used: B67, B54, B23, B25, B11, GV6 tail point, and KL1 bilateral. Day 4: No apparent change in condition; treatment repeated. Day 5: Patient able to stand. Bladder function improved. No further treatment. Day 9: Patient walking well. The value of acupuncture in this case is questionable because many such cases respond in similar manner without acupuncture therapy.

4. *Canine, 6-year-old spayed female Dachshund.* 5/28/75: Couldn't walk on back legs, right front paw

turning in. Symptoms were present on a previous occasion with other front leg affected. Tentative diagnosis: disc syndrome. Radiographic examination disclosed spondylosis deformans, and the animal was referred for acupuncture. Electroacupuncture treatment at 200 cycles AC. Trigger points were selected along the bladder meridian every other day for three treatments. The animal began walking after the second treatment, and results were considered excellent.

5. *Canine, 4-year-old female Mixed Breed.* Intervertebral disc lesion in the dog. The dog stood with its back arched and ears disinclined to move. She occasionally cried out when handled. She was paraplegic and showed a flaccid type paralysis dragging the hindleg. The muscle tone, reflexes, and sensation were all greatly diminished, although the dog retained control of defecation and urination. The pedal reflex was present, but appeared to be due to the local neural arc response, as there appeared to be no perception of sensation. The symptoms began with sudden onset 2 weeks before examination.

Diagnosis was based on the history and clinical features and was confirmed by radiologic examination. The lateral radiograph of the vertebral column indicated the presence of a disc lesion by the narrowing of intervertebral space between vertebrae L2 and L3. Also, there was a shadow in the intervertebral foramen. A guarded prognosis was given.

This case was treated by acupuncture alone and no medication was given. The dog was treated twice a week for 5 weeks using a sedating needling technique at the following points. The needles were inserted and left in place 30–40 min after initial insertion and rapid turning for 1 min. Acupuncture loci: GV4, B23 bilateral, B25 bilateral, B54, B67, ST36, and tail point.

During the first treatment, there was reflex response that involved the animal's perception on needling, but only for the right leg. This involved exaggerated flexing of the leg. The tail was also flaccid until the third treatment. Then, for a short period after needling of the special loci at the extremity of the tail, this resulted in 15 sec or so of tail wagging. The left hindleg showed slight flexing on needling BL67 and ST36 on the 6th day of treatment. After 2 weeks, the dog could stand for longer and longer periods. After 2½ weeks, the left hindleg made better progress, while the right hindleg seemed to regress. However, at 3½ weeks, the dog began to use the right hindleg in a willful, but uncoordinated manner. This was followed a week later by similar improvement in the left hindleg. The dog made gradual improvement for the next 2 weeks, and returned to

normal at the end of 5 weeks with no recurrence 6 weeks later.

Additional therapy included attempts at spinal adjustment during the second and fifth visits to remove any possible vertebral subluxation, and on each occasion a te shin was used on the bladder meridian from the cervical vertebrae to the sacrum bilaterally. In addition, the caretaker of the animal was instructed in massage techniques of the back and hindlegs to be done as often as time allowed. Although lumbar disc lesions followed by paraplegia require a guarded prognosis, some of these cases completely recover. One cannot say if acupuncture helped this case; recovery could have been spontaneous.

6. *Canine, 18-month-old female Dalmation.* Admitted on Day 1 after being hit by a truck. Signs on admittance: severe pain, shock, and paralysis. X-rays of spine showed no apparent findings. X-rays of hip showed a fracture of the ilium. Days 2–21: bowel and bladder incontinence. Paralysis was flaccid from the lumbar region posterior to the end of the tail. The animal could move its front legs involuntarily, but with no coordination of strength. It could lift its head to eat and drink. Initial therapy included antibiotics, steroids, physical therapy baths, and extensive massage. All to no avail.

Acupuncture therapy was initiated on Day 22. First treatment used the following points: GV4, bilateral B23, B24, ST36, and BL54. All pad points were bled. Pain points were not known, but bilateral near BL36 and BL38 points were used. All pain points: stimulation of sedation by twirling for 15–20 min. Pad points stimulated by tonification: quickly pricked deep and "woodpeckered"; then needles removed and bled. Three hours after acupuncture, the animal could support herself on her front legs.

Second acupuncture treatment: Same points and techniques used for 2nd treatment on Day 23, as in 1st treatment. The morning after the 2nd treatment (Day 24), the animal was found standing in her stall on all four feet. The back feet knuckled over, but she was up. Day 24–Day 30: No acupuncture given, but physical therapy continued with massage. Three times daily, the dog was taken on a forced walk, being supported by an assistant holding the dog's tail. Daily improvement in coordination was noted, and control of bowels slowly returned to normal control.

The dog was released to its owners' care during the 1st week of the next month for 2 weeks. She was still knuckling, and her owner was advised to wrap the back feet for protection. The dog returned and received two additional treatments. Pad points were used and bled. Points ST45 and B67 bilateral were tonified. Seven months later, the dog is perfectly normal and shows no lack of coordination or paralysis.

7. *Canine, 8-year-old male Miniature Schnauzer.* Ankylosing spondylitis of spine at L1 and L2 with spinal fusion in this area. I have been treating this dog for 2 years with steroids and Butazolidin® with only minimal relief. Dog is in pain on arising, drags back legs, and refuses to climb stairs. Dog admitted Monday–Friday for 3 weeks and treated three times each week. Points used for therapy: GV3, and GV4; bilaterally B23, B21, B54, and B47; also any sore points along spine in area of L1 and L2. Dog treated nine times using these points. Treatments 1–3: The needles in GV3, GV4, B23, and B21 were twirled fast and left in 30–40 min. The needles in B54 and B47 were twirled slowly and left in 10 min. Treatments 4–9: The same points were used and for approximately the same time as in the first three treatments, but moxibustion was used instead of needle manipulation. Moxa was applied until a response was observed. Moxa was used three times at GV3, GV4, B23, and B21. Moxa was used once at B54 and B47.

The dog improved after the first treatment and continued to improve with each succeeding treatment until he moved with ease. There was no evidence of the rear leg dragging, and pain was exhibited only when firmly palpated. I have given this dog one booster treatment 3 weeks after initial therapy, and so far he has been doing very well for 8 weeks.

8. *Canine, 3-year-old Dachshund.* Thoracolumbar disc. 2/27/75: Posterior paresis, anal reflex, and toe-pinch reflex. 3/3/75: Same; Rx–Azium®. 3/12/75: Dog lays in urine and stool. Weaker anal reflex. Extensor thrust reflex is medium. 3/14/75: Acupuncture treatment using GV4 and GV1, B23, B54, and K1. 3/15/75: GV4 and GV1, B23, 54, K1, and ST36. Good reaction to B23 and ST36 on left side. 3/17/75: GV4 and GV1, B11, B23, S36, and K1. Edema in hocks. 3/18/75: GV4 and GV1, B23, B67, GV54 (L), S36, and K1. Edema worse. Paresis worse. 3/22/75: GV1, B67, B30, B25, B23, B20, B17. Defecation as soon as removed needle from GV1. Edema gone. 3/26/75: A.M., GV4, GV13, B23, B11, B30 (R), and B62 (R). P.M., injected B-complex into SI3 bilaterally. Injected camphorated oil into B62 bilaterally. 4/7/75: More tone in rear legs. Trying to stand. Injected water into SI3 (R), B62 (R), and B11 (R). 4/15/75: Dog was able to pull up on rear legs. Trying to walk a couple of steps. Euthanasia. The dog never had any

pain from the disc and never had any sores on her hocks or posterior hips from being in the concrete runs all day. Control of urination and defecation was very good after acupuncture treatments were started.

9. *Canine, 4½-year-old female Dachshund.* Prolapsed disc, diagnosed by physical examination and X-ray. Since Day 1, no pain perception nor any reflexes in hindlegs. Only slight pain perception in forelegs. No anal sphincter reflex. Day 5: Dog in intense pain. Rx inserted and left needles in approximately 3 hours; used bilaterally BL23–25 and LI4; all hind toe pads right ST36. Day 7: Slight pain perception in hindlegs. Fifty per cent pain perception in front legs; dog in less pain. Rx same as 5/12/75. Day 9: Owner reports dog much better. Dog trying to erect itself, no longer in any pain. Pain perception in front legs was normal. Rx needles inserted in right: ST41, GB43, and ST36. Bilaterally B10, B23, B23, B25, and B28. Right BL67, GB43, and ST41. Day 16: Rx needles inserted and left in approximately 5 hours or until they slipped out. Bilaterally B10, B13, B23, B25, B28, B54, and B67 plus metacarpal pads. Left ST36, ST36, ST41, and GB43. Day 20: Dog able to walk on forelegs when hind end is supported, otherwise no change. RX needles inserted and left until they slipped out, or 6 hours. Bilaterally BL10, B13, B23, B25, B28, B54, and B67. Left ST36, ST41, and SP2. Day 21: Dog starting to drag herself with her forelegs. Rx same as Day 20. The dog has had a great improvement concerning the forelegs, but no improvement in the hindlegs.

10. *Canine, 5½-year-old male Collie.* 5/7/75: Presented down in rear, unable to stand, first day noticed. Dog had rough hair coat, was very thin, and had slightly pale mucous membrane. Fecal exam revealed hookworm ova; general exam revealed fleas. Temp., 102.6. Treatment: DNP® and Vermiplex®, Azium®, B-complex, flea spray, tetracycline, and Seletoc® capsule. 5/8/75: Dog still unable to rise, falls down immediately when released if propped up. Radiograph of pelvis: old (healed) fracture of ischium and mild dysplasia. The lumbar spine was normal. Medication: Azium® tablets. Seletoc® capsule, tetracycline.

Treatment: Multivitamin tablet, calcium and vitamin D tablet, Geri-Care® tablets, tetracycline. 5/10/75: Animal unimproved. Treatment as on 5/9/75. 5/11/75: Animal unimproved. Treatment as on 5/9/75. 5/12/75: Animal unimproved. Treatment: Acupuncture and moxibustion, using GB33, GB34, B23, B54, and ST36, all bilaterally. GV4, GV26. Animal able to stand on all four legs (when propped up) for approximately 3–5 sec immediately after treatment. Medication: tetracycline, Seletoc®, Geri-Care®, multivitamins. 5/13/75: Animal sitting up but unable to rise. Can stand for up to 10 min; walked around very slowly, stiffly, and hesitatingly, if propped up. Severe ataxia noted; dog unable to negotiate turns through doorways without falling. Treatment: Acupuncture (no moxa) same as on 5/12/75. Immediate improvement noted after acupuncture treatment. Animal walking faster with a freer gait; now able to negotiate turns. Dog allowed out in year, propped up and allowed to walk periodically. Medication: tetracycline, Geri-Care®, multivitamins.

5/14/75: Treatment, none. Medication: tetracycline, Geri-Care®, multivitamins. 5/15/75: Animal able to rise (slowly) unassisted from prone position. Moving loosely with a relatively free gait. Treatment: Acupuncture and moxibustion as previously. Dog seen moving around yard at a trot approximately 1 hour after treatment. P.M.: Dog sent home. Rx: multivitamins, Seletoc® every 3rd day. Four capsules total, flea spray. 5/19/75: Re-exam. Animal appears completely normal; chasing flying insects. 5/23/75: Presented for reworming, DNP®; animal remains normal.

11. *Canine, 4-year-old female Dachshund.* Day 1: Dog cried out in pain, reluctant to walk. Owner gave Azium® tablets. Better in 24 hours. Day 2: Dog unable to walk in PM after running and jumping in AM. X-ray: narrowed space at L1–2. Day 3: Injected 1 cc Seletoc® IM. Injected points with sterile water; B11, B20, and B21 (bilaterally), B54 (R), B67 (R), and S36 (R). Day 8: The dog was starting to use rear legs. Progressively got better over next 2 weeks.

12. *Canine, 4½-year-old male Dachshund.* April 9, 1975: No use of rear legs; paralyzed for 3 weeks showing no response with conventional treatment. Dog had a spinal operation at the University a year ago and recovered until present paralysis. 4/9/75: Point treated B23 right side, bilateral GB30, GB43, ST45, and LIV2. 4/12/75: No apparent response. Used same points as first treatment, adding pad point and tail point. 4/18/75: Dog could hold himself up if placed legs under him for a few seconds. Repeated same points as used on 4/12/75 plus moxa to needle at GV4. 4/25/75: Dog attempting to walk but staggering. No change in formula; all points used in #3. 5/4/75: Dog walking well and attempting to jump up. Treated B25, GB43, ST45, and LIV2. Told owner to bring back only if dog seemed to be slipping in-

stead of improving. 5/22/75: Left rear leg still slow in placing leg forward. Treated points B25 and ST36 bilateral using electrical impulse at 5 cps for 10 min. Progress evident; no further treatment needed.

13. *Canine, 4-year-old male Dachshund.* November 8, 1974: Complete posterior paralysis for 2 months. Legs flaccid and urinary incontinence. X-ray showed disc involvement at 11–12 thoracic vertebrae. No response in muscles to pinch but showed some evidence of pain. Acupuncture treatment: The following points used in treatment and changed slightly with each treatment and not all used at same time: all points bilateral B22, B23, B25, B27, B54, GB30, GB43, ST36, ST45, LIV2, pad points, and tail-stimulating points, GV4.

Treatment dates: November 8, 11, 14, 22, 27, 1974. December 4, 11, 18, 1974. January 3, 16, 23, 1975. February 5, 19. March 6, 20. April 2, 16. May 14, used electrical stimulator dense-dispersed for 10 min. Bilateral B23, ST36. On the eighth treatment, improvement in muscle tone was marked. On the tenth treatment, the dog could support his weight for a short time when legs placed under him, and able to control urine much better. The last time dog was treated was 5/14/75, and dog walking and running but with still some uncoordination, but muscles in back and legs have filled out and are back to normal size. The owners happy; they had the patience to keep going. At last treatment, I told them that I didn't think he would have to come back.

14. *Canine, 6-year-old male Miniature Schnauzer.* November 4, 1974: Dog in pain in region of 12th thoracic vertebra. Been down since 10/21/74. Getting worse under treatment at another hospital. X-ray had shown disc involvement in 11–12th thoracic intercostal space. Dog had so much pain that it had bitten owner when being brought in. 11/4/74: No sedative used. Treated trigger points on back corresponding to B14, B22, and B25 bilateral for 30 min. After needles were in 5 min, dog became calm and relaxed. When dog went home that evening, it could be picked up without snapping. This dog responded slowly. The following points were used in subsequent treatments but not all at one time: B22, B23, B25, B27, B54, GB30, GB43, ST36, ST45, LIV2, GV4, pad points, and tail-stimulating point. Moxa was used occasionally on B22, B23, B25, B27, GB30, and GV4. Treatment dates: November 7, 11, 14, 18, 21, 27, 1974; December 4, 11, 18, 1974; January 2, 1975; February 3, 25; March 3, 5, 10, 13, 20, 27; and

April 10. The first part there was a slight relapse, but responded quickly and after April 10, was released as was doing so well.

15. *Canine, male Basset.* This dog was a patient of a colleague, who referred dog to me with "hopeless" posterior paralysis. An x-ray revealed disc protrusion with calcification in L5-6-7. There was a sensitive response to the needle pricks from the atlas to this area. There was some tone in the bladder; however, he did some dribbling. Defecation was difficult. He moved himself around by dragging his legs behind him like a frog. Also the tail was paralyzed. The knee jerk was absent. Acupuncture was begun the first day at B23, B24, B48, B54, B60, and LI4. These points were treated 5 min with the Chinese electroacupuncture machine 71-1 at 15 cps each day. The muscles were severely atrophied, so we swam the dog in a figure eight in a tub of warm water each day after therapy. On the 6th day, we saw him reaching with his back leg as though he was trying to walk. On the 10th day, the dog was planting the left leg down as he walked and was drawing the right one forward and walking on the knuckle of the paw. The dribbling stopped after the 2nd treatment, and defecation was no trouble. We X-rayed again after the 10th treatment and the opaque discs had cleared. To date, we have treated 15 times, and the dog is able to ambulate in a simulated trot.

16. *Canine, 4-year-old female Pekingese.* 7/16/74: Admitted with severe pain due to back injury. X-rays showed a ruptured disc. Treatment was acupuncture with Gomenol®. Points used: GV4, bladder meridian. Released 7/19/74 in no pain. 1/4/74: Admitted with severe pain due to disc. Acupuncture treatment was repeated, and Gomenol® was used. Points used were GV4 and Bladder meridian. Released 11/4/74, PM. 4/18/75: Admitted with reinjured back. Treatment was repeated. Points used: GV4 and Bladder meridian (Gomenol®). Released 4/18/75 PM. June 5, 1975: The owner reports that since that time the dog is doing well and apparently has no pain.

Miscellaneous Diseases

1. *Canine, 7-year-old male Kerry Blue Terrier.* General pustular dermatitis, thickened skin, alopecia for more than 1 year. Treated elsewhere with usual baths, medicine, etc. Acupuncture and injected Gomenol® between all toes. Repeated in 1 week after three treatments; remarkable changes in skin; still under treatment.

2. *Canine, 4½-year-old male Doberman.* Severe diarrhea for 1 month, not responsive to Lomotil®, Kaopectate®, Neochal®, or Diathal®. Entered hospital, after seven negative stool analyses. Started acupuncture. BL25 bilateral, ST36, CV2, and ST25 left side. Repeated daily for 4 days. No bowel movement. for 4 days; on 5th day, normal formed movement. Discharged.

3. *Canine, 10-year-old female Dachshund.* Lipoma, right side of flank. Because animal was of placid disposition, used ST36 and GB34 for analgesia. Did not use electric stimulation but simply finger twirling; surgery was uneventful.

4. *Feline, 1½-year-old castrated male Domestic Shorthair.* Urinary lithiasis blocking penile urethra, on March 20, 1975, opened and flushed. Returned March 26, 1975, blocked again. Reopened and on antibiotics. Returned April 17, 1975; blocked again. May 7: blocked again, suggested acupuncture. Found B38 very sensitive, needled and injected Xylocaine®. May 14: found B38 and B40 or 41 sensitive, injected Xylocaine®. May 21: found B38 sensitive, needled and injected Xylocaine®. May 28: no sensitivity, needled and injected B38. Cat acting normal without medicine since start of acupuncture.

5. *Canine, 15-year-old spayed female Labrador.* After an apparent cerebral accident, the dog was able to walk with difficulty but was up on its toes with the front feet, and the large front foot pad was not touching the ground. Dog was also deaf for 6–9 months and would not respond to any noise or sounds. We treated the following points daily for 6 days: B8, B16, B67, B1; GV1, GV20, GV27; GB13, GB14, and GB15. After the first treatment, the dog was able to walk down on the front foot pads in a normal manner and the toe-up condition never returned. We treated the following ear points for deafness: GB2, SI19, TH21, and TH19. After the second ear treatment, the dog showed some small response to noise. We continued daily ear treatments. After the tenth treatment, the dog would immediately respond when her name was called. Dr. Nakatani advises against the use of the TH19 point for deafness now, and uses only the points in front of the ear. We will follow his advice on this in the future. He says that the use of the points behind the ear slow the progress greatly. In all cases, we treated each point once daily for 7 sec. We used a needle injector attached to our LC/Meter® with voltage at 12 and microamps at 200.

REFERENCES

1. Anon. 1972. *Chinese Veterinary Handbook.* (in Chinese). Pp. 587–670. Lan Chou Veterinary Research Institute. Gan shu, China: The People's Publishing Co.
2. Anon. 1973. Department of Physiology, Anhwei Medical College, Hofei, Anhwei. Effect of needling of the philtrum on hemorrhagic shock in cats. *Chinese Med. J.* 2:25.
3. Anon. 1975. *Acupunct. News Dig.* 5:4.
4. Anon. Unidentified newsclipping.
5. Antos, C. 1975. Acupuncture on Horses? *Rapidan River Farm Digest* 1:12–19.
6. Bachmann, G. 1966. Akupunkturbehandlung bei Haustieren. [Acupuncture treatment for domesticated animals]. *Dtsch. Z.f. Akupunktur* 15:109–10.
7. Braemer, C. 1968. Uber Akupunkturbehandlung beim Hund. [Acupuncture treatments for dogs]. *Dtsch. Z.f. Akupunktur* 17:115–16.
8. Chan, T. K. 1975. *Int. Vet. Acupunct. Newsl.* December.
9. Chen, S. H. 1976. *Veterinary Acupuncture.* Denver: University of Oriental Culture.
10. Cheney, M. W. 1975. Panel Report. *Modern Vet. Pract.* 56:798.
11. Kothbauer, O. 1973. Zur Behandlung von Gelenkschwellungen in Bereich des Sprunggelkes beim Rind durch Neuraltherapie. [Using Neural Therapy to treat Swelling in the Hock Joints of Cattle]. *Wien. tierärztl. Mschr.* 60:379, 381.
12. Lambardt, A. 1970. Zum Problem der Einfuhrung der Akupunktur in die Veterinarmedizin. [The problem of using acupuncture in veterinary medicine]. *Praktische Tierarzt* 51:185.
13. Lambardt, A. 1972. Akupunktur bei Einem Eber. [Acupuncture on a Boar]. *Der Praktische Tierarzt* 53:553–54.
14. Malapart. 1958. Akupunktur in der Veterinarmedizine. [Results with Acupuncture in Veterinary Medicine]. *Dtsch. Z.f. Akup.* 7:92–96.
15. Milin, J. 1956. Chapter XVII, Veterinary Acupuncture. In *Traite D'Acupuncture,* Tome I, ed. R. de la Fuye, pp. 473–89. Paris.
16. Milin, J. 1958. Veterinarmedizin und Akupunktur. [Veterinary Medicine and acupuncture]. *Dtsch. Z.f. Akup.* 7:15–20.
17. Milin, J. 1962. Die Akupunktur bei Tieren. [Acupuncture in animals]. *Dtsch. Z.f. Akup.* 11:38–45.
18. Milin, J. 1973. Acupuncture in gynecology of the dog. *Animal de Compagnie* 33:293–305.
19. Milin. J. Rheumatism in the Dog and Acupuncture.
20. Shin, S. H. 1975. Veterinary—anatomy and application. In *Compendium of Veterinary and Human Acupuncture,* ed. by H. E. Warner and R. S. Glassberg, pp. III, 1–III, 2. Anaheim, California: National Association for Veterinary Acupuncture.
21. Shiota, K. 1974. [Therapeutic Application of Acupuncture to Coughing in Canine Filariasis]. [In Japanese]. The 1974 Japan Clinical Veterinary Conference; Tokyo, Japan.

5

The Physiology
of Acupuncture

The scientific re-evaluation of acupuncture began in China in 1954; however, the number of reports and experiments in progress studying acupuncture increase logarithmically every year. These studies are picking away at the questions of acupuncture and are also adding a great deal to the store of knowledge on pain and pain control.

Advances in experimental procedures have enabled testing of the basic principles of acupuncture under controlled and clinical conditions. The mechanism of acupuncture's effects has not been clearly shown; however, evidence has been accumulating showing acupuncture's effectiveness, and several of its basic principles have been given credence through experiments (see also Chapter Six).

The following experiments deal with four major principles of acupuncture based on observations that are expressed in metaphysical terms in traditional Chinese medicine. A sound modern scientific basis has been established for each principle (see Chapter One for a complete discussion).

The first principle states that in successful needle therapy, a state of *te ch'i* results. The Yin-Yang Theory and the Meridian Theory explain that *ch'i* is the vital element of animal life, and that it flows in the meridians. For the needle insertion to achieve the desired therapeutic result, a state of te ch'i must be achieved. *Te ch'i* in Chinese means that the needle has contacted the ch'i, which must be manipulated in order to make the therapy effective, and that it was properly inserted into the meridian through the acupuncture point.

To the acupuncturist, *te ch'i* means a feeling of resistance or palpable motion of the needle in the tissue during insertion. The needle is felt to be caught or sucked in by something in the tissue.

In a human, the state of te ch'i is reported as a deep sensation of soreness, heaviness, tightness, or swelling. The animal responses reported to represent te ch'i are uneasiness, stamping the ground, swinging the tail, and a local muscle twitching at or around the insertion site.

The second principle states that there is a relationship between a specific meridian and a specific organ in the body.

The third principle states that when a specific point is stimulated, certain physiological changes occur. This implies knowledge of the functions of organs whose specific location and identity were not known; for example, the function of the adrenal gland was assigned to certain points on the kidney meridian. We know today that the adrenal is located near the kidney; they are separate organs but in the same dermatome.

The fourth principle states that acupuncture points have a specific, easily distinguishable location on the skin, related to the organ, and the points show changes when their related organs are functioning improperly or when they are stimulated.

The Phenomena of Te Ch'i

In 249 trials of needle insertion in humans, it was shown that there is a fairly good relationship between the muscle activity of the subject, as shown by electromyographic recordings (EMG), and the intensity of the manual feeling experienced by the acupuncturist. A similar relationship was shown between the muscle activity and the intensity of the subjective feeling of the subject. These seem to show the existence of a te ch'i type of response that is measurable.

It was thus assumed that the local muscular activity during acupuncture was a reflex activity. This was supported by the fact that both the subjective sensation and the acupuncturist's manual feeling, as well as electrical activity, disappeared entirely in patients under spinal anesthesia.[3] Because the lumbar spinal cord is thought to be involved in the transmission of the effect of acupuncture treatment, the spinal cord at the level of T–12 or L–1 of a rabbit was partially resected to test the effect of such a lesion on acupuncture analgesia.[11] With the unilateral or bilateral resection of the dorsal funiculus, including the dorsolateral fasciculus, needle insertion in ST36, or LI11 in rabbits significantly increased the pain threshold, compared with that of the control group. Unilateral resection of the lateral funiculus and needle insertion on points on the contralateral side failed to increase the pain threshold. Needle insertion on the ipsilateral side significantly increased the pain threshold.

A comparison of the degenerative fibers, using Marchi's method, suggested that the ventral portion of the lateral funiculus plays a significant role in transmitting the stimulus in acupuncture analgesia of the contralateral side. Because most of the ascending spinal fibers of the ventral funiculus project onto the reticular formation of the brain stem, central gray matter, and the thalamus, it is thought these structures may be closely related to acupuncture needle manipulation.

The preceding experiment suggests that the contralateral side of the spinal cord plays a special part in the te ch'i response. Furthermore, it is known that the nerve fibers involved with the flexor reflex can be excited only by stimuli from the contralateral side

and the ascending fibers for the flexor reflex are found in large quantities in the muscles and joints.[12] Therefore, a link was established between muscle reflex and nerve fibers in the spinal cord.

Further experiments were conducted to find out what specific nerve cells in the spinal cord were involved in the transmission of the te ch'i response. In another experiment, needling was done in the san li point in the rabbit. It was found that the results of this needling at a certain depth and angle of insertion were equivalent to or probably due to the stimulation of the common peroneal nerve. This was proven when resection or blocking of the perneal nerve by anesthetics caused the acupuncture effect to be lost.

An attempt was then made to trace the location of the peroneal nerve fiber at the cellular level in the spinal cord. This was done by damaging the nerve fibers and tracing the damage by a special staining method, which showed the degenerative fibers in the spinal cord.

Investigation by light microscopy revealed that degeneration of the peroneal nerve fibers went as far as six segments of the spinal cord via the ascending and the descending collateral branches of the somatic coarse fibers, entering the spinal cord at layer IV.[9] This indicates that acupuncture stimulation affecting the peroneal nerve would have to be relayed through the segments of the spinal cord using the same route of travel to the higher centers of the nervous system. Electron microscopic examination of the synapses in layers I to IV of the posterior horn of the lumbar spinal cord revealed that the synapse is characterized by an elliptical shape, a narrow synaptic cleft, and a minimal difference in thickness between the presynaptic membrane, and the synapse is the inhibitory type.[4]

As a result of these investigations, it was concluded that acupuncture stimulation excited the nerve cells and synapses in the spinal column that had an inhibitory effect on pain.

It is known that the spinothalamic tract is responsible for the transmission of the pain sensation from the periphery to the midbrain reticular formation, the nucleus parafascicularis, and the nucleus central lateralis of the thalamus.[1, 10, 14, 15] Experiments were conducted to prove that the inhibition of pain does not occur in the spinal column alone but also in the higher centers of the central nervous system.

Painful stimuli were applied to the body and reactions in the midbrain reticular formation and nucleus centralis lateralis of the thalamus were recorded.

The response of the midbrain reticular formation to pain stimuli applied to various parts of the body were entirely or partially inhibited by electroacupuncture of ST36 and GB34 in guinea pigs. These painful stimuli were measured as unit discharges and prolonged afterdischarges, and could be suppressed by intravenous morphine. Thus, the presence of pain-reacting cells was demonstrated in the medial reticular formation of the midbrain by their specific electrical discharges and subsequent suppression by acupuncture and morphine.[5]

Evoked and spontaneous single-unit responses of neurons in the nucleus centralis lateralis of the thalamus have been analyzed in 30 rabbits.[6] The responses to noxious stimuli were characterized by long latency (150–300 msec), prolonged high frequency after discharges and susceptibility to analgesics. Neurons of this particular type, distributed in the caudal region of the nucleus, are involved in the reception of pain impulses. By applying trains of electrical pulses to acupuncture points B60 and ST36, it was shown that characteristic responses produced by noxious stimuli could be inhibited. This inhibitory effect of the electric needling of the acupuncture point, with shortening of the duration of afterdischarges and/or lowering the discharge frequency, was usually not immediate but appeared 2.5 minutes after stimulation.

Furthermore, the neurons of the nucleus parafascicularis showed the same neuronal discharges as when the nucleus centralis lateralis was stimulated by a noxious substance. Pain-sensitive neurons were not found in other areas of the thalamus, such as the nucleus ventralis thalami.

Several conclusions can be drawn from these experiments: (1) What the traditional Chinese medicine called the *te ch'i* response is an observable, measurable phenomenon. (2) The te ch'i phenomenon is an expression of nerve-cell activity in the higher centers of the central nervous system. (3) A definite relationship exists between acupuncture and the central nervous system.

The Relationship of Specific Meridians to Specific Organs

Adrenalin was injected into a rabbit to alter the heartbeat. An acupuncture needle was then inserted and the effects observed. It was seen that needle insertion into P6 and ST36 induced an antiadrenergic effect that brought the heartbeat to normal. However, no significant effect was noted if the needle was applied to GB37 or nonacupuncture points on the lateral side of the tail.[8]

Other groups experimented on the effect of needle stimulation on experimental shock. Rabbit blood was injected into the femoral vein of a dog to induce shock. Needle insertion at the philtrum, GV26 brought the blood pressure, respiration, and heart rate back to normal significantly sooner than if the philtrum were not stimulated. Needle insertion at GV26 is prescribed for trauma in any part of the body.

Electroacupuncture of GV26 was shown to improve the physiologic status of cats in hemorrhagic shock by raising the blood pressure and increasing the rate and depth of respiration.[7] Acupuncture had no effect on normal blood pressure. During bloodletting (femoral artery), the time intervals for the blood pressure to drop from normal to 50 mm Hg (recorded in the common carotid artery) in acupuncture and control groups were 15.2 ± 6.1 min and 6.9 ± 2.6 min, respectively. The total volumes of blood loss to precipitate shock in the two groups were 21.8 ± 3.9 ml/kg and 15.8 ± 4.7 ml/kg, respectively, and these differences were statistically significant.

As for the fate of the cats in two groups that were not given blood transfusions after bleeding, the mortality rate in the acupuncture group was 25% within 3 hours, while that in the control group was 100%. In two other groups, blood transfusions were given as soon as bloodletting stopped and the blood pressure was kept at a level of 80 mm Hg for 1 hour. The amount of blood needed in the acupuncture group was 12.7 ± 3.3 ml/kg, while that in the control group was 32.7 ± 10.3 ml/kg. In cats anesthetized with pentobarbital sodium, no antishock effect was produced when acupuncture was used.

The following conclusions can be drawn from these experiments: (1) Evidence is accumulating indicating that stimulation of specific points may affect the function of an organ or system that is in a state of hyper- or hypofunction. (2) The successful stimulation of a point may be interfered with by anesthesia, showing a connection between acupuncture points and the central nervous system.

The Biochemical Responses

One experiment involved the use of acupuncture on lactogenic effects in women with inadequate lactation. The acupuncture point used was CV17. This meridian passes through the middle part of the brain, and in Chinese traditional medicine, it is supposed to affect all major organs. It is known that the pituitary gland secretes the lactogenic hormone prolactin, and the pituitary gland is located at the middle of the sagittal plane of the brain. After needle insertion, there was an increase in the level of prolactin in the blood parallel with clinical observation of mammary gland secretion.[18]

Experiments were performed to determine the effects of acupuncture on the increase in the number and modification in function of the white blood cells. The points stimulated were ST36 and P6. These two meridians are related to the blood in Chinese traditional medicine: the stomach nourishes blood and the heart controls blood flow. Blood itself is considered to be an organ responsible for transporting good and harmful substances in the body. Thus, if the stomach and heart are not working properly, the blood ceases to function efficiently. Furthermore, abnormal blood function may result in the domination of disease because the balance of harmful and good body substances is no longer maintained in the blood.

Needle insertion into the ST36 point of rabbits induced an immediate increase of white blood cells by more than 50%. The changes reached a plateau and, 24 hours after treatment the level was only 30–40% above normal. A differential count indicated a significant increase in neutrophils. Needle insertion into nonacupuncture sites did not produce significant changes. If procaine was injected at the sites before needling ST36, changes in neutrophils did not appear.

It was further observed that acupuncture of P6 and ST36 substantially increased the phagocytic activities of white blood cells to *Staphylococcus aureus*. The index of phagocytosis increased by 1.5 times after needle stimulation and by 50% after moxibustion. In an experiment using electroacupuncture, a relationship of the total number and differential count of white blood cells and phagocytic activities, and the role of the nervous system on the efficacy of acupuncture were also shown in rabbits.[16, 17]

The following conclusions can be drawn from these experiments: (1) Acupuncture produces a biochemical effect unrelated to the reduction of pain. (2) The assignment of a meridian to an organ does not limit it to the function of that organ alone. (3) Biochemical responses are also mediated through the nervous system.

The Location of the Acupuncture Points

The distributions of acupuncture points in man, horses, and cattle were used as references to locate and measure the skin electrical potential of dogs, rabbits, guinea pigs, and monkeys. The results showed that there are many high electrical-potential points widely distributed on the skin of these animals. The differences in electrical potential of surrounding areas are much smaller than at the particular point. The points found in the various species were: 84 points in dogs (34 unpaired and 50 paired); 53 in rabbits (20 unpaired and 33 paired); and 23 in guinea pigs (8 unpaired and 15 paired). It is especially interesting to note that the number, distribution, and location of points having a high electrical potential difference in the monkey are nearly equivalent to those of the acupuncture points in humans.

Differences in skin electrical potential at the acupuncture points, relative to the activity of the visceral organs, were also studied. It was shown that after subcutaneous injection of histamine in dogs, the changes in the electrical potential curve of GV20, B20, and LI11 are consistent with the electrical potential curves of the mucous membrane and changes in total stomach liquid volume and acidity. At the tip of the tail and unrelated to the stomach, a histamine injection did not alter the electrical potential. After feeding, the points of the stomach meridian of the monkey—ST36 and ST40—and of the spleen meridian—SP6 and SP8—had a higher skin electrical potential than they had before feeding. However, the electrical potentials of the acupuncture points of the pericardium meridian—P5, P6, and P7—do not show a consistent pattern of change.[2]

Auricular acupuncture is a division of acupuncture dealing with the relationships and therapeutic effects of various points of the ear to different organs of the body. The skin resistance of the ear shell of the rabbit, under conditions of experimental peritonitis, was studied. Tests were made on the concave surface of the external ear of three control and nine rabbits with induced peritonitis. The results revealed low resistance points around the external auditory meatus, along the crus helicis, the external surface of the tragus, the antitragus, and the incisura intertragica.

When peritonitis had developed, points of lower resistance appeared in the blood vessel area above the external auditory meatus, but they varied in distribution and number. They disappeared after 7 days when the rabbits recovered from the peritonitis. In the control rabbits, few or no low-resistance points were found in the blood vessel area. Statistical treatment of the data indicated that the electrical resistances of the points in the blood vessel area on the pinna were significantly lower during the period of experimental peritonitis than before—that is, the electrical resistances of these points during illness were significantly lower than those outside the blood vessel area. No such changes were observed in the control animal.[13]

The following conclusions can be drawn from these experiments: (1) Acupuncture points do exist and vary in electrical potential from other areas of the skin. (2) Organs of the body have corresponding acupuncture points. (3) Stimulation of the organ will produce an effect on its corresponding acupuncture point (see also Chapter Three).

REFERENCES

1. Anderson, F. D., and Berry, G. M. 1959. Degenerative studies of long ascending fiber system in the cat brain stem. *J. Comp. Neurol.* 3: 195–230.
2. Anon. 1959. Location of acupuncture points, in lecture notes of Acupuncture Editorial Board of Shanghai College of Chinese Medicine. Shanghai People's Press.
3. Anon. 1973. Electromyographic activity produced locally by acupuncture manipulation. Shanghai Institute of Physiology, Acupuncture Anesthesia Group. *Chinese Med. J.* 9: 532–35.
4. Anon. 1973. Preliminary experimental, morphological and electron microscopic studies of the connection between acupuncture points on the limbs and the segments of the spinal cord. Morphological Section of the Acupuncture Anesthesia Research Unit, Shenyang Medical College. *Chinese Med. J.* 3: 144–50.
5. Anon. 1973. The role of the midbrain reticular formation in acupuncture anesthesia. Acupuncture Anesthesia Coordinating Group, Shanghai College of Chinese Medicine, Shanghai Normal College and Shu Chung Hospital of the Shanghai College of Chinese Medicine. *Chinese Med. J.* 3: 136–38.
6. Anon. 1973. Electrical responses to noxious stimulation and its inhibition in nucleus centralis lateralis of the thalamus in rabbits. Shanghai Institute of Physiology. *Chinese Med. J.* 3: 131–35.
7. Anon. 1973. The effect of needling of the philtrum on hemorrhagic shock in cats. Department of Physiology, Anhwei Medical College. *Chinese Med J.* 2: 98–100.
8. Anon. 1974. The effect of needling various acupuncture points on the activities of the heart. Department of Physiology, Experimental Medicine Research Institute, Chinese Academy of Traditional Medicine. Abstracted in *Textbook of Acupuncture.* People's Press.
9. Azentagothai, J. 1964. Neuronal and synaptic arrangement in the substantia gelantinosa rolandic. *J. Comp. Neurol.* 122: 219–40.
10. Boivie, J. 1971. The termination of the spinothalamic tract in the cat, an experimental study with silver impregnation. *Exp. Brain Res.* 12: 331–53.
11. Chiang, C-Y., Liu, J-I., Chu, T-H., Pai, Y-H., and Chang, S-C. 1974. Spinal ascending pathway for the effect of acupuncture anesthesia in rabbits. *Gen. Sci.* 19:31–33.
12. Eccles, J. and Schade, J., ed. 1964. Physiology of the spinal cord. *Brain Res.* 12: 135–63.
13. Li, C-T., Chang, P-L., Hsu, L-H., and Yang, P-L. 1973. Survey of electrical resistance of rabbit pinna during experimental peritonitis. *Chinese Med. J.* 7: 428–33.
14. Lund, R. D., and Webster, K. 1967. Thalamic afferents from the spinal cord and trigeminal nuclei—an experimental anatomical study of the rat. *J. Comp. Neurol.* 130: 313–28.
15. Mehler, W. R. 1957. The mammalian "pain tract" in phylogeny. *Anat. Rec.* (Proc.) 127: 332.
16. Wong, F-C., Jen, I-B., Lin, T-C., and Szeto, L-M. 1955. The effect of electro-acupuncture on constituents of peripheral blood in rabbits. *Nat. Med. J.* 41: 417–20.
17. Wong, F-C., Jen, J-B., Szeto, L-M. and Lin, T-C. 1957. Effects of electro-acupuncture on phagocytic activity of white cells in rabbits. In *Electro-acupuncture Therapeutics.* Sansi People's Press.
18. Wu, Y-C., Wong, S-W., Kung. M-S., Chen, Y-H., Yang, E-S. and S. J. 1958. The effect of acupuncture on lactogenic hormone secretion. *Shanghai J. Chin. Med.* 12: 31–32.

6

Acupuncture Analgesia

The use of acupuncture to produce analgesia for painful procedures such as dental work, surgery, and parturition has caught the public's fancy. The use of acupuncture for analgesia has provided many dramatic articles and movies, popularizing the procedure and sustaining the public's interest in it.

Initially, there were very few details and very limited experimental information available in English; however, in the past few years much Chinese information has been translated and many neurophysiologic experiments have been done outside of China. These studies have attempted to provide a better understanding of pain and analgesia, and the possible mechanisms of action of acupuncture analgesia.

Experimental Results

A series of experiments were performed to test the validity of the hypothesis that acupuncture analgesia is essentially a function of the central nervous system resulting from the inhibitive interaction (in the brain, and especially in the thalamus) between the afferent impulses arising from the point of acupuncture and those from the site of pain.[32] Experiments performed using albino rats and rabbits showed that neurons in the nucleus parafascicularis and the nucleus cen-

tralis lateralis of the thalamus produced characteristic unit discharges in response to noxious stimuli, and these discharges could be prevented by morphine. The pain responses of these neurons were also inhibited by electrical stimulation of needles in certain acupuncture points, squeezing the Achilles tendon, or weak electrical stimulation of a sensory nerve. Too strong a stimulation, however, tended to exaggerate the response to pain. One kind of spontaneous rhythmic discharge of the nucleus parafascicularis neurons was demonstrated to be driven by the incessant inflow of pain impulses from surgical wounds in experimental animals. Spontaneous discharges of this kind, like the evoked pain discharges, could be enhanced by noxious stimuli and inhibited by innocuous stimuli—for example, the mechanical squeeze of the Achilles tendon or the needling of acupuncture points. The duration of inhibition of the spontaneous pain discharges of the parafascicularis neurons caused by an innocuous stimulus varied with the frequency of the progressing discharges at the moment of stimulation.

A study in rabbits showed that noxious stimuli produced single-unit responses of neurons in the nucleus centralis lateralis of the thalamus, characterized by long latency (150–300 msec), prolonged high-frequency afterdischarges, and susceptibility to analgesics.[19] Neurons of this particular type distributed in the caudal region of the nucleus are involved in the reception of pain impulses. The characteristic responses could be inhibited by trains of weak electric pulses applied to certain acupuncture points on the hindlimb. The inhibitory effect of the electric stimulation of the acupuncture point was seen as a shortening of the duration of afterdischarges and/or the lowering of the discharge frequency. This was usually not immediate but appeared 2–5 min after the onset of stimulation.

A series of studies has been reported showing that a humoral mechanism may be involved in acupuncture analgesia.[24] The cardiac and cephalic ends of the carotid arteries of two animals were cross-connected. Acupuncture was performed in one animal, while pain threshold was measured in the other. The results were compared with a control group in which neither of the pair had acupuncture. These experiments were done on rabbits, using potassium iontophoretic dolorimetry to determine the pain threshold on the ears. Pain thresholds of both the punctured and unpunctured animals of the acupuncture group, in 16 observations, were elevated markedly after 30 min of electric needling, and tended to decline after removal of the needle. No apparent trend of change was found in eight observations of the control group. Similar results were obtained in experiments with albino rats, using electrically heated wires coiled over the tails as pain stimuli and timing the duration from closure of the electric circuit to flapping of the tails as the pain threshold. The increment of pain threshold in the unpunctured rats of the acupuncture group was found to be highly significant. A humoral factor(s) therefore seems to be involved in acupuncture analgesia.

Vierck et al.[63] have suggested that increases in pain threshold produced by acupuncture may occur in waves—that is, they may or may not occur acutely during acupuncture stimulation—followed by a continuation of, or a return to, the normal threshold, with the appearance or reappearance of increased threshold in 48–70 hours.

In a study by Rabischong et al.,[60] serum was collected from rabbits in which acupuncture analgesia had been electrically produced and injected into the vein of another rabbit. Analgesia was produced in the recipients, with regional distribution similar to that in the donors.

The production of analgesia by electrical stimulation of specific areas within the brain and the mechanisms of this analgesia have been intensively investigated. Others have involved the site of action of narcotic analgesics such as morphine.

Analgesia can be produced by electrical stimulation of specific sites in the brain, especially the mesencephalic central gray matter and the periventricular gray matter.[52] Studies have been done in rats and cats.[52, 58] The analgesia produced was not related to the production of seizures, the production of electrolytic lesions, or to the rewarding properties of stimulation. An important finding was that the failure to respond to noxious stimulation could not be attributed to a general sensory, motivational, emotional, attentional, or motor deficit. Rather, electrical stimulation appeared capable of selectively reducing nociception. Studies with inhibitors or depletors of serotonin suggest that there is at least one serotonergic link in the pathway of analgesia production, both by electrical stimulation and morphine administration.[2]

Analgesia produced by electrical stimulation was diminished in rats given the serotonin synthesis inhibitor parachlorophenylalanine. This diminution of analgesia only occurred when the electrical stimulation was in the ventral central gray matter nearest to the serotonin-rich dorsal raphe nucleus. Analgesia produced by morphine is also diminished in the rat by parachlorophenylalanine.

A study done in rabbits showed that stimulation of acupuncture points feng lung (ST40) and yang fu (GB38) caused an increase in the serotonin levels of the medulla and thalamus. Intraventricular injections of serotonin produced increases in pain threshold.[8]

Recent studies have shown that analgesia produced by electrical stimulation can be reversed in rats, cats, and man by the parenteral administration of narcotic antagonists such as naloxone.

A series of studies done on rabbits adds some more information about the production of acupuncture analgesia.[50] Analgesia was produced by the manual or electrical stimulation of acupuncture needles placed at different sites. The area of analgesia was determined for the different methods of stimulation, for the different anatomic location of the needles, and for the different combination of connecting the positive and negative electrodes by pinching the skin with a clamp. The results are illustrated in Figures 6–1 to 6–4. Another part of this study evaluated the necessity for nerve conduction in relation to the production of analgesia. Electrically stimulating the sciatic nerve produced a given area of analgesia. If the nerve was severed or blocked with a local anesthetic, then either no analgesia or a very small area of analgesia was produced, showing that nervous

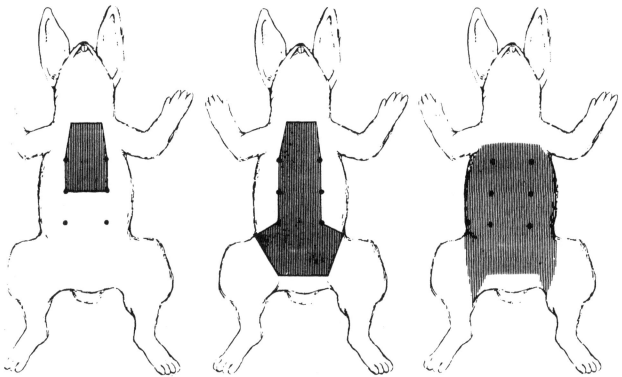

FIGURE 6–1. *Left,* area of local analgesia produced by manual stimulation with two needles on top of the head. *Center,* area of local analgesia produced by manual stimulation of the second or third web of the right forepaw and the top of the head. *Right,* area of local analgesia produced by manual stimulation of the second web of the right hindpaw and the top of the head. (From Matsumoto, T., *Acupuncture for Physicians,* 1974. Courtesy of Charles C Thomas, Publisher, Springfield, Illinois.)

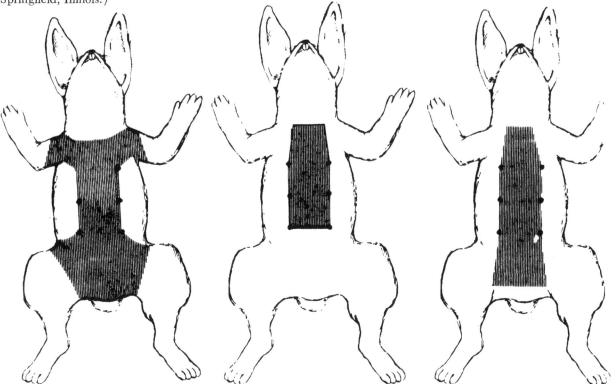

FIGURE 6–2. *Left,* area of local analgesia produced by electrical stimulation of the ears. *Center,* area of local analgesia produced by electrical stimulation of the second web of the right forepaw (positive) and the right thigh (negative). *Right,* area of local analgesia produced by electrical stimulation of the third web of the right forepaw (positive) and the top of the head (negative). Electrical stimulation: sine wave, 10 KHz, 200 μa. (From Matsumoto, T. *Acupuncture for Physicians,* 1974. Courtesy of Charles C Thomas, Publisher, Springfield, Illinois.)

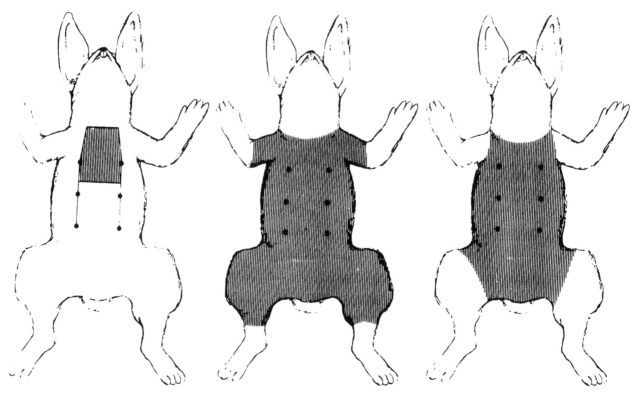

FIGURE 6–3. *Left,* area of local analgesia produced by electrical stimulation of the last web of the right forepaw (positive) and the top of the head (negative). *Center,* area of local analgesia produced by electrical stimulation of the second web of right hindpaw (positive) and the top of the head (negative). *Right,* area of local anaglesia produced by electrical stimulation of the second web of the right forepaw (positive) and the second web of the left forepaw (negative). Electrical stimulation: sine wave, 10 KHz, 200 μa. (From Matsumoto, T., *Acupuncture for Physicians,* 1974. Courtesy of Charles C Thomas, Publisher, Springfield, Illinois.)

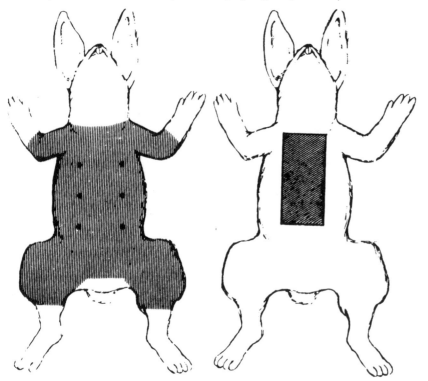

FIGURE 6–4. *Left,* area of local analgesia produced by electrical stimulation of the second web of the right forepaw (positive) and the top of the head (negative). *Right,* area of local analgesia following electrical stimulation of the top of the head (positive) and the second web of the right forepaw or hindpaw (negative). Electrical stimulation: sine wave, 10 KHz, 200 μa. (From Matsumoto, T., *Acupuncture for Physicians,* 1974. Courtesy of Charles C Thomas, Publisher, Springfield, Illinois.)

conduction between the site of the acupuncture needle and the spinal cord is necessary for the production of acupuncture analgesia.

Electricity has been used to diminish pain for at least 2000 years. In A.D. 46, Scribonius Largus advocated piscine electrotherapy specifically for the relief of pain: "For any type of gout, a live black torpedo (the torpedo ray, *Torpedo marmorata)* should, when pain begins, be placed under the feet. The patient must stand on a moist shore washed by the sea, and he should stay like this until his whole foot and leg, up to the knee, is numb."[34]

Uses of electricity for pain relief continues to be investigated, and some success has been achieved.[34, 41, 43, 45, 56, 61, 64]

Electricity has also been used to produce general anesthesia, but this state is completely different from that produced by acupuncture.[62] In electroanesthesia, the subject is unconscious; with acupuncture, sleep or unconsciousness is not produced.

The Use of Acupuncture Analgesia in China[5, 6]

In 1958 electroacupuncture and manual acupuncture were developed in China as alternatives for drug-induced analgesia. These methods were refined and standardized. Thus far, (1972) 255 case histories involving the testing of these methods on horses, donkeys, cattle, and pigs have been recorded and studied. The reported rate of success has been 95% (Table 6–1).

During the surgery performed under electroacupuncture analgesia, the animals calmly allowed operative procedures such as incisions, intestinal traction and suturing to proceed without appearing to be in pain.

Two methods of acupuncture analgesia are currently used in China. The first method is the electrical stimulation of the San Yan Lo Points. This method has been used in horses, mules, donkeys, cattle, and pigs. The second method is a special form of acupuncture analgesia and has been used only in donkeys and horses. It involves the stimulation of points in the ear. Electroacupuncture or manual stimulation may be used, depending on the skill of the practitioner, the number of points to be needled, and the time factor involved. In the stimulation of the San Yan Lo Points, local supplementary points are optional; in stimulation of the ear points, they are mandatory. Supplementary local points are points near the site of the operation that are in the same dermatome (these points have an asterisk in Chapter Three).

TABLE 6–1. *Effectiveness of Electroacupuncture Analgesia*
  Utilizing the San Yan Lo Points

ANIMAL	EXCELLENT	GOOD	FAILURE	TOTAL
Horse	172	33	4	209
Mule	24	7	1	32
Donkey	4	0	0	4
Cattle	1	2	0	3
Pig	7	0	0	7
TOTAL	208	42	5	255
Area of Surgery				
Head	5	0	0	5
Neck	4	1	0	5
Withers	2	0	0	2
Thorax	2	1	0	3
Abdomen	186	38	4	228
Gluteal region	1	0	1	2
Perineal region	3	0	0	3
Inguinal region	2	2	0	4
4 Limbs	3	0	0	3
TOTAL	208	42	5	255
PERCENTAGE	81.6	16.5	1.9	100

ELECTROACUPUNCTURE ANALGESIA USING THE SAN YAN LO POINTS

The Relationship Between the San Yan Lo Points and the Nervous System

The San Yan Lo Points consist of three acupuncture points (Fig. 3–39). They are san yan lo (FL23), yeh yan (FL24), and ch'ang feng (FL7). Electroacupuncture is actually the stimulation of a nerve that ultimately has an effect on the cerebral cortex. Anatomically, acupuncture needle insertion into FL7 is needle insertion on or near the radial nerve. For san yan lo and yeh yan stimulation, the needle is inserted into san yan lo through the arm, to yeh yan. In this case, the needle is inserted along the largest and the longest nerve trunk of the forelimb, the median nerve. Experiments were done with the nerve trunk bisected. They showed no analgesic effect if the nerve is stimulated on the distal end of the bisection, whereas stimulation of the proximal portion produces analgesia. The nervous system is the key to the success of the acupuncture analgesia.

Analgesic effects can be obtained by stimulating the nerve trunk anatomically related to a surgical area. The closer the needle is to the nerve trunk, the better the result. Best results can be obtained by stimulating the nerve trunk directly. During surgical procedures, continuous stimulation is essential to maintain a level of stimulation to the cerebral cortex to inhibit or diminish the pain reaction caused by surgery. Analgesic effects can also be obtained by stimulating the nerve trunk anatomically unrelated to the surgical area.

The sites of insertion for analgesia are as significant as they are in acupuncture therapy for diseases. The choice of needling points along the nerve trunk depends on the easy accessibility and convenience of position. As far as the level of stimulation is concerned, the analgesic effect depends solely on the level of stimulation and is unrelated to induction time. No matter how long stimulation is sustained, no effect is produced if it has not reached the optimum level of intensity. In critically ill animals, adequately strong stimulation is usually applied, and surgery commences with a minimum of induction time. If the nerve trunk is overstimulated, the animal will become agitated, with tachycardia and rapid respiration.

Different levels of stimulation are required at different acupuncture points. As a general rule, less stimulation is used if the point is located along a nerve trunk or plexus, and a large area of analgesia is produced; whereas at a point located in the area of a muscle belly, a higher level of stimulation is required and the area of analgesia is small.

Location of Points (See Chapter Three)

FL23. Three Yang Vessels, San Yan Lo (Figs. 3–37, 3–39). In the muscle groove, 2 tsun below the tubercle (of the radius) for the lateral ligament, lateral ligament, lateral to the forearm.
FL24. Night Eye, Yeh Yan (Fig. 3–39). Medial side of the forelimb, equivalent to the site of the "chestnut" (probably a little cranial to the chestnut).
FL7. Wind Chase, Ch'ang Feng (Figs. 3–28, 3–29, 3–37 to 3–39). Caudal and slightly ventral to the shoulder joint, in the depression between the long and lateral heads of the triceps brachialis at the caudal margin of the deltoideus.

Procedures for Acupuncture Analgesia

Needle: Two needles, Chinese numbers 18 and 19; lengths: 4 and 6 in., respectively. (In general, horses in the west are larger than those indigenous to China. The needle used for San Yan Lo and Yeh Yan will probably have to be 8 in. Choice of needle diameter is based on factors discussed in Chapter Two).
Apparatus: A semiconductor electroacupuncture machine.
Position of Animal: Standing, dorsal or lateral recumbency. The lateral position of the animal for the

operation is favored because the needle insertion can be on the same side as the operation. In a supine position, needle insertion can be done on the more convenient side.

Prescriptions

All three points are used simultaneously for each of the following surgical procedures.
Head region: Enucleation, resection, anastomosis of the tongue.
Neck region: Resection of the jugular vein, tracheotomy.
Wither region: Muscle resection and suture, closure of fistula.
Thoracic region: Rib resection, closure of pneumothorax.
Abdominal region: Abdominal hernia, intestinal anastomosis, cesarean section.
Urinary system: Nephrectomy, recanalization of the urethra, inguinal region surgery.
Extremities: Tumor resection of the feet, tendon release.

Method of Needle Insertion

FROM FL23 through FL24: The needle is inserted at an angle of 15–20 degrees from the skin at FL23 along the posterior margin of the radius slanting medially and ventrally toward yeh yan. After insertion, the needle point should be felt subcutaneously at FL24; care should be taken not to penetrate the skin.
FL24 (yeh yan) is absent in cows and pigs. In these animals, a corresponding area is used. The depth of needle insertion is slightly less in the pig than in horses and cattle, owing to the pig's smaller size.
FL7 Ch'ang Feng: Straight insertion for 3 tsun. The depth of needle insertion into ch'ang feng should vary according to the size and weight of the animal. The range is 2–3 tsun in average domestic animals.

Use of Apparatus

After needle insertion, the output wire of the electroacupuncture analgesic machine is connected to the handle. Starting from a low setting, the frequency and voltage are increased. The optimal frequency is about 30–50 Hz, and the optimal voltage is the highest tolerable for the animal (usually high enough to cause obvious local muscle contractions). The degree of analgesia can be tested by needle puncture over the area of the skin prepared for the surgical operation. If there is no pain response, the operation can start. The duration of electrical stimulation before surgery begins should be prolonged in individual animals with low pain thresholds. Electric current should be continually applied throughout the operation. The frequency and the output of the acupuncture analgesia machine should be consistent and meet minimum standards because they influence the analgesic effect. It will probably be necessary to increase the voltage and vary the frequency during the procedure as accommodation seems to take place with loss of analgesic effect.

Observable Results

Before the production of acupuncture analgesia, the animal is fully conscious, and there is sensation of pain at the site of the operation.

During analgesia, body temperature, pulse rate, and rate of respiration are increased initially and then return to normal after 20 min. The tranquilizing and analgesic effects of this method of acupuncture analgesia are reproducible.

Pain due to traction of the viscera is eliminated. However, in complicated cases, where there is much intestinal manipulation or twisting, slight pain is observed in some animals. This degree of pain does not interfere with the procedure. From practical experience, dorsal recumbency is somewhat more awkward than lateral recumbency. There is muscle spasm in the limb where needles are inserted. There is also mild muscle spasm in the contralateral limb. This usually does not interfere with the surgical procedure.

In severely ill animals, this may be the method of choice in emergency operations. Electroacupuncture analgesia does not affect cardiovascular function. Inotropic drugs may be given during the operation without interfering with the analgesic effect. Individual variations of analgesic effect exist in animals of different mental states, species, and sex. Mongolian horses react better than horses of mixed breeding. Mares and geldings have reacted better than stallions.

Assessment of Results (Table 6–1)

The parameters of assessment are given below. Movements considered pain response must be differentiated from spontaneous movements unrelated to the surgery.

Excellent: The animal appears calm on skin incision, dissection, suturing, or any other procedure.

Good: Mild muscle fasciculation and some movements observed that do not interfere with the operative procedure.

Failure: Electroacupuncture analgesia fails and drugs are used.

Discussion of the Principles of Electroacupuncture Anesthesia for Domestic Animals*

It is an objective truth that acupuncture as practiced in veterinary acupuncture anesthesia is effective as an analgesic. By first inserting needles at FL7 and FL23 of the sick animal, and then by applying pulsating electric stimuli from an electroacupuncture anesthesia machine, we have succeeded, without supplemental analgesic drugs, in conducting all forms of surgical operations on the completely conscious patient. By applying this technique, we have conducted 255 major and minor operations on horses, mules, donkeys, cattle, and swine, including cesarean section and more than 20 types of operations on the head, neck, chest, abdomen, buttock, perineum, and the four limbs. The rate of success is more than 95%.

The electroacupuncture effectiveness as a surgical anesthetic is due to the definite and real analgesic effect of needle stimulus. We know this to be true because without it, no matter what sedative is administered, if an anesthetic is not additionally administered, the animal will fail to withstand the pain caused by the surgery. They would proceed to struggle; their respiratory rates would increase, as would their pulse rates and body temperatures; and the animals would also sweat heavily and their muscles tremble. In some cases, shock or death would result.

It is well-recognized that without anesthesia, surgical objectives might not be realized in animal surgery, especially complicated major surgery. Thus, if under electroacupuncture anesthesia, the patient quietly accepts the incision, the pulling of intestines, suturing, and other surgical operations without exhibiting any reaction, we would have conclusively demonstrated that it is the definite and reliable analgesic effects of needle insertion that makes operations possible on sick animals under acupuncture anesthesia.

Anatomy of the San Yan Lo Points in domestic animals reveals that the ch'ang feng (FL7) insertion reaches the radial nerve and that the FL23 and FL24 insertions are made in the vicinity of the median nerve. Thus, both needles inserted in the San Yan Lo Points are located near nerve trunks, which means that the passing of a current through the two needles actually stimulates the two nerve trunks.

To further establish the function of the nerve trunks, we have selected the pelvic nerve trunk and the seventh cranial nerve on which to apply electroacupuncture stimulation. The results are identical to

* By the group from the Peking Municipal Veterinary Hospital.

those obtained by stimulating the forelimb nerve trunks. We have used surgical methods to expose the nerve trunks to which direct stimulation was then applied. Analgesic effects thus obtained were even more extensive and reliable.

Note, however, that the function of the nerve trunks in acupuncture anesthesia is only to provide transmission, while the real functioning processes take place in the central nervous system. As part of the experiment, we have applied local anesthesia to block the central nerve trunk of the forelimb and the pelvic nerve trunk. After that, we applied electroacupuncture to the distal portion of the nerves that have been blocked. No analgesic effects resulted, even when we increased the stimulus to ten times the strength necessary for normal electroacupuncture anesthesia. The same is true when we applied electroacupuncture to the distal portions of severed nerves, proving that success in electroacupuncture anesthesia hinges on the normal functioning of an intact nervous system. Once the nerve structures are destroyed, or when normal transmission is impaired, nerve excitation provided by needle insertion would fail to reach the central nervous system, and the objective of inducing anesthesia would be unattainable.

We have observed effective anesthesia despite an apparent lack of structural correlation between the surgical area and the area stimulated, nor do these two areas share the same or closely located nerves. This proves that without the central nervous system, electroacupuncture anesthesia is impossible.

In electroacupuncture anesthesia for domestic animals, continuous electric stimulation is necessary to maintain sufficient excitation of the central nervous system. In this way, reactions to the pain caused by surgery are continuously suppressed or weakened, resulting in continuous anesthesia. It is well born out by facts that the nervous system plays the central role in electroacupuncture anesthesia.

Different areas or points for needle insertion produce different anesthetic effects, characterized by the peculiarity of the areas or points concerned. Such peculiarity is, in turn, closely correlated with the distribution of the nerves.

We have conducted three sets of experiments. In the first set, needles were inserted at the traditional points and nonpoints along the nerve trunks. In the second set, needles were inserted at traditional points and nonpoints on muscular areas, where there are no visible nerve trunks beneath the needles. In the third set, needles were inserted at traditional points and nonpoints underneath the skin, where there are no visible nerve trunks passing beneath the needles.

The results are as follows: comparatively better analgesic effects were obtained from the first set; also, the intensity of stimulation needed was the lowest. From the second set, analgesic effects were obtained around the needle and in other individual areas, and the intensity of stimulation needed was higher than with the first set. The local analgesic effect obtained from the third set was still weaker, and the intensity of stimulation required was highest among the three sets.

Within the sets of the experiment, there were no discernible differences between insertions made on the points or nonpoints. Thus, we are of the opinion that whether or not one can obtain comparatively better results in electroacupuncture anesthesia for domestic animals depend on whether the needles are inserted along the pathways of the nerve trunks. The closer they are to the nerve trunks, the better the effects; better still it is to directly stimulate the nerve trunks.

Unlike therapeutic acupuncture, electroacupuncture anesthesia does not require accurate insertion at the points. It is sufficient to choose just any point along the passage of the nerve trunks. By connecting these points along the nerve trunks, we may call them, collectively, the name *anesthetic line*. Thus, when we talk about the peculiarity of an anesthetic point in electroacupuncture, we are not referring to a particular point, but to the anesthetic line that runs along a nerve trunk.

Choosing a point for insertion will be arbitrarily determined by practical considerations—that is, the point chosen should be easy to locate and remember, convenient for the surgical operation concerned, and the kind of restraint needed, and easy to popularize.

The San Yan Lo electroanesthesia technique has been developed on the basis of our country's traditional ching lo veterinary acupuncture theory. In clinical application, we have found that the convergence points of ching lo, as referred to in ching lo theories, are mostly located at the areas where nerves are densely distributed or areas that are close to nerve trunks. The central role played by the nervous system in electroacupuncture anesthesia is in agreement with a great part of that recorded in ancient documents about the functions of ching lo. For this reason, we should not treat ching lo and nerves as separate entities that are contradictory.

The anesthetic effects of acupuncture may be interpreted as the result of an action affected by the external factor of a stimulus of a certain intensity by means of the main internal factor of a nervous system inside the animal's body. Without that certain external factor that provides the nervous system with suitable stimulation, there can be no anesthetic effect. In acupuncture anesthesia for animals, we have tried a variety of stimuli, including twisting the needle by hand, drug injection, and electricity. We feel that whichever method is used, it must be able to provide a stimulation of sufficient and suitable intensity to the nervous system. Otherwise, satisfactory acupuncture anesthesia will not be attainable.

Scientific application has also made clear that the key to successful acupuncture anesthesia lies in the intensity of the stimulation, whether it is sufficient and appropriate, not whether the duration of induction is long or short. When the stimulation is weak, analgesic effects are not attainable, no matter how long the duration of stimulation is. It is only when stimulation reaches a certain level of intensity that satisfactory analgesic effects are obtained.

For animals in critical condition, we usually apply a stimulus of sufficient and appropriate intensity and proceed to operate immediately without recourse to an induction period. By saving crucial minutes, we may have saved many dying animals.

The nervous system can only withstand a certain level of stimulation. Overstimulation not only has no analgesic effects, but also may produce the opposite effect, causing pain. The animal responds by movement and physiologic changes. The heart and respiratory rates may go up. Thus, it is important that sufficient and appropriate stimulation be applied in electroacupuncture anesthesia.

Different areas and different points require varying degrees of stimulation. In the vicinity of nerve trunks, analgesic effects are extensive, even when the stimulation is comparatively weak. For muscular areas, analgesic effects are localized, even when the stimulation is comparatively strong. Subcutaneously, the necessary analgesic effects cannot be obtained, even when the intensity of stimulation exceeds either of the preceding cases, because much of the intensity of the stimulation is dissipated into muscular and subcutaneous structures. When stimulation of the nerve trunks decreases, a change in analgesic effect occurs. Thus, if we can find appropriate ways to provide sufficient and suitable stimulation to the nerves, we would be able to raise the effectiveness of acupuncture anesthesia.

VETERINARY ELECTROACUPUNCTURE MACHINE CIRCUIT DIAGRAM AND TECHNICAL CHARACTERISTICS

Clinical experience has shown a strong relationship between the effect of electroacupuncture and the functional characteristics of the electroacupuncture machine. After much experimentation and continual improvements, we have produced the veterinary model 71–5 electroacupuncture machine. This machine features high voltages, high frequencies, high adjustability, better effectiveness, simple circuitry, and ease of manufacture.

Technical Characteristics

Frequencies: 2–70 cycles/sec, continuously variable.

Voltages: Bidirectional (both positive and negative) pulse, maximum peak-to-peak voltage drops are 27 volts at a simulated load of 200 ohm, 260 volts at 5000 ohm, and 612 volts at open circuit. The voltage is continuously variable.

Electric consumption: This circuit draws a maximum of 160 milliamperes (ma)

Pulse width: 1 and ½ msec (the negative pulse width)

Circuit Diagram

See Figure 6–5.

Components and Specifications

Component specifications are already noted in the circuit diagram. T_1 is a B_{408} output transformer, T_2 is a 5-watt, tapped transformer made by the Tientsin Red Peak Radio Factory. The secondary of this circuit connects to a 2000-ohm impedance; this can be connected according to the attached instruction booklet (Translator's note: I suspect this refers to the instruction booklet for T_2). The 3AD12 transistor can be replaced with a 3AD30. The power source of 18 volts is from #1 batteries.

Maintenance and Notes

If the output adjustment control is functioning only intermittently, poor contact because of corrosion at the positive terminal of the battery may be the cause. To correct this, prevent dampness, and sand down the positive terminal or the case of the battery.

The 3.3 kilo-ohm potentiometer should be a high-voltage, humidity-resistant, sealed type. Otherwise, this component can be easily damaged, resulting in loss of control over output voltage.

After 8 to 10 uses (of about 3 hours each) in abdominal cavity surgery, if it is found that insufficient excitation is produced, examine the battery to see if the voltage has dropped below 14 volts or has been weakened or become damp. If so, replace with a new battery.

The output voltage is 260 volts, so the output post must not be replaced with the power or earphone

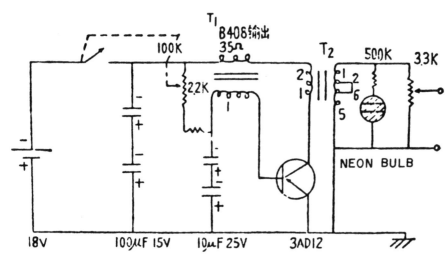

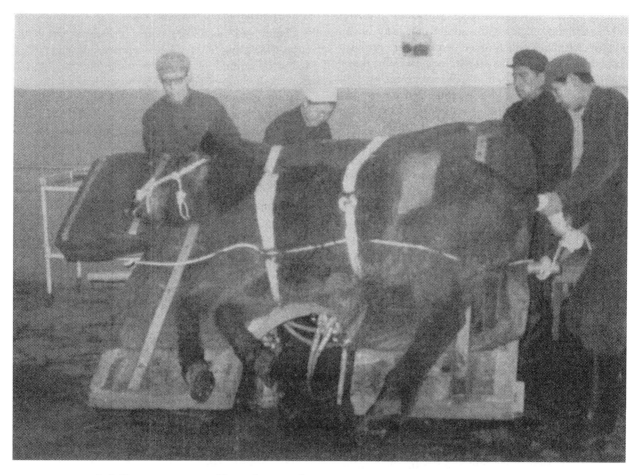

FIGURE 6–5. Circuit diagram of a Chinese veterinary acupuncture electric stimulator.

plugs commonly found in transistor radios. The best choice is probably banana plugs, leading separately to the two terminals, and this is also convenient to use.

In 1975, Dr. O. Kothbauer, a veterinarian, and other health scientists from Austria visited China and saw many demonstrations of acupuncture including surgery (exploratory laparotomy) on a horse, utilizing acupuncture analgesia produced by electrical stimulation of the San Yan Lo Points with a Chinese 71–5 stimulator. Pictures taken by Kothbauer are reproduced in Figures 6–6 to 6–13.

FIGURE 6–6. Demonstration in China: horse tied to operating table. (Courtesy of Dr. O. Kothbauer.)

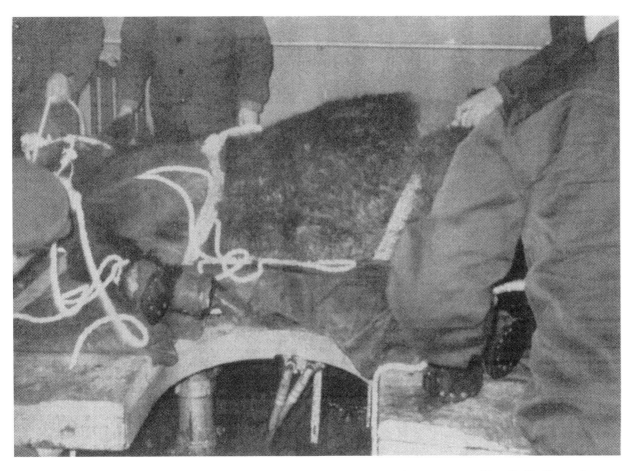

FIGURE 6–7. Demonstration in China: horse tied to operating table. (Courtesy of Dr. O. Kothbauer.)

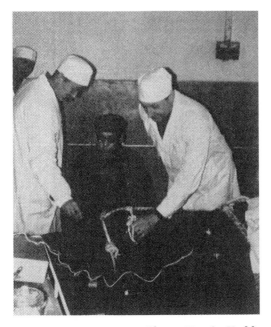

FIGURE 6–8. Demonstration in China: Dr. O. Kothbauer examining horse. (Courtesy of Dr. O. Kothbauer.)

Horse and Donkey Ear Acupuncture Anesthesia[6]

STRUCTURE OF THE EAR (FIGS. 6–14 TO 6–17)

The anatomic description will be based on the position of the ears being an intermediate one—that is, not directed forward or back, but to the lateral side—with the inner surface of the ear facing a lateral direction.

The external ear of the horse and donkey consists of the auricle, which has a medical convex side and a lateral concave side. Three cutaneous ridges are located on the lateral convex surface, which runs parallel to the edges of the ear, but the ridges do not reach the apex. They are called the *rostral, middle,* and *caudal earfolds.* The middle and the caudal ear folds extend slightly ventral to joint at the ear base to form the common earfold. There is also a longitudinal furrow between the middle and the caudal earfold called the *interfold furrow.*

The rostral and the caudal surfaces of the ear join to form the ear margins. They are called, according to their position, the *rostral* and *caudal ear margins.*

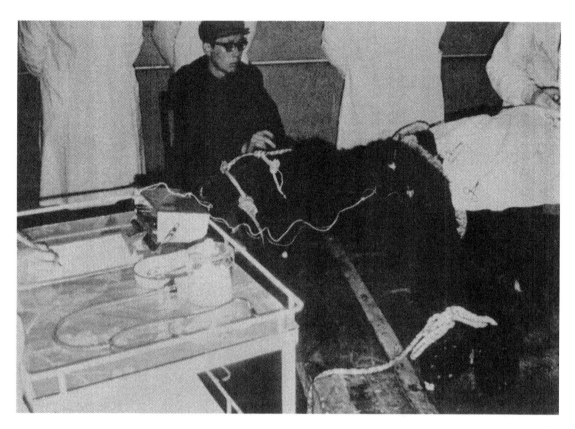

FIGURE 6–9. Demonstration in China: electric stimulator connected to two needles in the foreleg of the horse (FL7 and FL23), and surgery is beginning. (Courtesy of Dr. O. Kothbauer.)

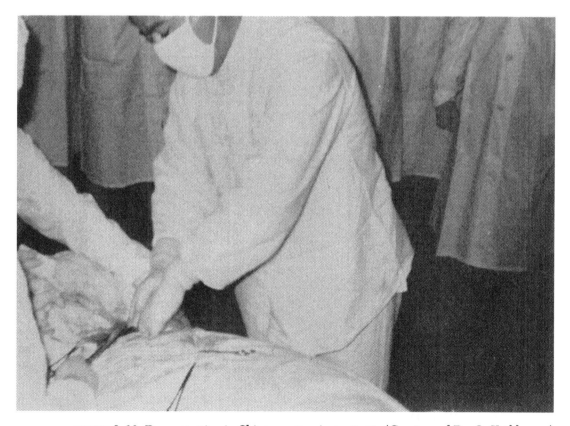

FIGURE 6–10. Demonstration in China: surgery in progress. (Courtesy of Dr. O. Kothbauer.)

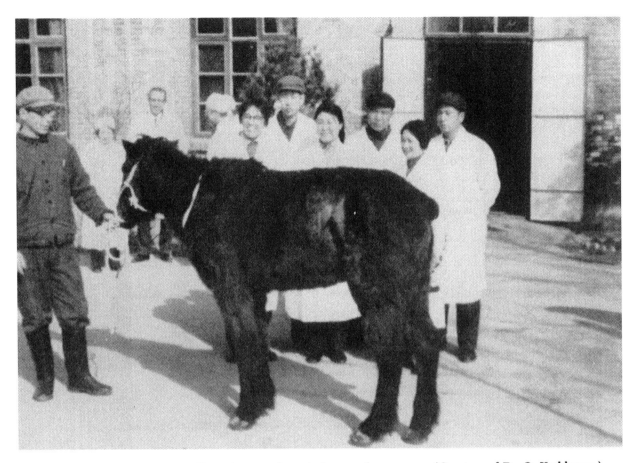

FIGURE 6–11. Demonstration in China: horse and surgical team after surgery. (Courtesy of Dr. O. Kothbauer.)

The dorsal end of the rostral and caudal ear margins join to form the apex. Ventrally, they come together to form the *incisura intertragica*. The rostral ear margin extends downward and branches off into two branches—the *medial* or *base of the middle ear margin* and the *lateral ear margin*. These two bases form a triangular fossa, the *interbase fossa*.

At the lower end of the rostral ear margin, close to the incisura intertragica, there is a small protuberance called the *tragus*. At the lower end of the caudal ear margin, and close to the incisura intertragica, there is another protuberance, the *antitragus*. Straight down below the medial side of the lower fold of the antitragus, there is a horizontal skinfold called the *lower fold of the antitragus*. Lying in between the navicular fossa and the external orifice of the external auditory meatus, it is a funnel-shaped structure along the crus helicis. The longitudinal axis of the funnel is longer than the horizontal axis, and the base is divided by three skinfolds into four shallow fossa. They are called, according to position the *rostral*, *middle*, *caudal*, and *lateral fossae*. The middle fossa is the largest; the caudal, the smallest. The lower end of the lateral fossa is the *external auditory meatus*.

LOCATION OF THE AURICULAR ACUPUNCTURE POINTS (FIGS. 6–14 TO 6–17)

Collective Wisdom (Ch'ing Wei). Located on the rostral margin of the caudal earfold, 3 tsun from the tip of the ear.

Sympathetic (Chiao Chien). At the upper terminal end of the middle earfold.

Heavenly Gate (Shen Men). In the interfold furrow, 3 fen above the bifurcation of the common earfold.

Kidney (Shen). Two fen rostral to the bifurcation of the common earfold.

Abdomen (Fu). At the rostral margin of the point between the upper third and the middle third of the common earfold.

Thorax (Hsiung). At the junction between the lower middle third of the common earfold.

Triple-burner (San Chiao). At the junction of the upper and middle third of the longitudinal axis of the lateral fossa at the orifice of the external auditory meatus.

Lung 1 (Fei 1). At the midpoint of the horizontal line drawn toward the rostral earfold from the junction of the lower and middle third of the base of the middle ear margin.

Lung 2 (Fei 2). At the rostral margin of the lower end of the rostral earfold.

Occiput (Chen). Five fen rostral and 1 tsun below the incisura intertragus.

PROCEDURES FOR ACUPUNCTURE ANALGESIA

Needles

The Chinese number 21 acupuncture needle is used; length varies according to size of the animal and the depth of insertion, usually 10–15 mm inserted into both ears.

Prescriptions

Abdominal surgery—The heavenly gate, lung 1, abdomen, and triple-burner points are used (the triple-burner point may be blocked by 2% procaine). All supplementary points are local acupuncture points at or near the site of surgical incision, and

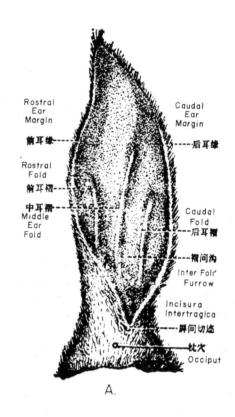

FIGURE 6–12. Anatomy of horse ear.

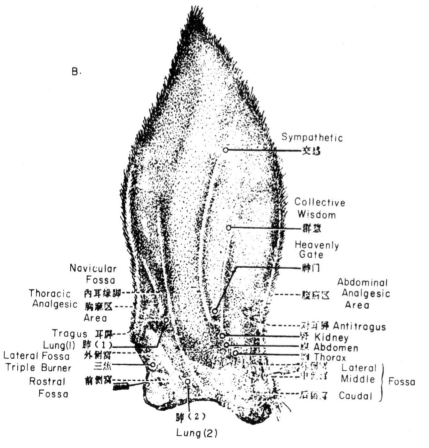

FIGURE 6–13. Acupuncture analgesia points in the ear of the horse.

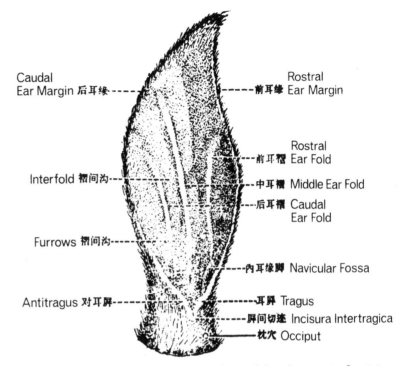

FIGURE 6-14. Anatomy of the mule ear.

Caudal Ear Margin 后耳缘

Rostral Ear Margin 前耳缘

Rostral Ear Fold 前耳褶

Middle Ear Fold 中耳褶

Caudal Ear Fold 后耳褶

Interfold 褶间沟

Furrows 褶间沟

Navicular Fossa 内耳缘脚

Antitragus 对耳屏

Tragus 耳屏

Incisura Intertragica 屏间切迹

Occiput 枕穴

they are commonly used points with high needle sensation. These acupuncture points are marked by an asterisk in the description of acupuncture points (see Chapter Three).

Joint space surgery—The heavenly gate and lung 1 points are used. All supplementary points are local acupuncture points indicated for the particular joint.

Fistula of parotid gland—The heavenly gate and lung 1 points are used, supplemented by electrical or manual stimulation of acupuncture points at and around the site of operation.

Thoracic surgery—The heavenly gate, and lung 1,

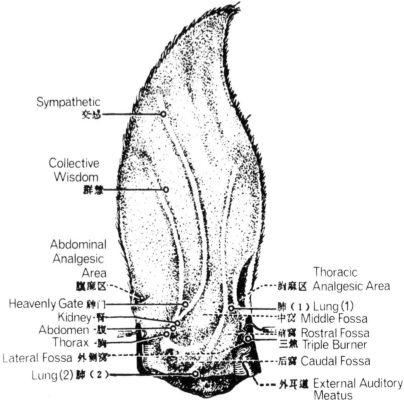

FIGURE 6-15. Acupuncture analgesia points in the ear of the mule.

Sympathetic 交感

Collective Wisdom 群慧

Abdominal Analgesic Area 腹腔区

Heavenly Gate 神门

Kidney 肾

Abdomen 腹

Thorax 胸

Lateral Fossa 外侧窝

Lung (2) 肺 (2)

Thoracic Analgesic Area 胸腔区

Lung (1) 肺 (1)

Middle Fossa 中窝

Rostral Fossa 前窝

Triple Burner 三焦

Caudal Fossa 后窝

External Auditory Meatus 外耳道

and thorax points are used, all supplemented by electrical or manual stimulation of local acupuncture points at the site of the operation.

Reduction of bone fractures of the limbs—The heavenly gate, occiput, and kidney points are used, supplemented by local acupuncture points.

METHODS OF NEEDLE INSERTION

Difficult insertions are done first. The needle is inserted in a slanting direction and is whirled during insertion. The needle should go through the cartilage of the ear but should not pierce through to the other side of the skin. The bony structure may be reached along the base of the crus helicis.

The needle is whirled 150–180 times/min, or electrical stimulation is used as described below.

General induction time is 15–20 min. The needle is whirled at regular time intervals. For heavy induction, 15 min is used for the heavenly gate, lung, and other corresponding points. For example, in abdominal surgery, heavy induction is performed on the ear and abdominal points. After the induction, the operation proceeds. During the operation, the needles are continually whirled to maintain the analgesia until the operation is over.

ELECTRICAL STIMULATION

There are two types of stimulators—the standard type, and the square-wave stimulator. The standard apparatus has an electric potential of 9–12 volts and an effective current of 6–7 ma (maximum of 8–9 ma).

In the square-wave stimulator, the smooth square-wave amplitude is 4 volts and the rough square-wave amplitude is 7.5 volts, both with a frequency of 3.8 times/sec.

During the first few minutes of needle manipulation, there is a slight increase in respiration and pulse rate. They returned to normal 3–5 min later. Pupil dilation then follows. After 20 min of needle whirling, there are signs of excitement and anxiety. Thirty minutes later, respiration becomes deep, pupil size becomes normal, and the lips and eyelids droop. There is a delayed response of the corneal reflex. These signs indicate successful analgesia. At this point, there is a loss of pain sensation, and the operation may proceed.

RESTRAINT

Depending on different surgical sites, different methods of restraint are used. For example, in lower abdominal surgery, scrotal hernia, penis resection, limb and trunk surgery, and resection of the jugular vein, the lateral position may be used. Many procedures may also be done in the horse standing.

ASSESSMENT OF RESULTS

There are no great detectable physiologic changes during surgery using ear analgesia. Sometimes, the heart rate may increase slightly. Ear analgesia acupuncture may be used in both depressive and excitable types of horses and donkeys.

The standards of assessment of results are the same as stated before (see Electroacupuncture Using the San Yan Lo Points in Animals, p. 261).

A CASE HISTORY

The following case history presents abdominal surgery done on a horse using ear acupuncture analgesia. It was performed by a veterinary medical team in Tu P'ung Commune in Lan Chou, February 29, 1971.

History: Male, red horse, four years old, with constipation.

Diagnosis: Lacerated rectum.

Prescription: Lung 1, occiput, and ear root points were used. The deepest depression of the rostral fossa was used as the needling point, one on each side. It was located by pulling the ear flat to expose the rostral and caudal fossae and its bone. Acupuncture points on both ears were used. This prescription, using the ear root point, is an alternative to the standard prescriptions listed on page 6-22.

Method: The animal was adequately restrained. The needle used was number 21 with the appropriate length of 2.5–3 inches. For the ear root point, the needle was inserted perpendicular to the ground until the horny structure was reached. Electrical stimulation was used.

Reaction: During abdominal incision, muscle separation, and peritoneal incisions, the animal remained calm. On manipulation of the intestines, the hindleg flexed three times. The pulse ranged around 52 beats per minute; respiration varied between 12 and 20 breaths per minute. The animal remained calm when the intestine, muscles, and skin were sutured. Duration of the operation was 4½ hours.

Acupuncture Anesthesia
in Various Animals

HORSE

A study in Japan that has repeated the work of the Chinese, wherein analgesia of the trunk of the horse was produced by stimulation of the San Yan Lo Points (FL23, FL24, FL7).[33] The points were stimulated by an electric device that delivered an electrical stimulus at a frequency of 0.5 cycle/sec, 2.5 volts, and 20 ma. The head drooped, the animal salivated, and there were definite analgesic effects on the trunk. No mention was made of the manner in which the electrodes were connected—that is, which were positive and which were negative—or the shape of the waveform. Also there was no description of the method by which analgesia was assessed.

CATTLE

A most important achievement in acupuncture analgesia is the work done by Dr. O. Kothbauer.[38] Some of the work done studying acupuncture analgesia was done in rabbits, and many people question the validity of subjective observations in this species regarding analgesia and immobility during pain production. The use of the cow as an experimental animal is efficacious because cows usually don't relate well to strangers—it is unlikely that a stranger could have a calming or any other positive effect on a cow that would cause it to withstand pain without reacting.

The nipple is very sensitive, quite accessible, and because Kothbauer's veterinary practice for 20 years dealt mainly with cattle, he understood the responses of this species to injections around the nipple (with local anesthetic), and surgery of this area is well known.

The work was done over several years and in several phases. The responses of the cows were graded *no effect, slight analgesia, moderate analgesia,* and *complete analgesia.* These were determined subjectively by observations of the animal's responses to the testing procedure. The three parts of the test were (1) insertion of a large hypodermic needle completely through the nipple; (2) an incision of 4 cm that entered the teat cistern; and (3) suturing the incision. The responses observed were: (1) no response—that is, no change in the normal attitude of the cow; (2) rapid movements; (3) other signs of annoyance; (4) lifting of the hindlegs; (5) kicking; and (6) attempts at escape.

The first trial involved mechanical rotation of needles inserted into conception vessel 17 and liver 14 or 15.

The liver point used was on the same side of the body as the nipple that was used. This produced analgesia for needle insertion into the nipple but not for incision or suturing. The addition of the point liver 2 added analgesia for incision but not suturing.

In the human, point liver 2 is between metatarsal 1 and 2, and stomach 44 is between metatarsal 2 and 3. The metatarsals in the cow are 3 and 4; therefore, it is not clear where the liver and stomach meridians might be in the cow. Kothbauer calls the point liver 2, but it could be stomach 44.

The use of electrical stimulation and bilateral liver points made analgesia production more consistent and better, but there was still response to suturing. Trial 4 was conducted by adding stimulation to bladder 30. This still did not provide analgesia for suturing. Then the waveform was changed, and two more needles were added along the base of the udder. This provided analgesia for suturing of the incision (Fig. 6-18, Table 6-2).

The cows had been restrained with nose leads. To determine whether this method of restraint was producing the lack of response to the procedures, several cows were restrained in this manner and tested for analgesia; there was no analgesia seen. Then acupuncture was performed in the same cows, producing analgesia.

The final trials were done using placebo points, inserting the needles about a handsbreadth from where they should have been placed. No analgesia was produced. Then the needles were put in the proper positions, and analgesia resulted. From this simple but very significant study, it could be concluded that (1) acupuncture analgesia can be produced in the cow; (2) that the analgesia is not due to restraint or hypnotism; and (3) that accurate placement of the needle is important.

Acupuncture analgesia has been produced in the cow, enabling the performance of cesarean sections.[39] The points used were liver 14 and bladder 30 as described previously and in Table 6-2. Stimulation was with the Chinese SB 71–72, frequency set at 180–2400 cycles/min (probably a misprint in the journal and should be 180–240 cycles/min or 3–4 Hz). Voltage was increased until the skin began to twitch. Stimulation was applied for 20 min before surgery began. The site of surgery was the left paralumbar fossa.

DOG

There have been many reports of the production of acupuncture analgesia in dogs.[1, 22, 29, 36, 37, 47, 48, 57, 59] One of these reports says that bilateral placement of needles in ST36 and GB34, with electrical stimulation of an intensity such that localized tetany occurs, will produce analgesia for surgical oophorectomy in dogs after an induction period of 20 minutes.[22]

In another study in the dog, needles were placed bilaterally at TB23, H5, B22, B23, and K6. These needles were not connected to an electrical device but were left alone in position. Analgesia for a test incision (deep, 3-in. surgical incision in the cranial lateral quadrant of the abdomen) was produced in

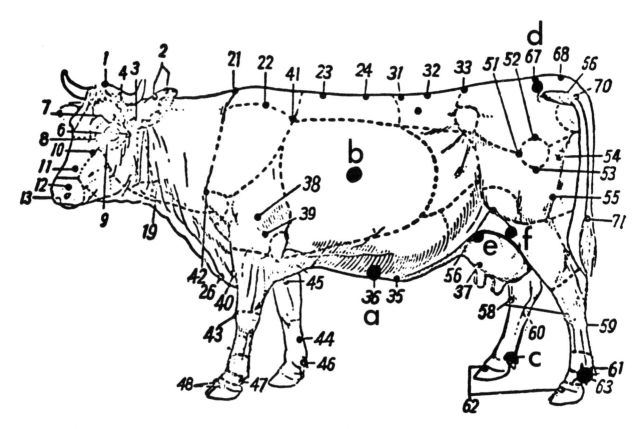

FIGURE 6–16. Acupuncture points for the production of analgesia of the udder teat (a–f). (Courtesy of Dr. O. Kothbauer.)

TABLE 6–2. *Acupuncture Analgesia of the Udder Teat of the Cow*

TRIAL	ACUPUNCTURE POINTS	TYPE OF STIMULATION	RESPONSE		
			TEAR PERFORATION WITH NEEDLE	TEAR INCISION (4 CM)	SUTURING OF INCISION
1	a, b	A	+	0	0
2	a, b, c	A	+	+	0
3	a, b, c	B	+	+	0
4	a, b, c, d	B	+	+	0
5	a, b, c, d, e, f	C	+	+	+
6	x = only restraint with nose leads	—	0	0	0
	y = a, b, c, d, e, f	C	+	+	+
7	x = Placebo points	C	0	0	0
	y = a, b, c, d, e, f	C	+	+	+

a = C17 = on the midline 3 in. cranial to the xyphoid process.
b = LIV14 or 15 = at the level of the shoulder joint between the 8th and 9th ribs.
c = LIV2 = caudal and medial to the medial condyle of the metatarsal bone, cranial to the deep digital flexor (stomach 44?)
d = B30 = above the last sacral foramen about 2½ in. from the midline.
e and f = 2 × 10 cm needles subcutaneously along the base of the udder.

A = Rotation of needles for 1 to 10 min.
B = Electroacupuncture: 8V, 5–6 Hz, for 20 min, rectangular wave form.
C = Electroacupuncture: 8V, 5–6 Hz, for 25 min, sawtooth wave form.

+ = complete analgesia
0 = no effect

(Courtesy of Dr. O. Kothbauer)

all of 20 dogs tested. These dogs received no drugs and did not meet the acupuncturist until the time of the study.[47, 48]

A French group produced acupuncture analgesia by using the points san lang lo and tsiang fong—probably san yan lo (TB8) and ch'ang feng (see Chapter Three, horse FL7, FL23, FL24).[29] They reported performing, in the dog, hysterectomies, femoral head resections, perianal tumor resections, umbilical hernia repair, and fracture repairs, with no adverse pain or other reactions from the dogs.

There are several reports from Japan concerning the production of acupuncture analgesia in the dog.[1, 36, 37, 59] In one study, eight points were electrically stimulated: LI11 and Yanhoudian (?) on one forelimb; H3 and P6 on the other forelimb; ST36 on one hind limb; SP6 on the other hind limb; and between the 3rd and 4th middle foot bones (bilaterally on hind limbs). A bipolar pulse wave was applied having a frequency of 15–50 cycles/sec with 4–6 volts. Some of the dogs were sedated; most were not. Analgesia was produced on the four limbs, and the trunk except for the scrotum, labia, and anus. Muscle tone was increased.[36]

Another Japanese group produced analgesia of the body except for the scrotum, labia, anus, tail, and head by electrical stimulation (4.5–5.5 volts, 2.5–4.5 ma, 15–30 cycles/sec) of LI11 and Yanhoudian(?) on the forelimbs and ST36 and Banggu(?) on the hindlimbs. The negative terminals were connected to LI11 and ST36, and the positive terminals to Yanhoudian and Banggu.[59]

The next report to appear was on the relationship between the area of analgesia produced and the points that are used.[37]

When forelimb points are used the following areas of analgesia are produced: 1) LI11–Yanhoudian combination: analgesia extending upward from the outside of the elbow of the treated limb over and crossing the back of the neck centerline and downward to the outside of the elbow of the untreated limb. The trunk and the abdomen may also be affected; 2) H3–Yanhoudian combination: analgesia extending upward from the outside of the elbow of the treated limb over and crossing the centerline of both the back of the neck and the front of the neck (throat?) and downward to the area around the carpus of the untreated limb; 3) H3–P6 combination: analgesia from the left side and the right side of the neck, extending to the ribs, the abdomen, and the buttock; 4) TB5–Yanhoudian combination: Similar to 3; 5) ch'ang feng–TB8 combination: analgesia of the entire trunk and the four limbs (except the portion of the front limbs beneath the elbows.)

When hind limb points are used the following areas of analgesia are produced: 1) ST36–Banggu combination: analgesia spreading from the outside of both the left and the right hind limbs (except the very tip) to the rear of the body. Occasionally, analgesia is also found on the shoulders; 2) SP6–Banggu combination; analgesia spreading over the thighs and the rear of the body.

When head points are used (two pairs): SP10–TB17 combination: analgesia spreading over all four limbs (except for the very tip) and the entire trunk.

In all the preceding cases, analgesia is not established at the scrotum, the labia, around the anus, and the tail.

The last of this series of reports from Japan also tried to determine the electrical parameters of stimulation, sites of points, and areas of analgesia produced in dogs.[1] The points they used were: the base of the ear, LI4, TB8, B49, SP6, GB20, GV4, LI11, H3, ST36, SP10, and SP9. The voltage varied between 1.5 and 6; the current varied between 3 and 8 ma. The waveform was a transformed square wave, the frequency used was roughly the patient's pulse rate plus 100. After 20 minutes of stimulation, insensitivity to pain was established for all areas other than the head, four limbs, and the tail. Twenty-nine dogs were tested: 10.4% (3) had almost no pain at all; 65.5% (19) had numbness; and 24.1% (7) had no effect.

One group from the United States reported on the successful use of acupuncture analgesia in 15 dogs.[57] The procedures were all abdominal and included such things as overaiohysterectomy, cesarean section, splenectomy, and bowel resection. The points used were ST36 and SP6. A square wave was used to stimulate the points through needles at a frequency of 125 Hz. The periods of stimulation were 2 seconds long followed by a pause of 2 seconds. Analgesia was achieved in 10 minutes.

Acupuncture Analgesia in Man

There have been many reports (written, television, movie) on the use of acupuncture for the production of surgical analgesia in humans. [18, 20–22, 24, 26–28, 30, 46, 49] The most common and dramatic are about thoracic surgery in a patient who is awake and smiling. The patient is not intubated or mechanically ventilated. During surgery, the patient drinks tea or eats orange slices. These reports have stirred much interest in acupuncture, but they have also produced much controversy. The people who thought that acupuncture could not produce analgesia for surgery fell into two main groups—those who said acupuncture analgesia was really hypnotism and those who said that the preoperative medication, which was often given, provided the analgesia. A mystical power has also been attributed to Chairman Mao, and this is said to give the patients the moral strength to withstand the pain from surgery.

It is known that surgery can be performed under hypnotism, but generally a great deal of rehearsing and practicing must be done to be successful.[40] Katz *et al.* concluded that hypnotizability was related to the successful use of acupuncture—that is, patients who are easily hypnotized are more likely to respond positively to acupuncture.[35] There is no question that a positive mental attitude and a great trust in one's physician can influence patients and perhaps even raise their threshold of pain. However, it is unlikely that patients could be convinced to not respond to or feel pain during major surgery. The section on acupuncture analgesia in animals (p. 259) adds weight to the arguments against the pain relief being due to hypnosis or suggestion.

The preanesthetic medication usually reported are low doses of a barbiturate or narcotic analgesic. The narcotic can certainly provide pain relief, but it is not likely to provide analgesia for major surgery in the doses reported.

The production of acupuncture analgesia by western physicians without presurgical analgesics is evidence against political sources for analgesia.

Acupuncture analgesia has been used for surgery from one end of the body to the other, but the most commonly reported and most successful cases have been those of the neck and chest. Success rates have varied from 10 to 100%.

REFERENCES

1. Akamatsu, S., *et al.*, 1974. Acupuncture anesthesia in dogs. Proceedings of the 1974 Japan Clinical Veterinary Conference.
2. Akil, H., and Mayer, D. J. 1972. Antagonism of stimulation-produced analgesia by p-CPA, a serotonin synthesis inhibitor. *Brain Res.* 44:692–97.
3. Akil, H., Mayer, D. J., and Liebesking, J. C. 1972. Psychophysiologie: comparaison chez le rat entre l'analgesie induite par stimulation de la substance grise peri-aqueducale et l'analgesie morphinique *C. R. Acad. Sci. Paris* 274:3603–5.
4. Andersson, S. A., Ericson, T., Holmgren, E., and Lindqvist, G. 1973. Electroacupuncture: Effect on pain threshold measured with electrical stimulation of teeth. *Brain Res.* 63:393–96.
5. Anon. 1972. Electro-acupuncture anesthesia in animals using the San Yan Lo points. Peking Municipal Veterinary Hospital.
6. Anon. 1972. *Chinese veterinary handbook.* Pp. 664–69. Lan Chou Veterinary Research Institute. Gan shu, China: The People's Publishing Co.
7. Anon. 1973. The role of midbrain reticular formation in acupuncture anesthesia. Acupuncture anesthesia

coordinating group of Shanghai College of Traditional Chinese Medicine, Shanghai. *Chinese Med. J.* 3:32.
8. Anon. 1973. The relation between acupuncture analgesia and neurotransmitters in rabbit brain. Acupuncture anesthesia research group. Hunan Medical College, Changsha. *Chinese Med. J.* 8:105.
9. Anon. 1973. Electrophysiologic study of spinal reflexes under acupuncture anesthesia. Acupuncture anesthesia research unit, Hsu Yi County People's Hospital, Hsu Yi County, Kiangsu. *Chinese Med. J.* 3:33.
10. Anon. 1973. Effect of acupuncture on pain threshold of human skin. Research group of acupuncture anesthesia, Peking Medical College, Peking. *Chinese Med. J.* 3:35.
11. Anon. 1973. Acupuncture anesthesia in splenectomy: report of 305 cases. Ch'angshan County People's Hospital, Chiangshan, Chekiang. *Chinese Med. J.* 2:22.
12. Anon. 1973. Acupuncture anesthesia in neurosurgery. Department of anesthesiology, Hsuan Wu Hospital, Peking. *Chinese Med. J.* 2:15.
13. Anon. 1973. Acupuncture anesthesia for operations in shock and critical cases. Department of anesthesiology, Teaching Hospital of Anhwei Medical College, Hofei, Anhwei. *Chinese Med. J.* 2:24.
14. Anon. 1973. Acupuncture anesthesia in pediatric surgery. Department of surgery, Peking Children's Hospital, Peking. *Chinese Med. J.* 2:23.
15. Anon. 1973. Laryngectomy under acupuncture anesthesia. Eye, Ear, Nose and Throat Hospital of Shanghai First Medical College, Shanghai. *Chinese Med. J.* 2:18.
16. Anon. 1973. Observations on analgesic effect of needling *Chuanliao* point in neurosurgery: report of 619 cases. Hua Shan Hospital of Shanghai First Medical College, Shanghai. *Chinese Med. J.* 2:16.
17. Anon. 1973. Acupuncture anesthesia in thyroidectomy. Shanghai First People's Hospital, Shanghai. *Chinese Med. J.* 2:17.
18. Anon. 1973. Pulmonary resections under acupuncture anesthesia. Shanghai First Tuberculosis Hospital, Shanghai. *Chinese Med. J.* 2:19.
19. Anon. 1973. Electrical responses to nocuous stimulation and its inhibition in nucleus centralis lateralis of thalamus in rabbits. Shanghai Institute of Physiology, Shanghai. *Chinese Med. J.* 3:31.
20. Anon. 1973. Acupuncture anesthesia in cardiac surgery. Thoracic section, acupuncture anesthesia group of Second Teaching Hospital of Hunan Medical College, Changsha, Hunan. *Chinese Med. J.* 2:21.
21. Anon. 1973. Acupuncture anesthesia in thoracic surgery: clinical analysis of 818 cases. Section of thoracic surgery of Peking Acupuncture Anesthesia Coordinating Group. *Chinese Med. J.* 2:20.
22. Anon. 1974. Veterinary application of acupuncture anesthesia in small animals. In *Acupuncture Anesthesia Textbook,* International Acupuncture Anesthesia Coordinating Group with W. P. Loh. LaPorte, Ind.: Century Medical Publications.
23. Anon. 1974. *The Principles and Practical Use of Acupuncture Anesthesia.* Hong Kong: Medicine & Health Publishing Co.
24. Anon. 1975. Acupuncture anesthesia: an anesthetic method combining traditional Chinese and western

medicine. Shanghai acupuncture anesthesia coordinating group, Shanghai. *Chinese Med. J.* 1:13–27.

25. Anon. 1975. Acupuncture anesthesia. A translation of a Chinese publication of the same name. U.S. Dept. of Health, Education and Welfare Publication No. (NIH) 75–784.

26. Bonica, J. J. 1974. Acupuncture anesthesia in the People's Republic of China: implications for American medicine. *JAMA* 229:1317–25.

27. Brown, P. E. 1972. Use of acupuncture in major surgery. *Lancet* 1:228.

28. Bull, G. M. 1973. Acupuncture anaesthesia. *Lancet* 2:417–18, 973.

29. Cazieux, A., et al. 1974. Analgesie acupuncturale [Acupunctural analgesia]. (in French, English summary). *Rev. Med. Vet.* 125:1487–89.

30. Chang Ching-tsai, Chu Hsiu-ling, and Yang Lian-fang. 1973. Peripheral afferent pathway for acupuncture analgesia. *Scient. Sinica* 16:210–17.

31. Handwerker, H. O., Iggo, A., and Zimmermann, M. 1975. Segmental and supraspinal actions on dorsal horn neurons responding to noxious and nonnoxious skin stimuli. *Pain* 1:147–65.

32. Hsiang-tung, Chang. 1973. Integrative action of thalamus in the process of acupuncture for analgesia. *Scient. Sinica* 16:25–60.

33. Kameya, T., Ikeda, S., and Watanabe, H. 1974. A survey of acupuncture literature and the analgesic effect in race horses produced by acupuncture of the San Yan Lo group of points. Proc. of the 1974 Japan Clinical Veterinary Conference, Tokyo, Japan.

34. Kane, K., and Taub, A. 1975. A history of local electrical analgesia. *Pain* 1:125–38.

35. Katz, R. L., Kao, C. Y., Spiegel, H., and Katz, G. J. 1974. Pain, acupuncture, hypnosis. *Adv. Neurol.* 4:819–25.

36. Kitazawa, K., et al. 1974. An investigation of electric acupuncture anesthesia, I. Proc. of the 77th Japan Veterinary Conference.

37. Kitazawa, K., et al. 1974. An investigation of electric acupuncture anesthesia, III: relationship between analgesic area and points used, on dogs. Proc. of the 78th Japan Veterinary Conference.

38. Kothbauer, O. 1973. Uber die Analgesierung einer Euterzitze des Rindes mittels Akupunktur. [On producing an analgesic effect in the nipple of the cow's udder with acupuncture]. *Osterreich. Arztezeitung* 18:1037–39.

39. Kothbauer, O. 1975. Ein Kaiserschnitt bei einer Kuh unter Akupunkturanalgesie. [A cesarean section done on a cow under acupuncture analgesia]. *Wien. Tieraerztl. Mschr.* 62:394–96.

40. Kroger, W. S. 1973. The scientific rationale for acupunctural analgesia. *Psychosomatics* 14:191–94.

41. Kross, M. E., et al. 1972. Induction of local electroanesthesia in dogs. *Lab. Animal Sci.* 22:515–17.

42. Liebeskind, J. C., Mayer, D. J., and Akil, H. 1974. Central mechanisms of pain inhibition: studies of analgesia from focal brain stimulation. *Adv. Neurol.* 4:261–68.

43. Lindblom, U., and Meyerson, B. A. 1975. Influence on touch, vibration, and cutaneous pain of dorsal column stimulation in man. *Pain* 1:257–70.

44. Linzer, M., and Van Atta, L. 1974. Effects of acupuncture stimulation on activity of single thalamic neurons in the cat. *Adv. Neurol.* 4:799–811.

45. Long, D. M., and Hagfors, N. 1975. Electrical stimulation in the nervous system: the current status of electrical stimulation of the nervous system for relief of pain. *Pain* 1:109–23.

46. Lowe, W. C. 1973. *Introduction to Acupuncture Anesthesia.* Flushing, N.Y.: Medical Examination Publishing Co.

47. Lynd, F. T. 1975. Animal acupuncture. *Southwest. Vet.* 28:119–21.

48. Lynd, F. T. 1975. Report on acupuncture investigations in animals. Personal communication, May 26.

49. Mann, F. 1974. Acupuncture analgesia: report of 100 experiments. *Brit. J. Anaesth.* 46:361–64.

50. Matsumoto, T. 1974. *Acupuncture for Physicians.* Pp. 101–22, 171–79. Springfield, Ill.: Charles C. Thomas.

51. Mayer, D. J., and Hayes, R. L. 1975. Stimulation-produced analgesia: development of tolerance and cross-tolerance to morphine. *Science* 188:941–43.

52. Mayer, D. J., and Liebeskind, J. C. 1974: Pain reduction by focal electrical stimulation: an anatomical and behavioral analysis. *Brain Res.* 68:73–93.

53. Mayer, D. J., and Murfin, R. 1975. Sites and mechanisms of action of morphine-like analgesics and analgesia produced by focal electrical stimulation of the brain. 6th International Congress of Pharmacology; Helsinki, Finland.

54. Mayer, D. J., Price, D. D., and Rafii, A.: Acupuncture hypalgesia: evidence for activation of a central control system as a mechanism of action. *Proceedings of the 1st World Congress of the Association for the Study of Pain.* New York: Raven Press (in press).

55. Mayer, D. J., Wolfle, T. L., Akil, H., Carder, B., and Liebeskind, J. C. 1971. Analgesia from electrical stimulation in the brainstem of the rat (abstract). *Science* 174:1351–54.

56. Melzack, R. and Wall, P.D. 1965. Pain mechanisms: a new theory. *Science* 150:971–79.

57. O'Boyle, M., and Vajda, G. K. 1975. Acupuncture anesthesia for abdominal surgery. *Mod. Vet. Pract.* 56:705–7.

58. Oliveras, J. L., Redjemi, F., Guilbaud, G., and Besson, J. M. 1975. Analgesia induced by electrical stimulation of the inferior centralis nucleus of the raphe in the cat. *Pain* 1:139–45.

59. Oono, K., et al. 1974. [An investigation of electric acupuncture anesthesia, II: the electrical effect]. Proc. of the 78th Japan Veterinary Conference.

60. Rabischong, P., Niboyet, J. E. H., et al. 1975. Bases experimentales de l'anaglesie acupuncturale. [Experimental basis of acupuncture analgesia]. (In French, English summary). *Nouv. Presse Med.* 4:2021–26.

61. Shealy, C. N., Taslitz, N., et al. 1967. Electrical inhibition of pain: experimental evaluation. *Anesth. Anal.* 46:299–305.

62. Smith, R. H. 1963. *Electrical Anesthesia.* Springfield, Ill.: Charles C. Thomas.

63. Vierck, C. J., Lineberry, C. G., Lee, P. K., and Calderwood, H. W. 1974. Prolonged hypalgesia following acupuncture in monkeys. *Life Sciences* 15:1277–89.

64. Wang, J. K. 1976. Stimulation-produced analgesia. *Mayo Clin. Proc.* 51:28–30.

7

The Present Status
of Veterinary Acupuncture
in the United States
and Canada

In 1971 and 1972, there were many reports published in the United States by people who visited China, about the uses of acupuncture for medical therapy and surgical analgesia.[1-4, 6-9] Since that time, much research has been started, and clinical experience in acupuncture in humans and animals has accumulated.

In January 1973, the California Veterinary Medical Association Committee on Acupuncture met for the first time in Palo Alto, California, to make recommendations to the California Veterinary Medical Association and the Board of Examiners in veterinary medicine regarding what, if any, place acupuncture should have in veterinary medicine.

The conclusion reached at that meeting was that although each member had certain information regarding acupuncture, the committee did not know enough to make recommendations to anyone, and that the committee should recess for three months to gather information. During that meeting, the committee was informed about the work being done at the University of California at Los Angeles under the direction of Dr. David Bressler. Members of the committee exchanged information, including many articles on veterinary acupuncture written in Chinese. Dr. Norman Sax and Dr. Richard Glassberg con-

tacted Bressler at UCLA and proposed a veterinary acupuncture project. Bressler, who was also director of research for the National Acupuncture Association, was excited about the idea and obtained the services of two acupuncturists to work with the veterinarians involved. Dr. Sang Hyuck Shin, a graduate of Dong Yang Oriental Medical College, Korea, and John Ottaviano, who studied for four years with master acupuncturist, Dr. Gim Shek Ju.

An acupuncture chart, obtained from Dr. Wolfgang Jochle, was translated from Chinese to English by Margaret Tan, an acupuncturist working at the University of California at San Francisco Medical School. Dr. Alice De Groot, a veterinarian in Southern California, offered to let the investigators treat some of her equine cases. All the veterinarians involved were quite amazed at the success Shin and Ottaviano had in treating the cases presented to them. Many of the cases had been treated using western therapy with no success, and they were thought to be hopeless. A veterinarian from Covina, California, Dr. Michael Gerry, brought a dog from his practice with long-standing hip dysplasia. The dog responded dramatically to treatment, and Gerry offered to let the project use his office to treat small animals. The group then continued to treat large and small animals referred to them. The project at that time was being carried out under the auspices of the National Acupuncture Association.

As time progressed, a seminar for veterinarians was held at UCLA in March 1974 to bring the profession up to date in veterinary acupuncture.

In 1973, the California Board of Examiners in Veterinary Medicine ruled that acupuncture could be performed by a nonlicensed person only under the direct visual supervision of a licensed veterinarian at a school of veterinary medicine. They further stated that if any grievances were received against a veterinarian practicing acupuncture, they would most likely find the veterinarian guilty of incompetence.

The Board of Examiners informed the veterinarians involved that they could no longer donate the use of their clinics, and that if the project was to continue it would have to do so under the direction of a faculty committee from the University of California Veterinary School at Davis, and in a separate facility for acupuncture only. They also advised that a nonprofit organization with veterinarians on the board of directors would have to be formed to handle any funds involved; thus, the National Association for Veterinary Acupuncture (NAVA) was formed with R. S. Glassberg, DVM, as its first president. While these requirements were being fulfilled, the acupuncture project was halted for several months. Ultimately, the Dean at the University of California School of Veterinary Medicine appointed a faculty committee on acupuncture that was willing to supervise the practitioners involved in the research in Southern California.

An equine/small animal hospital needed to carry on the research became available in Anaheim, California. The facility was leased, and the project resumed in January 1975.

By the summer of 1976, approximately 600 animals had been treated. A review of the first 300 cases showed that approximately 100 animals were cured or markedly improved, 100 showed some improvement, and 100 showed no improvement.[5]

On April 26–28, 1974, a symposium was presented in Kansas City, Missouri, entitled "Acupuncture for the Veterinarian." The responses of the veterinarians who attended were varied. Some were interested; some completely rejected the material. However, many continued their interest and tried to find more information and attempted to treat some animals.

On December 16, 1974, the International Veterinary Acupuncture Society (IVAS) was incorporated in Georgia. Formation of this society was the cul-

mination of the work of many people, but the two driving forces behind it were H. Grady Young, DVM, and Marvin J. Cain, DVM. Young had for some time stimulated interest in veterinary acupuncture and acted as a source of information for veterinarians in the United States. With the formation of IVAS, a series of seminars was set up as a joint venture of IVAS and Dr. Edward C. Wong (APP Technique Seminars, Inc., and Chinese Academy of Medicine). Wong is a sixth-generation acupuncturist, educated in China. He left a lucrative practice in Singapore to emigrate to the USA. Here he was with one of several groups that held acupuncture seminars throughout the country, teaching acupuncture to physicians.

The series of veterinary seminars presented by IVAS and the Chinese Academy of Medicine, beginning on January 30, 1975, were set up as follows. The first seminar lasted four days, and the other four seminars were three days each. They were given at monthly intervals. The first four were held at the College of Medicine, University of Cincinnati, in Ohio. The last seminar was held at the continuing Education Center of the University of Georgia, at Athens. Approximately 50 veterinarians attended the series of seminars. An examination was given at the end of the series and a certificate given to veterinarians who successfully completed the examination, attended 100 hours of the seminars and submitted five acupuncture case reports. A second series was given by the same sponsoring groups and arranged the same way. This series, beginning October 16, 1975, and ending April 1976, was held at the Continuing Education Center, Purdue University, West Lafayette, Indiana. Another series was given in 1977.

IVAS periodically publishes a newsletter containing much information on veterinary acupuncture, including seminar notices, reprints of important recent publications, and copies of some of the papers presented at the seminars. A series of lectures was given by NAVA at the NAVA Clinic in Anaheim, California. It was held one weekend a month for five months beginning October 25, 1975. Since that series, the officers of NAVA changed the format for their seminars to a single three-day course. The NAVA staff printed a compendium that includes the basic concepts of acupuncture, charts, formulas for treatment, and reprints of past NAVA lectures. The compendium provides information on large animals, small animals, and humans, and is sent to participants far in advance of the seminar so it can be read before the seminar.

The professional and government control of acupuncture as a treatment in humans varies from state to state. Most states consider acupuncture the practice of medicine because it always requires a diagnosis and usually involves a needle piercing the skin. Acupuncture may therefore be practiced only by physicians, osteopaths, and in some cases by dentists. Some states require attendance for a certain number of hours and/or the passing of an examination before allowing an individual to practice acupuncture. A few states will allow anyone with credentials of training who can satisfactorily pass an examination to perform acupuncture on individuals who are referred to them by a licensed physician or osteopath with a diagnosis.

In veterinary medicine, the situation has not yet been well-defined. Most states consider acupuncture the practice of veterinary medicine and therefore can only be performed by a veterinarian licensed to practice in that state. Some states have not considered the question of acupuncture. In 1975, a questionnaire was sent to the State Veterinary Medical Associations and the State Veterinary Licensing Board of each state concerning the control and practice of veterinary acupuncture in that state. Twenty-eight of 50 state associations did not respond, nor did 14 of 50 licensing boards.

The American Veterinary Medical Association has two policy statements concerning acupuncture. The first, concerning advertising, was formulated by the Council on Biologic and Therapeutic Agents and approved by the House of Delegates in 1974:

The Council determined that acupuncture is an experimental method of therapy in American veterinary medicine. Acting in its assigned role as advisor to the advertising manager of the Journals, the Council advised that advertisements for acupuncture equipment and instruction are not acceptable.

The principal policy statement was first formulated by the Council on Veterinary Services and approved by the House of Delegates in 1974. This statement was modified and approved by the House of Delegates in 1976:

The AVMA has serious concern about acupuncture, regarding it as entirely experimental until strong evidence is available that the procedure has therapeutic value in animals and additional cases have been evaluated. Experimental controlled studies under the supervision of veterinarians must be conducted in conjunction with cases handled therapeutically.

The public must be protected from those who make claims for acupuncture without adequate controlled experiments or research and the veterinarian must be aware of the legal responsibilities when acupuncture is used.

The administration of an acupuncture needle should be regarded as a surgical procedure under the state veterinary practice acts.

The opinion of the American Veterinary Medical Association Professional Liability Insurance Trust, as of April 1975, on coverage for the use of acupuncture is as follows:

As a professional activity, the use of veterinary acupuncture would be covered under the AVMA Trust's Professional Liability insurance and the veterinarian would be protected if a claim should arise out of the use of this procedure.

The American Association of Equine Practitioners (AAEP), through a committee chaired by Dr. Leonard Gideon, drafted a statement in 1975:

1. The AAEP considers the use of acupuncture as experimental until clinical efficacy has been proven by sound research and clinical investigation.
2. The AAEP recommends that each state support the position of the AVMA on acupuncture:
   a. That it is a part of the practice of veterinary medicine,
   b. That it is experimental and not for widespread use at present, and
   c. That it be regulated by the State's Veterinary Practice Act.
3. The AAEP further recommends that veterinary school personnel, other academic personnel, and practicing veterinarians that are interested in equine acupuncture investigation should identify themselves to a coordinating committee within the AAEP. This would serve to expedite the gathering and evaluation of equine acupuncture information. An annual report would be made to the Executive Board and Association.

The Canadian Veterinary Medical Association's opinion concerning acupuncture in veterinary medicine is as follows: "The subject of acupuncture is a practice matter and would be in the jurisdiction of provincial associations in Canada. The CVMA has not formulated any policies or guidelines relative to this procedure."

Letters sent to the ten provincial associations resulted in seven answers. Alberta, Newfoundland and Labrador, New Brunswick, and Saskatchewan reported that they have no policy or guidelines at this time. Prince Edward Island is revising their Veterinary Act and they may include guidelines on acupuncture.

The Ontario Veterinary Association has considered the question for some time. Its present opinion is that

TABLE 7–1. *Totals, by State, of IVAS-Certified Individuals*

Connecticut	1
Florida	3
Georgia	3
Illinois	11
Indiana	16
Louisiana	2
Massachusetts	1
Michigan	8
Mississippi	1
Missouri	2
Nebraska	1
New York	3
North Carolina	1
Ohio	13
Oklahoma	1
Pennsylvania	3
South Carolina	1
Texas	2
Virginia	2
Wisconsin	1
	76
Ontario, Canada	6
Mexico	1
TOTAL	83

the public and members must be informed about the uncertainty of the value of acupuncture in veterinary science. The Association cautions its members that normal discipline and procedures will be applied including those concerning specialty advertising.

The British Columbia Veterinary Medical Association recently issued (August 19, 1976) the following directive:

DIRECTIVE TO PRACTITIONERS ON ACUPUNCTURE:

It is the opinion of B.C.V.M.A. that Acupuncture is a surgical procedure that is still under investigation. If Veterinarians are using this procedure in their practice the Association feels it is necessary that the Client agree to the use of it after being duly informed and signing a release form suggested by Council. The opinion of Council was reached after both large and small Animal Committees researched the topic and found other Medical and Veterinary groups had reached a similar opinion, the Client form be used until further study has been completed.

Council will strive to inform its Membership of further developments in Veterinary Acupuncture procedures.

The question of who may practice acupuncture is a difficult one. The approaches of the two veterinary acupuncture societies have been different. IVAS requires the successful passing of an examination, the submission of five case reports, and attendance of at least 100 hours at their seminars before receiving a certificate. Eighty-three individuals from the United States, Canada, and Mexico have received a certificate (Table 7–1). NAVA does not offer a certificate at the present time (summer, 1976). The AVMA has no policy statement concerning the training or regulation of individuals administering acupuncture. AAEP considers it part of the practice of veterinary medicine and so is regulated by the States' practice act. Of the states responding to the questionnaire, thirty consider acupuncture the practice of veterinary medicine, and so acupuncture is covered by the State practice act.

REFERENCES

1. Dimond, E. G. 1971. More than herbs and acupuncture. Americans in China, II. *Saturday Review.* Dec. 18.
2. Dimond, E. G. 1971. Acupuncture anesthesia: Western medicine and Chinese traditional medicine. *JAMA* 218:1558–63.
3. Dimond, E. G. 1971. Medical education and care in People's Republic of China. *JAMA* 218:1552–57.
4. Dimond, E. G. 1972. Medicine in the People's Republic of China. *JAMA* 222:1158.
5. Glassberg, R. 1976. Personal communication.
6. Reston, J. 1971. A view from Shanghai. *New York Times.* August 22.
7. Signer, E., and Galston, A. W. 1972. Education and science in China. *Science* 175:15–23.
8. Snow, E. 1971. Report from China, III: Population care and control. *New Republic* 164:20–23.
9. Tkach, W. 1972. A firsthand report from China: "I have seen acupuncture work," says Nixon's doctor. *Today's Health* July, pp. 50–56.

8

The History of Veterinary Acupuncture

Prehistoric Chinese Veterinary Medicine

At the dawn of the Paleolithic society (early part of the 40th to 21st centuries B.C.), the technical knowledge and means for basic acupuncture and moxibustion existed.[15] Weapons and tools made of stones, including flints and small, hard, sharp stones, were in frequent use and may have been used for pain relief, possibly by bloodletting or direct pressure on the skin. The *Nei Ching* (*The Yellow Emperor's Classic of Internal Medicine*), the classic ancient Chinese text of medicine and acupuncture published not later than A.D. 220, mentioned early attempts in acupuncture during this period (Anon., 220). Although fire was also used at this time, there are no written records to indicate the use of moxibustion (see Chapter Three).

The Neolithic period (latter part of the 40th to 21st centuries B.C.) saw an improvement in toolmaking. Archeologic discoveries in North China suggested the use of polished stone, bamboo, bone, and fire. There is no proof that these were used for acupuncture or moxibustion.[15]

If medicine was practiced at all during this period, it was limited to man, and the practice was arbitrary and individualized.

Ancient Chinese Veterinary Medicine

SHANG DYNASTY (C. 1766 B.C. TO 1122 B.C.)

The earliest verified record of Chinese veterinary medicine can be traced to this period. Priests, at this time, were considered to possess healing powers because it was thought that only they could placate what was believed to be the cause of disease—evil spirits. These priests were called "priest doctors" and those that treated animals were called "horse priests."[3] There is no written evidence that acupuncture or moxibustion was used in animals or humans at this time. Excavations at An-Yang in Honan Province between 1922 and 1923 brought to light records in the form of primitive characters on turtle shells and animal bones of a formal body of medical knowledge and a specific class of medical practitioners. Among the 160,000 pieces of turtle shells and animal bones collected, archeologists found the names of thirty-six different diseases. These records also mentioned the healing power of priests and their control of moxibustion-like techniques in their divination practices, which included fortunetelling based on the way bones and shells cracked after being exposed to fire.

As economic productivity and social organization became more stable and more complex, the govern-

281

ment was able to establish a separate Department of Veterinary Medicine.[4]

CHOU DYNASTY (1122 B.C. TO 222 B.C.)

The *Shih Ching (Book of Odes)*, a collection of folk songs and prayers compiled at this time, recorded the interest and observations by the people of their animals.[5]

The earliest recorded doctor of veterinary medicine was Chao Fu. He was identified as an expert in animal diseases and a chariot warrior in legends, classics of history, and in classics of Chinese veterinary medicine at the time of Emperor Mu Huang (947 B.C. to 928 B.C.) of the Chou dynasty.[82]

SPRING AND AUTUMN AND WARRING STATES PERIODS (403 B.C. TO 221 B.C.)

The technologic advances of this period were based on the use of iron, and acupuncture needles of this period were made of iron. The *Nei Ching* recorded, "With the use of the tiny metal needles, poisonous drugs and flints became obsolete."[6]

During this period, compilation of two of the most important Chinese medical text began and with them the development of the philosophic basis of Chinese medical practice.

The *Huang-ti Nei Ching Su Wen* or *Nei Ching (The Yellow Emperor's Classic of Internal Medicine)* is the single most important medical text in traditional Chinese medicine. The exact date of completion is not known; however, it is believed that its compilation began during the Warring States Period. Some supplementary information was added during the Western Han Period. The Book consists of two parts, the Su Wen (Plain Talk) and the Ling Shu (Needle Classic).[8]

The Ling Shu is known as the Book of Acupuncture and Moxibustion, or "The Needle Classic," although acupuncture was extensively covered in the Su Wen. The purpose of the book was "to set standards of acupuncture for the benefit of later generations."[9] The principles and practices of acupuncture as outlined 1000–3000 years ago have not been seriously challenged since (by practitioners of acupuncture). This book holds the prestige of antiquity as well as current scientific interest and has been translated into English.[78] It has survived political changes and revolution, and is a timeless work to which each successive generation has left its mark.

The major contributions of the *Nei Ching* to the practice of acupuncture and moxibustion were: (1)

The establishment of the Meridian Theory: the location, origin and termination points of the twelve "ching," and fifteen "lo" and the "ch'i ching pa mo". (2) The size and shape of each needle, its use, and the methods of manipulation. (3) The determination of the names and locations of the acupuncture points. A total of 365 acupuncture points were described, and the distance between each was measured. (4) The prescription of each of the acupuncture points for a variety of diseases: malaria, paralysis, epilepsy, infectious diseases, fever, and others. (5) The distribution of "forbidden" acupuncture points. These are the points located in anatomic areas in the vicinity of vital organs for which incorrect needle manipulation would result in injury or death.

The *Nan Ching (The Treatise of Difficulties Concepts)*, another text on acupuncture and moxibustion, second only in importance to the *Nei Ching*, was published a little later than the *Nei Ching*. A large portion of its contents were based on the *Nei Ching*. However, a question-and-answer form was used to explain the theory and practice of acupuncture, including the Meridian Theory, acupuncture points, and methods of needle insertion. This book is believed to have been written by Pien Ch'ueh, a physician of the Warring States Period, and it is in existence today in complete form.

By the end of this period, Chinese medicine fully adopted the Yin-Yang Theory, which explained and developed acupuncture techniques. This undermined the authority of priests and enabled the creation of a profession specialized in acupuncture. The theoretic basis of the Yin-Yang Theory (see Chapter One) gave acupuncture a more legitimate and widespread appeal and greatly influenced Chinese veterinary medicine, as evidenced by the widespread acceptance of the theory in Chinese veterinary classics.

Shun Yang, whose other name was Pao Lo, (birth approximately 480 B.C.) was the first full-time practitioner of Chinese veterinary medicine. He is considered the father of Chinese veterinary medicine.[73]

CH'IN AND HAN DYNASTIES (221 B.C. TO A.D. 220)

During the Ch'in and Han Dynasties, medical science flourished because better and more efficient methods of communication facilitated the pooling of knowledge. The first book of pharmacy, *Shen Nung Pen Ts'ao Ching (The Shen Nung Book of Medicinal Herbs)* was completed. Several editions of *Nei Ching* and *Nan Ching* were used as standard textbooks of medicine; however, titles of books on veterinary medicine from this period are known.

The practice of veterinary medicine was verified by archeologic findings in 1930, providing a prescription written on a wood strip in the early Han Dynasty. It showed in detail the kinds of herbs used and the quantities given. Before the invention of paper (A.D. 97), written records were found on wood or bamboo strips that were bound together with strings to serve as a book. These scripts were excavated in the desert area of Kansu Province in western China.[36]

Chang Chung-ching (circa A.D. 140–220), the Hippocrates of China, was the father of differential diagnosis and therapy. In his immortal contribution to medicine, *Shang Han Lun (The Treatise on Typhoid)*, he analyzed cases of fever, distinguished between chronic and acute diseases, tracing out their causes, and laid down methods of treatment and proper prescriptions.

Chang's book contains twelve chapters on acupuncture and seven chapters on moxibustion, and it established a very important principle influencing the practice of Chinese medicine, both human and animal. Acupuncture is to be used for yang type diseases, and moxibustion is to be used for Yin diseases. In modern medical terminology, if the defense mechanism of the body is at its peak, acupuncture is more suitable; if it is functioning at a decline, moxibustion is the choice. This was a general principle and individual conditions were always considered in reaching a diagnosis. Chang indicated what should be expected if the wrong diagnosis and treatment are used. It was also the first book of Chinese medicine to combine the use of herbal medicine and acupuncture in order to achieve a better therapeutic result.

THREE KINGDOMS, CHIN DYNASTY, NORTHERN AND SOUTHERN DYNASTIES (A.D. 220 TO 618); AND T'ANG DYNASTY (A.D. 618 TO 907)

The post-Han, pre-T'ang period (A.D. 220–618) was marked by warfare and power realignments. However, there were several significant developments in acupuncture. Huang-Fu Mi (A.D. 215–282), the author of *Chia I Ching (The Treatise of A, B, C)*, using his own practical experience as a framework, edited the materials from several books available to him, resulting in 12 volumes and 128 sections. His major contributions to the advancement of acupuncture were: the systematic organization of the information into sections on physiology, pathology, diagnosis, and methods of treatment; and the organization and standardization of the various techniques and precautions during needle insertion.

Chia I Ching was the foundation for the development of acupuncture and moxibustion in the T'ang dynasty and had an important influence on the practice of acupuncture in Japan, France, and Korea. Further advances were described in the book *Ch'ien Ching Fang (Golden Prescriptions)* by Sun Ssu Miao (A.D. 590–682). In it was discussed the concept of "tender points". According to this concept, although tender points do not have a permanent location, they are effective points in the treatment of diseases. The diseased organ is associated with physical changes at the tender point (see Chapters Two and Three for changes detectable as electrical resistance. In this book, a very convenient way of measuring the distance between acupuncture points was introduced. The unit of measurement, called the *tsun* (inch), is broken up into tenths, each of which is called a *fen*. The same method, first used in people, was also used in animals (see Chapter Three).

Fragmentary information on veterinary medicine in the pre-T'ang period may be found in books on agriculture and human medicine (Chia, Kao, A.D. 618). According to *Shui Shu Ching Chi Chih (The Bibliography of Treatise and Books in the Shui Dynasty)*, there were nine books specializing in veterinary medicine. These books are not available today. They were: (1) *Liao Ma Fang (Prescriptions for Horses)*, one volume; (2) *Pai Le Chih Ma Jan Pinn Ching (Treatise on Treatment for Sick Horses by Pai Le)*, one volume; (3) *Yu Chi Chih Ma Ching (Treatment of Horses by Yu Chi)*, three volumes; (4) *Chih Ma Ching (Treatment of Horses)*, four volumes; (5) *Chih Ma Ching Mu (Lists of Books on the Treatment of Horses)*, one volume; (6) *Ma Ching K'ung Hsueh T'u (Acupuncture Points and Meridians for Treatment of Horse Diseases)*, one volume; (7) *Jan Chen Ma Ching (Treatise on Horse Disease)*, one volume; (8) *Chih Ma Niu T'o Lu Ching (Various Treatises on the Treatment of Horses, Cattle, Camels and Donkeys)*, three volumes and one-volume index; (9) *Chih Ma Ching (Treatment of Horses)*, three volumes (there was one volume solely devoted to the treatment of diseases of horses using acupuncture).

This period is also one in which many horses were raised for military requirements on the northern front. The T'ang government established a Department of Veterinary Medicine and a School of Veterinary Medicine.[10] This was the first time in China that the practice of and education for veterinary medicine were formalized.

During the closing years of the T'ang dynasty, Li Ssu reviewed the literature on veterinary medicine. He edited *Ssu Mu An Chi Chi (A Collection of Ways to Relieve Suffering Horses)*. This important work provided considerable detail. In the chapter "Chao Fu 81 nan Ching" (81 questions and answers by Chao Fu), 72 serious diseases and 36 etiologies of diseases were classified. This was the earliest work in differential diagnosis in veterinary medicine.

SUNG AND YUAN DYNASTIES (A.D. 960 TO 1368)

During the Sung dynasty (A.D. 960–1279), the government established the Pien Chi Yuan (Office of Collection and Editing). This department edited and corrected the books published before the period. This government was the first to establish the storage of honey and medicine. The federally appointed officials were responsible for the supplies to veterinarians.[11] This was the first drug store for veterinary medicine in China.

At the beginning of the Sung dynasty, *Shih Mu An Ch'i Chi (A Collection of Ways to Relieve Suffering Horses)* had a total of four volumes of basic theory and prescriptions. At the end of the Sung dynasty, this book had eight volumes as a result of incorporation of materials from major publications of the period, as for example, *Fan Mu Chuan Yen Fang (Tested Prescriptions of Nomad Origin)*, edited by Wang Yueh of the northern Sung period; *Huang-ti 81 Wen (81 Questions of Huang-ti)*; and still later, *72 We Han Pin Yuan Ke (72 Etiologies of Evil Diseases)*. Information was taken from various veterinary texts of the period. All these contributed to advances in the diagnosis and treatment of animal diseases.

In the Yuan dynasty (A.D. 1271–1368), K'a Kuan Lou edited *Chuan Chi T'ung Hsien Lun (A Description of the Treatment of Sick Horses)*. This publication is an important work on the diagnosis and treatment of horses.

MING DYNASTY (A.D. 1368 TO 1644)

During the time of the Emperor Chia Ch'ing, the famous veterinarians Yu Pen-Yuan and Yu Pen-Heng, after 60 years of practice, published *Liao Ma Chi (The Treatise on Horses)*. After Ting Ping wrote a preface to this book in 1608, the book was called *Yuan Heng Liao Ma Chi*. This book was not only a collection of the practical experience of the Yu brothers, but a masterpiece synthesizing veterinary medical information through the Ming dynasty. The book is the most widely distributed and the most influential text in the last 300 years of Chinese veterinary medicine. Treatment using acupuncture and herbal medicine outlined in this book forms the basis of modern Chinese veterinary medicine. More than 30 citations of earlier books on veterinary medicine were included. In the Ming dynasty, there were three major publications of veterinary medicine: Yang Shih-Ch'ao edited the *Ma Shu (The Book of Horses)* in 14 volumes, and the *Niu Shu (The Book of Cattle)* in 12 volumes. The government also edited *Lei Fang Ma Ching (Prescriptions for Horses)*. The *Niu Shu* was lost. Only 12 volumes of the *Ma Shu* and Chapters 6 and 7 of *Lei Fang Ma Ching* exist today. These were found in *Shih Mu An Ch'i Chi*, *Yu Ch'i T'ung Hsien Lun*, and *Yuan Heng Liao Ma Chi*. Other citations of earlier dynasties are also found in *Yuan Heng Liao Ma Chi*.

CH'ING DYNASTY (A.D. 1644 TO A.D. 1912)

During the reign of Emperor Ch'ien Lung, Li Tzu Yu re-edited *Yuan Heng Liao Ma Chi*, and Hsu Chiang wrote another preface. The title of the book then became *Yuan Heng Liao Niu Ma T'o Chi (The Treatment of Cattle, Horses, Camels by Yuan and Heng)*. The content and chapters are not the same as those in the Ming edition. In the Ming edition, *Yuan Heng Liao Ma Chi* has four sections entitled, respectively, "Spring," "Summer," "Autumn," and "Winter." It included the following chapters: "On a discussion of the viscera," "Thirty-six postures," "Chao fu 81 nan ching," and "Pai Le songs of cauterization." In the Ch'ing edition, the contents of these sections were enlarged and enriched. However, the twenty-fourth discussion of "Tung Hsi Shu Wen's forty-seven discussions" was deleted. There were other changes in titles and content.

Advances in the diagnosis and treatment of cattle diseases were made. In 1800, Fu Shu Feng wrote *Yang Ken Chi (A Record of Feeding and Ploughing)*, a representative publication of the period. During the years of the Ch'ing dynasty, pig diseases became epidemic. *Chu Ching Ta Ch'uan (A Complete Collection of Pig Diseases)*, in 1900, contained the diagnosis and treatment of pig diseases and had 63 examples of complete prescriptions.

The Modern Development of Chinese Veterinary Medicine

During the final years of the Ch'ing dynasty and the early years of the Republic, there was no opportunity for formal training in medicine, nor government policy regarding the standard of the practice.

In 1917, the first School for Chinese Medicine patterned after western models was established in Shanghai. It was privately financed and was the first school of its kind to offer a formal program leading to a diploma and a license in Chinese medicine. At the same time, Chinese veterinary medicine was not integrated into any formal structure. Instead, there were western-style schools leading to a degree in veterinary medicine. However, in 1956, there were 159,000 practitioners of Chinese veterinary medicine providing essential services in rural China, where 90% of the population was concentrated.[81]

The modern Chinese Government policy on Chinese veterinary medicine was formulated in 1944, when Mao Tse-Tung wrote, ". . . if the modern practitioners of human and veterinary medicine do not unite with the more than one thousand traditional practitioners in this region and help them progress in knowledge and ability, they are in fact helping evil and letting many humans and animals die of diseases."[56] At this time, wartime conditions prevented the formal implementation of this directive, so that it was the graduates of schools of veterinary medicine from Universities in the north that implemented it. They trained personnel in veterinary medicine and learned acupuncture and moxibustion themselves.

In March 1947, the School of Agriculture of the Northern University was established; the section of veterinary medicine of the School was devoted to the development of Chinese veterinary medicine.[16] This was the beginning of modern Chinese veterinary medicine in China.

In 1955, Kim Chung-Tze published *Hsing Yue Ma Ching (New Treatise on Horses and Cattle)*. It was based on *Yuen Heng Liao Ma Chi*, and was the first book of Chinese veterinary medicine to use modern veterinary terminology.[47]

In January 1956, the government issued the official policy on veterinary medicine, emphasizing the development of Chinese veterinary medicine. In September of the same year, the Department of Agriculture sponsored the First National Conference of Chinese Veterinary Medicine in Peking. At this conference, the experience and knowledge of most of the well-known practitioners of Chinese veterinary medicine in the country were brought together. Many research projects were initiated. Two journals started publication in the same year. They were: *Chung-kuo Shou-i-hsueh Tsa-chih (Chinese Journal of Veterinary Medi-*

cine) and *Hsu-mu and Shou-i (Herdsmen and Veterinary Medicine)*.

Two years later, from June 25 to July 4, 1958, the Chinese Academy of Agriculture sponsored the first National Research Conference of Chinese Veterinary Medicine in Lanchow. This was also the occasion marking the founding of the Research Institute of Chinese Veterinary Medicine in Lanchow. The 74 participants represented 37 independent institutes throughout China. Those identified were: 7 research institutes, 5 schools of veterinary medicine, 2 provincial veterinary medicine continued education centers, 12 provincial veterinary medicine clinics, and 2 county hospitals of veterinary medicine.

Proceedings of the meeting reported the use of Chinese veterinary medicine in treating 110 animal disorders; acupuncture was used in 39 of these. Furthermore, a three-year plan was drafted and won the endorsement of the participants. The goals of the three-year plan were:

1. Publication of a book on Chinese veterinary medicine.

2. Publication of a book on the herbal medications used in Chinese veterinary medicine.

3. A review of the methods for castration of fowl and other domestic animals.

4. A study of the therapeutic efficacy of treating various diseases using Chinese veterinary medicine.

5. Publication and editing of the various ancient classics of Chinese veterinary medicine.

6. Study of the history of Chinese veterinary medicine.

According to the record, there are more than 70 classics of Chinese veterinary medicine. However, only 16 were found to be in existence in 1958. To re-edit these medical classics for publication, seven research units were assigned. The seven institutions are: Peking University of Agriculture, Nanking College of Agriculture, Nanking Research Institute of History of Agriculture, Nanking University of Agriculture, Sze-Chuen Institute of Agriculture, Chiang-si Institute of Chinese Veterinary Medicine, and Kim-su Herdsman Institute. A classic of Chinese veterinary medicine published in Japan, the *Liao Ma Hsin Lun (New Treatise of Treating Horses)* and another one from Korea, *Hsin Pien Char Shing Ma Niu Yi Fang (New Collections of Prescriptions for Horses and Cattles)* were also studied.[17]

The two journals, the *Chung-kuo Shou-i-hsueh Tsa-chih* and *Hsu-mu and Shou-i*, have many articles on the history of Chinese veterinary medicine and the theory and diagnosis in Chinese veterinary medicine for the period 1956–1958. The results of many scientific studies were first reported in the First National Conference of Chinese Veterinary Medicine in 1958. At least eight of these reports were published in the two journals in 1959.

The Hei-lung-ch'iang Domestic Animal Sanitary Institute reported a study on disorders treated using acupuncture with good results. These disorders included paralysis of the intestine, paralysis of the neck muscle secondary to rheumatism, rheumatism affecting the musculoskeletal system, encephalitis, abrasion and soft tissue injury, arthritis, keratitis, postpartum paralysis, and bronchitis.[17] Another group reported on the efficacy of treatment in 616 cases of diseases of domestic animals by using electroacupuncture. The study was performed over a period of 3 years. The disorders treated included crippling, facial nerve palsy, diaphragmatic spasm, overwork, epilepsy, paralysis of the penis, paralysis of the bladder, nerve paralysis of other etiologies, induced labor, and tetanus.[33] Several others reported on treatment of viral pneumonia and rheumatism by using acupuncture or a combination of acupuncture and other methods.[18, 34, 35, 44, 54, 68, 71]

This was a period when the ancient methods were systematically collected and edited. The methods were then used and their efficacy examined. Methods having good therapeutic efficacy were then used in practice. This was therefore a period of modification and standardization of the practice of Chinese veterinary medicine. Furthermore, the Schools of Veterinary Medicine in the Institute of Agriculture in the Universities have their students trained in both Chinese and Western methods of veterinary medicine.[17] This period was then followed by the development of new applications of acupuncture—for example, acupuncture anesthesia.

Acupuncture anesthesia was first developed in humans in 1958, and was first applied in horses and donkeys in 1969. Both body points and auricular points were developed for large animals.[27] Furthermore, scientific experiments using dogs, cats, and other small animals showed the effectiveness of some acupuncture points in acupuncture anesthesia.[50] Chinese veterinary medicine in China has never developed a small-animal practice. The demand of the public for the treatment of pets is insignificant because of cultural differences between East and West. However, acupuncture treatment of wild birds and wild animals has been recorded in veterinary classics, and acupuncture treatment of domestic fowl is widely practiced today.[19, 81]

From 1959 to 1972, many books on Chinese veterinary medicine were published.[20–25, 82] In 1972, the Lanchow Institute of Veterinary Medicine edited the book *Shou-i Shou-chai (Handbook of Veterinary Medicine)*, the first book published in China in which Western and Chinese methods of veterinary medicine were combined. This is expected to be the book used by students of veterinary medicine in China for the decade to come. Textbooks for schools of medicine and other technical colleges are re-edited in China once every 10–15 years.

Veterinary Acupuncture Outside China

JAPAN AND KOREA

There have been many periods of exchange between Japan, Korea, and China, including some specific ones involving veterinary medicine, which probably included acupuncture. During the reign of Empress Jingu-Kogo (202 B.C.), Chinese religion, literature, art, and domestic animals were brought to Japan. The fiftieth emperor of Japan (482–507) sent Kuwajima Nakakami to China to learn veterinary medicine; on his return, Nakakami taught the subject.[42] During the reign of the 33rd emperor of Japan (598–628), a priest who trained veterinary officers emigrated from Korea to Japan.

Chinese medicine had been introduced into Korea as early as the Chou dynasty (1111–249 B.C.). The art of acupuncture found its way into Japan by way of Korea during the period 531–571, which coincided with the introduction of Buddhism. Subsequently, more than 17 scholarly delegations were sent to Korea and China; these have had a great effect on incorporating acupuncture as part of medical practice in Japan. The subsequent prosperity of Buddhism had much to do with the popularization of Chinese medicine among the Japanese. In the Heian period (794–1198) particularly, many famous Japanese physicians utilized traditional Chinese medicine and acupuncture. During that time, Tamba Yasuyori, a doctor and acupuncturist, wrote the oldest Japanese medical treatise *Ishimpo (The Spirit of Medicine)*.

The subsequent rise of Zen Buddhism in Japan paved the way for further interchange between noted Chinese scholars and Japanese priest-scholars. As a result, some of the Japanese priests rendered great services as men of medicine. The native medicine in the Kamakura period (1199–1339) drew chiefly upon the Chinese medicine of the Sung dynasty. Acupuncture was given official support in the Tokugawa period (1611–1867). A school was established by

Tokugawa Tsunayoshi, the fifth shogun, who at the same time encouraged the popularization of acupuncture by appointing Dr. Sugiyama Waichi in charge. At one time there were as many as 45 acupuncture schools in Yedo (now Tokyo) alone. During this period, Sugiyama Waichi devised the steel-tube acupuncture instrument still in common use in Japan.[28]

Several very old Japanese books describe the ancient art of Chinese veterinary medicine:

Kuna-Ankishu (Notes on Hippology), in six volumes, was written by Dohaso in 1604 (Yedo). Volume I contained (a) 81 questions by Kotei (Chinese emperor, ca. 3000 B.C.) on horse diseases; and (b) Chinese prophylaxis. Volume II contained (c) studies of the exterior of the horse; and (d) 81 problems dealing with treating equine diseases, by Sofu (Chinese hippologist, ca. 300 B.C.). Volume III contained (e) 72 poems on the art of recognizing diseases in horses through examining their sweat; and (f) the pulse theory. Volume IV contained (g) Hakuraku's methods of acupuncture; and (h) 36 questions from Kotei on the origin of diseases. Volume V: (i) prophylaxis according to seasons. Volume VI: (k) special pathology and therapy of the horse; and (l) pharmacology.

Ryoyaku-ba-ryu-benkai (Selected Medical Methods for Treating Diseased Horses) by Zisanshi: 1st Edition, Kyoto, 1759; 2nd Edition, Yedo, 1859. The work contains five fragments: (1) general hippology, (b) exterior of the horse, (c) theories of medical treatment, (d) physiology of the horse, and (e) specifics concerning various diseases of the horse, with selected prescriptions.

Both these sets contained information on animal acupuncture and charts locating acupuncture points. *Kuna-Ankishu* contains an illustration of the horse with single points for maximal influence on diseased organ functions.

There is an older Japanese book—*Bakyo Taizen (A Complete Collection of Equine Classics)*, after the Latter Daigo Emperor, 1339—purported to contain information on meridians in the horse.[45, 64] This same title was known in China—*Ma Ching Ta Ch'uan (A Complete Collection of Eqyine Classics)*—during the Yuan dynasty 1271–1368, but was lost. It was reimported from Japan after World War II. During the 19th and first half of the 20th centuries, Japanese medicine, human and veterinary, was largely influenced by Europe and America.

Since the late 1950's, interest in acupuncture has risen again in Japan. Some present-day investigators include Dr. Yoshio Nogahama, Chiba University

School of Medicine; Dr. Masao Maruyama, Showa University School of Medicine; Dr. Yoshio Manaka, Kyoto University School of Medicine, who founded a very formal branch of acupuncture based on ryodoraku in 1953 (see p. 22). Dr. Meiyu Okada runs the Meishin School, which furnishes clinical training in acupuncture and moxibustion. When Okada served in the military (1943–1945), he was in the Asahikawa Transport Corps. During this time, he had the opportunity to study horses and subsequently wrote his *Distribution of Keiraku (meridians) Branches in the Horse*. Okada has published an acupuncture chart of the horse (see p. 134). Further impetus was added to the study of acupuncture by the shortage of drugs during the war.[28]

In 1974, Dr. Masayashi Kirisawa, a veterinarian who runs an equine clinic in Tokyo, came to the USA and reported the following: He uses acupuncture on about 50 racehorses a day. Inflammation and rigidity of the muscles of the neck and shoulder can incapacitate a horse, and it is for these conditions that he uses needle acupuncture. Another form of horse acupuncture is done with bigger, knifelike needles, used to produce bleeding (exhausted horses accumulate "bad blood", and purging restores their health).[51]

At present in Japan, there are several people pursuing the study of acupuncture in animals. Dr. R. Nakamura has written a book on therapeutics in veterinary medicine, and in it is a chapter on acupuncture and moxibustion.[62] This is the only Japanese veterinary book containing information on this subject. Nakamura is also doing research on adapting the methods of ryodoraku to dogs.[63]

There have been several reports from Japan during the last few years on veterinary acupuncture primarily related to surgical analgesia.[1, 2, 45, 48, 49, 63, 66, 72] The Society of Japanese Veterinary Anesthesiology is an organization with more than 600 members that publishes the *Japanese Journal of Veterinary Anesthesiology* and holds several seminars a year; the President is Dr. H. Kimata. This society has recently established a Veterinary Acupuncture Committee, and Dr. T. Kita is the chairman.[75]

There have been about five reports on the efficacy of moxibustion in dogs, cattle, and a goat since 1949.[63]

FRANCE

Jesuits led by Matteo Ricci went to Macao in 1582; Chao Ch'ing, Kuantung Province in December 1582; and Peking in 1600. This established the first communication between China and the West. The first work in a European language on acupuncture was by the Jesuit P. P. Harvieu, published in 1671. France became a stronghold of acupuncture. It was recognized and sponsored by distinguished French physicians such as Rene T. H. Laennec (1781–1826), the inventor of the stethoscope: Pierre Bretonneau (1771–1862), the first descriptions of typhoid fever; and Bretonneau's pupil, Armand Trousseau (1801–1867). The leading French anatomist of his time, Jules-Germain Cloquet (1790–1883) was a practicing acupuncturist. Acupuncture became even more prevalent in France in 1927, when Georges Soulie de Morant, who was French consul at Shanghai for 20 years, returned to Paris. He had become a master *acuponcteur* and with the backing of Dr. Paul Ferreyrolles, the chief of staff of the Hospital Bichat, wrote a book on acupuncture.[31, 72]

France's involvement in Indochina again presented acupuncture and spawned interest in its application in veterinary medicine.

The first mention made of acupuncture in the French veterinary literature was in 1836.[14, 58] It describes a case of a paraplegic, feverish ox treated by the implantation of 30 needles, 3 in. long, in two rows, to the right and left of the lumbar spine. These needles were driven in with the aid of a mallet and left in place 48 hours.

An army veterinarian published information showing how acupuncture theory could be used as a diagnostic aid in treating diseases of the horse—for example, ". . . the injection in the pastern causes, in normal horses, a normal reflex, and that the latter is exaggerated at the left in gastrics and at the right in cardiacs. These phenomena are caused by an irradiation in the brachial plexus, of the visceral irritation, and advises, at the time of limpings which are not improved by local cocainization, taking action by treating the viscera."[58, 69, 70] In 1943, M. and C. Lavergne, in their Abstract of Acupuncture, cited cures for lameness in animals through the application of needles.[58] Five theses on veterinary acupuncture have been written at the National Veterinary School in Alfort, France, during the 1950's and 1960's.[30, 53, 57, 61, 77]

Several papers have been published by French authors on this subject in French and German publications.[58-60] Milin came to the United States and lectured on veterinary acupuncture at a seminar presented by the International Veterinary Acupuncture Society in 1976.

AUSTRIA

Some of the stepping stones of the advancement of acupuncture in the western world have come from Austria. One of the major forces in that country is the Ludwig Boltzmann Acupuncture Institute and its head, Dr. Johannes Bischko. The Institute is a non-profit organization supported by a private foundation, the Ludwig Boltzmann Society, which also supports approximately 35 other Ludwig Boltzmann institutes with a wide range of medical interest, including leukemia, neurochemistry, experimental surgery, and veterinary endocrinology. The Acupuncture Institute has a team of members, all working on a voluntary basis, who either work at the out-patient clinics of the Policlinic Hospital of the City of Vienna or at their own hospitals or institutes, carrying out research in the frame of their specific fields, such as obstetrics, gynecology, dentistry, and anesthesiology. The institute also trains doctors.

As acupuncture is a recognized medical method of treatment in Austria, the city-run Policlinic Hospital provides an out-patient clinic in which the patients are treated by the institute's members free of charge under a socialized medical system. They treat approximately 65 patients per morning in the out-patient clinic, and are always completely scheduled many months in advance.

Their patients are treated for the most diverse illnesses. In the out-patient clinic, they perform therapeutic acupuncture only, including special forms such as ear or scalp acupuncture. Surgery with acupuncture analgesia is performed at the Institute of Anesthesiology of the University of Vienna. Tooth extractions with acupuncture analgesia are performed in the Dental Department of the Policlinic.

Through courses and practical training in the adjoining out-patient clinic of the Policlinic, 1000 physicians were taught acupuncture, some with intensive, specific training. These physicians were the founders of specialist clinics in various university clinics and hospitals in Austria and other countries. Through this, a network of scientifically recognized associates comprising practically all medical and veterinary fields was formed, making the Ludwig Boltzmann Acupuncture Institute a center for information on acupuncture in the Western world today.

Two veterinarians, Dr. Oswald Kothbauer (large animals) and Dr. Ferdinand Brunner (small animals), are members of the institute. Both carry out their research in their private offices. Kothbauer, a private practitioner (primarily a cattle practice) in the little town of Grieskirchen, Austria, is one of the few veterinarians in the western world who has been involved with animal acupuncture for the past 20 years. He has written at least 11 scientific publications on the subject and has significantly advanced animal acupuncture in several ways. First was his work utilizing acupuncture to accurately localize diseased organs in the cow. He was the first person in the western world to produce acupuncture analgesia in the cow and published information on this in 1973 (see p. 271), and he produced a movie of those studies. Kothbauer significantly increased interest in animal acupuncture in the United States during trips there in 1974 and 1975. He lectured at the International Acupuncture Congress in 1974 and at seminars of the International Veterinary Acupuncture Society and the National Acupuncture Veterinary Association in 1975 and 1976.

Dr. Bischko, the head of the Institute, is one of the most influential proponents of acupuncture in the world today. He studied in Vienna, receiving his MD degree in 1947, and he has been interested in acupuncture since the early 1950s. After his training in Paris, he was in close contact with related departments in Germany (Munich, Dr. Bachmann).

In 1958, Bischko began a small out-patient clinic in the Policlinic Hospital of the City of Vienna in the ear, nose, and throat department (Head. Professor E. H. Majer, MD), which was especially helpful in therapy-resistant cases, and rapidly expanded.

On March 6, 1972, the first complete acupuncture analgesia for a tonsillectomy in the western world was performed by Bischko in that department. This operation was the breakthrough for acupuncture, not only in Austria, but also probably in the entire western world.

On July 1, 1972, Bischko was appointed by the Ludwig Boltzmann Society to found an acupuncture institute, which has since involved an ever-increasing number of scientists and physicians who wish to learn and study this method.

Closely connected with the Ludwig Boltzmann Acupuncture Institute is the Austrian Acupuncture and Auricular Therapy Society, also a nonprofit organization with more than 400 members. The society sponsors courses given by members of the Ludwig Boltzmann Acupuncture Institute, and supplies its members with the newest reprints of published articles written by institute members and course calendars. This society was formed in 1953, and Bischko has been president since then.

GREAT BRITAIN

Acupuncture was introduced into England on February 18, 1821, when Edward Jukes, a surgeon-accoucheur to the Westminster Medical Institution,

applied the needles to a Mr. Scott, who suffered from severe pains in the loins.[31]

The following quotation was taken from a British Veterinary Journal published in 1828:[13]

On the whole, these experiments have been very unsatisfactory. One case of chorea in the dog was cured by acupuncturation, and another relieved. The attempt to reduce a schirrous testicle utterly failed. Two cases of supposed rheumatism were cured, but not in short a time as that in which we generally succeed in removing a rheumatic affection by other means. In strain of the extensor muscles of the forearm, M.C. laboured hard for nearly three months, and, although, at last, the lameness was removed, the cure is to be traced to the state of rest in which the animal was suffered to remain so long, more than to the influence of the needles. In paralysis of the hinder extremities, acupuncturation was totally useless.

From so few facts, however, we cannot draw any satisfactory conclusion. Two things, however, are sufficiently evident, that the sudden and magical relief which the human being has sometimes experienced has not been seen in the horse; and that, probably form the thickness of the integument, the animals suffered extreme torture during the insertion of the needles.

In 1822 and 1828, two books were written by J. M. Churchill describing some history and case histories of patients treated by acupuncture.[38, 39] From these books the following quotes were taken.

Nearly five years have elapsed since I published my little Treatise on Acupuncturation: in which will be found the following passage, "It remains for the medical profession to ascertain its claims to attention by the test of experience, and having undergone the ordeal of experimental enquiry, it, I have no doubt, so fully develope its merits, as to obtain a conspicuous rank in medical estimation, as a valuable curative measure."

Without the fostering care of a great name, my prophecy has been verified, and acupuncture is now employed, not only in the Eastern Hemisphere, in France, and in America, but throughout the British dominions, and in our London hospitals, under the auspices of men, who stand deservedly high in the ranks of literature and science.

Novelties in the curative art, are generally received in opposite extremes; some espousing them in the warmest manner, with, or without, the requisite knowledge, while others are satisfied with their present attainments, and purse the even tenour of their way, without tormenting themselves by the acquirement of further information. Thus, it has been with the subject under consideration, for while many have never practised it, others have expected too much from it, and after a few indiscriminate trials, have abandoned it as useless. But I am happy to produce confirmation of its magical powers, from the pens of men, whose veracity and disinterestedness cannot be doubted. For the part I took in advancing the practice, I have been assailed by some with unmerited abuse, while others have pitied me as a visionary, and considered the relief ascribed to it, to be the result of mental influence over the corporeal sufferings of those, whose understandings are weak.

William Morgan, a young man in the employment of a timber merchant, felt a violent pain suddenly attack the loins whilst in the act of lifting a very heavy piece of mahogany. The weight fell from his hands, and he found he was incapable of raising himself. He was immediately cupped and blistered on the part; but two days had passed and he was still labouring under considerable pain, augmented violently by every motion of the body. On the third day the operation of Acupuncturation (by a needle of an inch and a half in length) was performed upon the part of the loins pointed out as the seat of the injury, which, as in the former case, dissipated the pains in five or six minutes, and restored the motions of the back. He returned, however, the next day, with the same symptoms at first, but in a mitigated degree. A needle was now passed to the depth of an inch on each side of the spine, which, as I expected, terminated the disease in a few minutes, and it was with pleasure that I understood the next morning, that the man had gone to his usual employment.

Another report from 1858 contains an interesting quote:[80]

Acupuncture is a remedy that seems to have its floods and ebbs in public estimation; for we see it much belauded in medical writings every ten years or so, even to its recommendation in neuralgia of the heart, and then it again sinks into neglect or oblivion; and it is not unlikely that its disuse may be occasioned partly by fear of the pain, and partly by the difficulty the patient finds so trifling an operation can produce such powerful effects. Another reason for its neglect may be, that, like every other remedy, it fails occasionally, and the practitioner, disgusted at having persuaded his patient to submit to a pain, which, though slight, has been attended with no benefit, will not again undergo such a disappointment. However this may be, its use is not as frequent as it deserves; and now that we know the rationale of its operation, I venture to bring forward a few cases in illustration of its remedial powers, in order that others may be induced to give it a more extensive trial, and thus ascertain its true value in the treatment of neuralgia or rheumatic pains.

CASE I. A middle aged labourer came to me with a chronic rheumatism of the parts about the right shoulder, particularly in the deltoid, which was so painful that he could not raise his arm horizontally. I inserted two needles into the muscle, one just below the head of the huemrus, and the other near the insertion of the muscle, and in about a quarter of an hour he could lay his hand

on his head, and in a few days was suite well, without a second operation.

CASE II. An elderly labourer, suffering from rheumatic pain and stiffness of the rectus and other muscles in front of the right thigh, so that he dragged the limb in walking, was enabled to walk without much limping, after the insertion of three needles down the front of the thigh for a period of twenty minutes; and he required no further treatment.

CASE III. An old clergyman, very liable to sciatica, having been advised to try acupuncture, was in the habit of using daily, previous to dressing himself, two or three needles inserted along the course of the nerve, to enable him to walk down stairs with comfort.

CASE IV. A lady of middle age, suffering so much from lumbago and sciatica, that she could not rise from her chair without assistance, after trying hip baths and mustard poultices in vain, was induced to apply the needles to the most painful parts, when, to her astonishment, the pain was much relieved, and after three applications, was entirely removed.

Britain continued to maintain an interest in acupuncture and one of the most prolific authors on the subject, in English, is Felix Mann. There are also several British veterinarians interested in the subject at the present time.

UNITED STATES AND CANADA

Acupuncture had apparently slipped across the Atlantic and began to appear in medical publications in the early 19th century.

The first written report may have been a review of the British booklet written by J. M. Churchill, *Treatise on Acupuncturation.*[12] In 1825, Francklin Bache, translated and published Morand's "Memoir on Acupuncture."[61] In 1829, there was a three-page section in a surgery textbook on acupuncture and electropuncturation.[76] Other articles continued to appear and then during the second half of the 19th century there were very few articles on acupuncture.[32]

References to the use of acupuncture as therapy appeared in two standard textbooks of human medicine in the early 20th century.[41, 67]

From Sir William Osler, ". . . for lumbago acupuncture is, in acute cases, the most efficient treatment. Needles of from 3–4 inches in length (ordinary bonnet needles, sterilized, will do) are thrust into the lumbar muscles at the seat of the pain, and withdrawn after 5–10 minutes. In many instances, the relief is immediate, and I can corroborate fully the statements of Ringer, who taught me this practice, as to its extraordinary and prompt efficacy in many instances ..."

From A. R. Edwards, "Myalgia . . . Deep injection of water into the muscles of the back may relieve pain. Ringer's method of acupuncture with long needles which are pushed 3 inches into the back and left there for from 5–10 minutes is beneficial, but is usually vigorously opposed by the patient. Very energetic massage, with the application of heat, probably gives the best results. The actual cautery, the application of the constant current, and the use of Tesla's coil give good results."

Harvey Cushing's biography of Osler describes a disappointing experience with acupuncture:

The patient was none other than old Peter Redpath, the wealthy Montreal sugar refiner, who, being on the M.G.H. (Montreal General Hospital) Board, had hopes that the newly appointed physician might be able to cure him of intractable lumbago . . . in due course, they proceeded to treat him by acupuncture, a popular procedure of the day, which consists in thrusting a long needle into the muscles of the small of the back. At each jab, the old gentleman is said to have replied out a string of oaths, and in the end get up and hobble out, no better of his pain—this, to his (Osler's) great distress, for he had expected (the patient) to experience immediate relief which, as he said, "meant a million for McGill."[31]

REFERENCES

1. Akamatsu, S., *et al.* 1967. The Use of Skin Electricity Measurement in Dogs. (In Japanese). Proceedings of the 140th Japan Clinical Veterinary Conference.
2. Akamatsu, S., *et al.* 1974. Acupuncture Anesthesia in Dogs. (In Japanese). Proceedings of the Annual Meeting of the Japanese Society for Clinical Veterinary Science.
3. Anon. 1112 B.C. (a). *Chou Li. (Rites of Chou).* Written in the Chou dynasty. In the chapter "Hsia kuan" (Official title of Hsia): "Horse priests are responsible for the treatment of animal diseases." The title may have originated in the Shang Dynasty.
4. Anon. 1112 B.C. *Chou Li. (Rites of Chou).* In the chapter of "T'ien kuan" (Official titles) it states: "Veterinarians are responsible for the treatment of animal diseases, pyoderma, and injuries." This is the first time the term *veterinarian* is used, and is an official title in the Chou dynasty. Veterinarians were responsible for the care of horses for military purposes.
5. Anon. 249 B.C. *Shih Ching (Book of Odes).* In the chapter "Mu yang P'ien" (On goats): "If the ears and horns are shiny, moist and warm, and the animal is apparently not skinny and have no skin disease, these are signs of good health. If the ears and horns are cool, dried and dull, and the animal is skinny and frequently has skin diseases, these are signs of poor health."
6. Anon. 220 A.D. *Nei Ching (Yellow Emperor's Classic of Internal Medicine).* It states: "Huang-ti, or the Yellow Emperor, said to Ch'i Pai, 'We govern the people. We wish they would not have to take drugs that may be poisonous, nor do we want them to use rough and unrefined stone flints. We should provide them with fine, delicate metal needles to clear up the meridians, and regulate their Ch'i and blood.'" Ch'i Pai was the chief medical officer.
7. Anon. 220 A.D. *Nei Ching (Yellow Emperor's Classic of Internal Medicine). Nei Ching* specified nine types of needles used in ancient times. The needle included tools for massage and "surgery." They were described as follows: (1) Ch'an chen (chisel needle): Its blade was shaped like an arrowhead. It was used in treating skin diseases. (2) Yuan chen (round needle): It had an egg-shaped tip and was used for massage. (3) Shih chen (spoon needle): The blade was round. It was used for pressing on the skin. (4) Feng chen (lance needle): The blade was prism-like, sharp on three sides. It was used for blood-letting. (5) Pi chen (stiletto needle). The blade was shaped like those of a curved sword, and was used to drain pus in purulent infections. (6) Yuan li chen (round, sharp needle): It was used to relieve pain with quick insertion and strong stimulation. (7) Hao chen (soft hair needle): It had the widest use. It was used to relieve pain or to treat other diseases. (8) Ch'ang chen (long needle): It was used in areas with thick fascia and muscle. (9) Ta chen (big needle): It was called the "fire needle" later, and was heated for use. Its present-day name is "hot needle". It was obvious, therefore, that at the time of *Nei Ching*, acupuncture had a wider definition than today. However, the hao chen, or the so-called acupuncture needle of today, was the most important tool of acupuncture then. Through the ages, the other types of needles were replaced by more refined instruments. These nine needles were all made of iron.
8. Anon. 220 A.D. The *Nei Ching*, consisted of two parts: "Shu wen" (9 volumes or twenty-four volumes, depending on how the divisions are made) and "Ling shu" (9 volumes or 12 volumes). The *Han Shu (Book of Han),* the most reliable history of Han dynasty, written by Ssu-Ma Ch'ien states: *"Huang-ti Nei Ching* has a total of 18 volumes." Huang-Fu Mi, a doctor of the state of Ch'in, who studied *Nei Ching* ascribed 9 volumes to the "Needle classic", or "Ling shu", and 9 volumes to the "Shu wen", for a total of 18 volumes. Many of the references quoted in the "Shu wen" can be found as "Ling shu", but not vice-versa. Therefore, the "Ling shu" may have been published before the "Shu wen". Whereas the "Ling shu" is the so-called "Needle classic", 70% of chapters in the "Shu wen" discuss acupuncture.
9. Anon. 220 A.D. *Nei Ching* states: "In order to record knowledge as it progresses from generation to generation, it is necessary that the rules and principles are clearly spelled out. Thus, students and scholars will find it easy to learn and difficult to forget. This is why the "Needle classic" was written."
10. Anon. 618 A.D. *Chiu T'ang Shu (History of the Early*

T'ang Dynasty). In the chapter "Chih kuan chih" (Royal officials and staffs): "In the Ta Fu Chih (The branch of the government in charge of veterinary medicine) . . . 600 veterinarians, 4 scholars of veterinary medicine, and 100 students."

11. Anon. 618 A.D. *Wen Hsien T'ung K'ao. (Identification and Interpretation of Documents of the Generations).* It states: "Honey and drugs were kept in storage in the capital of the Sung dynasty; two supervisors were appointed from among the federal officials to provide supplies for horse doctors."

12. Anon. 1822. Review of J. M. Churchill's Treatise on Acupuncturation. *Med. Deposit.* 7:441–49.

13. Anon. 1828. On Acupuncturation in Veterinary Practice. *The Veterinarian* 1:203–5.

14. Anon. 1836. Abstract of an article by M. Flammens, Acupuncture–Pratiquée dans le cas paraplégie, etc. (in *Journal de Médicine Vétérinaire Pratique.* August 1836). *Recueil de Médicine Vétérinaire* 13:599.

15. Anon. 1926. Archeologists unearthed "Peking Man", an ancient human inhabitant of China of more than 500,000 years ago. He used simple stone tools, bone tools, and fire.

16. Anon. 1958. Review of the first national research conference of Chinese veterinary medicine. Chinese Academy of Agriculture. *Chung-kuo Shou-i-hsueh Tsa-chih (Chinese J. Vet. Med.)* 6:488–92.

17. Anon. 1958. Editorial Communication. The great cooperation and great leap forward in research in Chinese veterinary medicine. *Chung-kuo Shou-i-hsueh Tsa-chih. (Chinese J. Vet. Med.)* 6:493–95.

18. Anon. 1959. Department of Medicine, Chinese Academy of Agriculture report on acupuncture treatment of viral pneumonia in pig. *Hsu-mu Shou-i. (Herdsman Vet. Med.)* 5:205–8.

19. Anon. 1959. Chiang-hsi Agricultural Research Institute, Kan-nan Agriculture College. *Chung-kuo Shou-i-hsueh Tsa-chih (Chinese J. Vet. Med.)* 12:368–74.

20. Anon. 1959. Shui-Yuan Herdsman and Veterinary Medicine Research Institute and Shui-Yuan College of Herdsman and Veterinary Medicine. *Acupuncture and Moxibustion of Pig Diseases.* Peking: Higher Education Press.

21. Anon. 1960. Chinese Academy of Agriculture. *Lecture Notes of Diagnosis and Treatment in Chinese Veterinary Medicine.* Peking: Agriculture Press.

22. Anon. 1970. *Selected Topics of Recent Advances in Chinese Veterinary Medicine.* Peking: Agriculture Press.

23. Anon. 1972. Chiang-hsi Provincial Animal and Plant Disease Control Station. *Acupuncture in Veterinary Medicine.* Shanghai: Shanghai People's Press.

24. Anon. 1972. Research Institute of Chinese Veterinary Medicine of the Chinese Academy of Agriculture. *Physical Diagnosis in Chinese Veterinary Medicine.* Peking: Agriculture Press.

25. Anon. 1972. Ann-fai College of Agriculture. *Diagnosis and Treatment in Chinese Veterinary Medicine.* Ann-fai Province: Ann-fai People's Press, Hofai.

26. Anon. 1973. *Veterinary Acupuncture.* Modern Veterinary Practice. 54:37–42.

27. Anon. 1974a. University of Veterinary Medicine, People's Liberation Army, Clinical application and basic principles of acupuncture anesthesia in veterinary medicine. *Selected Topics of National Acupuncture Anesthesia Study Conference,* 3:229–33.

28. Anon. 1974b. Booklet entitled *International Institute for Acupuncture Treatment.* Atami, Japan.

29. Bachmann, G. 1966. Akupunkturbehandlung bei Haustieren [Acupuncture Treatment for Domesticated Animals]. *Dtsch. Z. Akupunktur* 15:109–10.

30. Bernard, J. 1954. Contribution a l'etude de l'acupuncture chez les carnivores. Doc. Thesis, National Vet. Sch., Alfort, France.

31. Bowers, J. Z. 1973. Acupuncture. *Proc. Amer. Philosoph. Soc.* 117:143–57.

32. Cassedy, J. H. 1974. Early uses of acupuncture in the United States. *Bull. N.Y. Acad. Med.* 50:892–906.

33. Chai, C. T., *et al.* 1959. Therapeutic efficacy of clinical application of acupuncture in veterinary medicine. *Chung-kuo Shou-i-hsueh Tsa-chih. (Chinese J. Vet. Med.)* 3:71–75.

34. Chang, F. T. 1959. Efficacy of injection of strynine into the paihui point of the donkey in treatment of lumbar paralysis secondary to rheumatic arthritis. *Chung-kuo Shou-i-hsueh Tsa-chih (Chinese J. Vet. Med.)* 3:85–86.

35. Chang, W. H. 1959. The application of acupuncture in treatment of rheumatism of pig. *Hsu-mu Shou-i (Herdsman Vet. Med.)* 5:205–8.

36. Chen, C. V. 1968. *History of Chinese Medical Science.* Pp. 28–29. Hong Kong: Chinese Medical Institute.

37. Chia, S. H. A.D. 618. In *Ch'i Ming Yao Shu (Important Techniques for Farmers).* The chapter "Yang yang p'ien" (On raising goat): "To determine whether a goat is sick, a ditch of 1 foot, 4 inches deep and 2 feet, 8 inches, wide is dug. If the goat can jump from one side of the ditch to another, it is healthy. Otherwise, the sick goat is separated."

38. Churchill, J. M. 1822. A Treatise on Acupuncturation; Being a Description of a Surgical Operation Originally Peculiar to the Japanese and Chinese, and by Them Donominated Zin-King, Now Introduced into European Practice, with Directions for its Performance, and Cases Illustrating its Success. London: Simpkin and Marshall.

39. Churchill, J. M. 1828. Cases Illustrative of the Immediate Effects of Acupuncturation, in Rheumatism, Lumbago, Sciatica, Anomalous Muscular Diseases, and in Dropsy of the Cellular Tissue; Selected from various Sources, and Intended as an Appendix to the Author's Treatise on the Subject.

40. Cushing, H. 1925. *The Life of Sir William Osler.* Oxford, England.

41. Edwards, A. R. 1907. *Principles and Practice of Medicine.* Philadelphia: Lea Bros.

42. Froehner, R. 1953. Zur Altchinesisch-japanischen Pferdeheilkunde. [A Discussion of Ancient Chinese and Japanese Equine Medicine]. (In German). *Deutsche Tierarztliche Wochenschrift/Tierarztliche Rundshau,* 51:272–76.

43. Harview, P. P. 1671. Les Secrets de la Medicine Des Chinous. At Grenoble, Chez Phillipes Charvys Marchand Libraire, en la Place de Mal-Confeil.

44. Jim, S., and Chou, P. 1959. Treatment of viral pneumonia of the pig by using acupuncture. *Chung-kuo Shou-i-hsueh Tsa-chih (Chinese J. Vet. Med.)* 12: 357–59.

45. Kameya, T., Ikeda, S., and Watanabe, H. 1974. A Survey of Acupuncture Literature and the Analgesic Effect on Race Horses by Acupuncture on the Sanyo Raku (San Yang Lo) Group of Points (in Japanese). Proceedings of the 1974 Japan Clinical Veterinary Conference. Tokyo, Japan.

46. Kao, H. A.D. 618. In *Chou Hou Fang (Prescription for Emergencies)*. "In cases of constipation of various causes, for example, chronic enteritis, in horses, the therapeutist should trim the fingernail and clean the solid secretion in the rectum."

47. Kim, C. T. 1955. *Hsing Yue Ma Ching (New Treatise of Horses and Cattles)*. Shanghai: Financial Economic Press.

48. Kitazawa, K. 1974. An Investigation of Electric Acupuncture Anesthesia III: Relationship Between Analgesia Area and Points Used in the Dog (in Japanese). Proceedings of the 78th Annual Meeting of the Japanese Society of Veterinary Science.

49. Kitazawa, K., et al. 1974. An Investigation of Electric Acupuncture Anesthesia, I (in Japanese. Proceedings of the 77th Annual Meeting of the Japanese Society of Veterinary Science.

50. Kung, S. H. 1976. Basic sciences and clinical applications of acupuncture. In press.

51. Lal, G. B. 1974. Pinning your hopes on horse acupuncture. *San Francisco Examiner*. Dec. 19.

52. Lee, W. M. 1836. Acupuncture as a remedy for rheumatism. *South. Med. Surg. J.* 1:129–33.

53. Lepetit, J. 1950. Essais d'Acupuncture Practique sur les Animaux. Doc. Thesis, National Vet. Sch., Alfort, France.

54. Lo, T. L., and Yen, S. T. 1959. Preliminary report on combined Chinese medicine and western medicine in treatment of viral pneumonia of the pig. *Chung-kuo Shou-i-hsueh Tsa-chih (Chinese J. Vet. Med.)* 10:297.

55. Lu, H. C. *The Yellow Emperor's Book of Acupuncture*. Academy of Oriental Heritage, Vancouver, B.C., Canada, 1974.

56. Mao, T. T. 1953. *Quotations of Mao Tse-Tung*, vol. 3, pp. 1032. Peking: People's Press.

57. Metivet, J. M. 1963. Contribution a l'ètude comparée de la Resistance Electrique Cutanee. Application a la Therapeutique Cher urgicale Veterinaire. Doc. Thesis, National Vet. Sch. Alfort, France.

58. Milin, J. 1956. L'acupuncture veterinaire (in French). In *Traite d'acupuncture, Tome I*, ed,. R. de La Fuye pp. 473–89. Paris: Librairie E. Le Francois.

59. Milin, J. 1958. Veterinarmedizin und Acupunktur [Veterinary Medicine and Acupuncture]. *Dtsch. Z. Akupunktur* 7:15–20.

60. Milin, J. 1962. Die Akupunktur bei Tieren [Acupuncture in Animals]. *Dtsch. Z. Akupunktur* 11:38–45.

61. Molinier, F. 1972. Contribution a l'études des potentiels du tissu conjunctif, sous cutane et relations avec l'acupuncture. Doc. Thesis, National Vet. Sch., Alfort, France.

62. Morand. 1825. *Memoir on Acupuncture*. Trans. F. Bache. Philadelphia: Desilver.

63. Nakamura, R. 1975. *Therapeutics in Clinical Veterinary Medicine* (in Japanese). Tokyo: Yokendo.

64. Nakamura, R. 1975. Personal communication.

65. Okada, T. 1975. Personal communication.

66. Oono, K. 1974. An Investigation of Electric Acupuncture Anesthesia II: The Electrical Aspect (in Japanese). Proceedings of the 78th Annual Meeting of the Japanese Society of Veterinary Science.

67. Osler, W. 1917. *Principles and Practice of Medicine*. St. Louis: Mosby.

68. Poon, S. Y. 1959. Treatment of diseases of pig by needle retention method. *Chung-kuo Shou-i-hsueh Tsa-chih (Chinese J. Vet. Med.)* 10:291–92.

69. Roger, J. 1921. Les coliques de cheval, diagnostic et traitment [Colics of the Horse, Diagnosis and Treatment]. Paris: Le Francois Editeur.

70. Roger, J. 1926. Le reflexe phalangien et le reflexe de flexion du boulet [The Phalangeal Reflex and the Reflex of the Flexion of the Fetlock Joint]. *Revue Veterinaire (Veterinary Reciew)*, p. 260.

71. Shek, M. S., and Chang, C. K. 1959. Report on treatment of 616 cases of diseases of domestic animals by using electro-acupuncture. *Chung-kuo Shou-i-hsueh Tsa-chih (Chinese J. Vet. Med.)* 12:351–52.

72. Shiota, K. 1974. Therapeutic Application of Acupuncture to Coushing to Canine Filariasis (in Japanese). Proceedings of the 1974 Japan Clinical Veterinary Conference. Tokyo.

73. Soulie de Morant, G. 1934. *Precis de la Vraie Acuponcture*. Paris.

74. Sung T. 1958. The great veterinarian Shun Yang (Pa Lo), a painting showing treatment of horses. *Chung-kuo Shou-i-hsueh Tsa-chih (Chinese J. Vet. Med.)* 1:26–27.

75. Takeuchi, A. 1975. Personal communication.

76. Tavernier, A. 1829. *Elements of Operative Surgery*, ed. and trans. S. D. Gross. New York: Collins and Haunay, Collins, Roorbach. Pp. 55–57.

77. Viet, F. 1963. Contribution a l'étude de l'acupuncture en pathologie osteoarticulaire. Doc. Thesis, National Vet. Sch., Alfort, France.

78. Veith, I. 1966. *The Yellow Emperor's Classic of Internal Medicine*. Berkeley: University of California Press.

79. Wang, F. 1953. *Hsien Ch'in Yi Hsueh Shih Liao Yi Pan (Some Aspects of the History of Chinese Medicine of the Early Ch'in Dynasties)*. Shanghai: Shanghai People's Press.

80. Ward, T. O. 1858. On acupuncture. *Brit. Med. J.* 28:728–29.

81. Wu, S. C., and Yu, S. 1958. Important contributions of ancient Chinese veterinary medicine. *Chung-kuo Shou-i-hsueh Tsa-chih (Chinese J. Vet. Med.)* 2:73–76.

82. Yang, C. T. 1959. *Methods of Veterinary Acupuncture*. Peking: Agriculture Press.

83. Yu Shen: The earliest doctors of the Chinese veterinary medicine. *Chung-kuo Shou-i-hsueh Tsa-chih (Chinese J. Vet. Med.)* 6:240–41.

Index

circulation–sex. *See* pericardium
cold, common
    cattle, 217–218
    dog, 217–218
    horse, 217–218
colic
    horse, 224, 232–233
conjunctivitis
    pig, 229
constipation
    cattle, 216
    horse, 216
    pig, 228
contusion
    pig, 229
cough
    dog, 230, 240
cystic ovaries
    cattle, 218
    dog, 218
    horse, 218
    swine, 218
cystitis
    cattle, 218
    horse, 218

deafness
    dog, 247
dermatitis
    dog, 247
diarrhea
    cattle, 217
    dog, 217, 247
    horse, 217
    swine, 217, 226
digit pain
    horse, 221
dongs, 55
dysmenorrhea
    dog, 229–230

elbow joint, injury
    horse, 220
electroanesthesia, 259
epilepsy
    dog, 231, 240–243
epistaxis
    cattle, 217
    dog, 217
    horse, 217
equipment
    electric point finders, 37–38
    electric stimulators, 38–40, 57–66
    importation, 55–56
    needles, *see* needles

fatigue
    horse, 219
fen, 68
fetlock joint twist
    horse, 221
flexor tendonitis
    horse, 221

Food and Drug Administration
    (FDA), 55–56
fu organs, 1

gallbladder, 6
gas releasing needle *see* needle,
    gas releasing
gastroenteritis
    cattle, 216
    horse, 216
    pig, 216, 227
glossitis
    cattle, 215
    horse, 215
glossoplegia
    horse, 224

hao chen. *See* needle, hao chen
heart, 3
heart–constrictor. *See* pericardium
heaves
    horse, 233, 236–237
hip dysplasia
    dog, 231
hoof and mouth disease
    pig, 227
hot needle. *See* needle, hot

inch. *See* tsun
indigestion
    cattle, 217
    dog, 217
    horse, 217
    pig, 217, 227
influenza
    pig, 226–227
International Veterinary Acupuncture
    Society (IVAS), 278
intervertebral disc syndromes
    dog, 231

kidney, 6

lameness
    carpus
        horse, 225
    elbow
        horse, 225
    hip
        horse, 225
    hock
        horse, 225
    shoulder
        horse, 225, 236
    stifle
        horse, 225, 236
laminitis
    cattle, 215
    horse, 215, 225, 234, 236–238
large intestine, 8
laryngitis
    pig, 227
liver, 3

lumbago
    dog, 239
lung, 5
lung epidemic hemorragic disease
    pig, 226

mastitis
    cattle, 219
measurement. *See tsun*
Meridian Theory, 2, 16–19
moxibustion. *See* acupuncture points,
    stimulation
muscle spasm
    horse, 225
myalgia,
    dog, 238
myositis
    horse, 225, 236–237
myotonia
    cattle, 215
    horse, 215

National Association for Veterinary
    Acupuncture (NAVA), 278
navicular disease
    horse, 225, 235–237
needle
    composition, 30–32
    gas releasing, 29
    hao chen, 22–23
    hot, 26–27
    insertion, 23–26, 34
    manipulation, 35
    piercing jaundice, 28–29
    prism, 28
    source, 32–33
    sterilization, 33–34
    wide, 27–28
needle feeling. *See* te ch'i
Nei Ching, 1, 281–282
nephritis
    pig, 227–228

obesity
    horse, 224
organ, 2–3, 249, 251–252

pain
    carpus
        horse, 233
    lumbar
        horse, 232–235
paralysis
    brachial plexus
        horse, 220
    esophageal
        cattle, 216
        horse, 216
    facial
        cattle, 212
        dog, 231
        horse, 212, 223–225

Milton Keynes UK
Ingram Content Group UK Ltd.
UKHW030629020824
446397UK00001B/1